MW01428308

A Colour Atlas of
CONTACT LENSES & PROSTHETICS
Second Edition

Montague Ruben
DOMS, FRCS, FCOph.

Honorary Consultant Ophthalmologist
and formerly Director of the Contact Lens Department
Moorfields Eye Hospital, London

Formerly Distinguished Professor of Vision Science
University of Houston, Texas

Wolfe Medical Publications Ltd

Copyright © M. Ruben, 1989
Second edition published by Wolfe Medical Publications Ltd, 1989
Printed by Smeets–Weert, Holland
ISBN 0 7234 1502 1

First edition published 1982

All rights reserved. No reproduction, copy or transmission of this
publication may be made without written permission.

No part of this publication may be reproduced, copied or transmitted
save with written permission or in accordance with the provisions of the
Copyright Act 1956 (as amended), or under the terms of any licence
permitting limited copying issued by the Copyright Licensing Agency,
33-34 Alfred Place, London, WC1E 7DP.

Any person who does any unauthorised act in relation to this
publication may be liable to criminal prosecution and civil claims for
damages.

A CIP catalogue record for this book is available from the British
Library.

This book is one of the titles in the series of Wolfe Medical Atlases,
a series which brings together probably the world's largest systematic
published collection of diagnostic colour photographs.
    For a full list of atlases in the series, plus forthcoming titles
and details of our surgical, dental and veterinary atlases, please
write to Wolfe Medical Publications Ltd, 2-16 Torrington Place,
London WC1E 7LT.

Contents

Preface	5
Abbreviations	6

1 Lens material — 7
- Physical properties — 7
- Measurement of properties — 7
- Gas permeability — 12
- Chemical formulae — 15

2 Lens design — 17
- Basic priciples — 17
- Curves — 18
- Computerized lens design — 20
- Lens thickness distribution and gas flow — 27
- Reduced front optics — 29
- Pseudo-conic surfaces — 30
- Toric back surface junction — 30
- Best (optimal) lens forms — 31

3 Manufacture of lenses — 32
- Lathe cutting — 32
- Pressure grinding — 34
- Moulding — 34
- Scleral lens manufacture — 36

4 Checking of lenses — 38
- Standards — 38
- Magnifyers and microscopes — 38
- Shadowgraphs — 40
- Lens curvature — 41
- Thickness gauges — 43
- Power — 43
- Size of hard lenses — 44
- Water content of soft hydrophilic lenses — 45
- Specific gravity of HGP lenses — 46

5 Care and spoilage — 47
- Contamination of the lens — 47
- Heat disinfection — 48
- Chemical disinfection — 49
- Cleaners — 50
- Lubricant drops — 51
- Lens spoilage — 51
- Damage to the ultrastructure — 52
- Polymer damage — 55
- Fungal and bacterial contamination — 62
- Soft lenses for disposal — 64

6 Fitting of contact lenses — 66
- General principles — 66
- Lens stability — 67
- Finding the fitting curve from eye models — 67
- Fitting corneal hard lenses — 68
- Lens power — 71
- Trial lens fitting — 71
- Assessment of fit — 72
- Interpalpebral lens fit — 74
- Hard lens centration — 74
- Corneal intermediate sized lenses — 77
- Lid-lens adhesion — 78
- Toric surfaced lenses — 79
- Lens stabilization — 81
- Multi-vision lenses — 83
- Soft lens fitting — 87
- Scleral (haptic) lens fitting — 96
- Preformed geometric scleral lenses — 99
- Electrodiagnostic scleral lenses — 99
- Writing of prescriptions — 100
- Computer programs — 101

7 Fitting lenses for the abnormal eye — 102
- Indications for fitting — 102
- Myopia — 103
- Binocular vision indications — 105
- Occlusion therapy — 106
- Anisometropia and aniseikonia — 107
- Congenital hyperopia — 109
- Regular and irregular astigmatism — 110
- Subnormal vision aids — 111
- Albinism and aniridia — 112
- Nystagmus — 113
- Aphakia — 113
- Keratoconus — 121
- Hard corneal lenses — 122
- Keratoglobus — 128
- Marginal dystrophy — 128
- Heredokeratodystrophies — 128
- Keratoplasty — 129
- Radiokeratotomy — 133
- Therapeutic bandage lenses — 134
- Bullous keratopathy — 135
- Recurrent erosions — 137
- Mesodermal dysplasia — 138
- Acne rosacea — 138
- Marginal inflammatory ulceration — 138
- Pathological dry eye — 139

Stevens-Johnson syndrome	141	Corneal reactions	165
Benign mucus membrane atrophy	142	Endothelium and lens wear	167
Ocular burns	143	Animal histology—stromal changes	171
Drug dispensing gel lenses	146	Neovascularization	173
Ocular myopathies	148	Infection	176
		Lids and conjunctival problems	180
8 Adverse reactions	**150**	Optical problems	182
Causes of the pathological response to lenses	151	**9 Prosthetics**	**183**
Gaseous exchange	151	Corneal prosthetic lenses	183
Epithelium and lens wear	153	Scleral hard prosthetic lenses and shells	186
Tear film	157	Orbital prostheses	189
Dk/L values	160		
Punctate keratitis	162	**Index**	**195**

Preface

Since the first edition of this atlas was published in 1982 there has been increasing emphasis on the fitting of hard gas permeable lenses. Over the same period much more knowledge has accumulated from research on the function of the cornea when submitted to the stress of a contact lens. New material has therefore been added to illuminate these areas. At the same time, in this new edition the grouping of the subject matter has been changed and obsolete material removed.

The text is completely new, with introductory paragraphs within each section. Where clarification is necessary, more than one illustration is used to make a point. There are more tables and graphs included in this edition, especially to explain results of research findings. In addition, histology is given more extensive treatment in a chapter on adverse reactions to the wearing of contact lenses.

My aim has been to make the atlas attractive to students and teachers: emphasis throughout is on pictorial representation. The subject matter is directed specifically to practitioners and students working in an ophthalmological environment, so the major part of the atlas deals with eye abnormalities. A chapter on prosthetics covers the basic ground for what in most instances is a simple procedure. Another development is the increasing use of coloured cosmetic contact lenses in the word of fashion. Contact lens practitioners and technicians who work with ophthalmologists may find this book of value, especially if they have not encountered eye disease during their training.

I gratefully acknowledge the help of all contributors (the source of all material other than my own is stated in the captions), and I am entirely responsible for the comments and interpretations made upon their photographs. I also thank my publishers for being so cooperative and the late Peter Wolfe for encouraging me to write this second edition.

Abbreviations

AEL—Axial edge lift

BK—Bullous keratopathy

BMMA—Benign mucus membrane atrophy; an ocular pemphigoid

BVD—Back vertex distance or trial lens distance from the cornea (measured to the shut lid with 2mm allowed if not measured with the refractor head)

C3, C2, C1—Respectively tri-, bi- and single-cut back surface

CL—Contact lens

d.—Dioptre

$Dk \times 10^{-11}$ (ATVP)—Gas diffusion constant; the rate of gas (oxygen) transmission through a material is expressed as $= Dk \times 10^{-11} \times cm^2/s.ml. \ O_2$ mmHg abbreviated to $Dk \times 10^{-11}$ (ATVP)

Dk/L—Rate of diffusion of a gas through a specified thickness of material. It is the gas permeability measure of a contact lens for specific zones of known thickness or, when given for total Dk/L, is for an average thickness. Dk/L units are 10×10^{-9} (ATVP).

d1, d2, d3 etc—Diameters of succeeding peripheral curves (preceded by the back or front surface of the lens)

d_o—Diameter of the base curve zone

E—Eccentricity

EKP—Epikeratoplasty

EW—Extended wear

f—Focal length

F_e—Equivalent spectacle lens power

F_o—Ocular refraction (calculated from the spectacle or trial lens power and BVD)

FOD—Front optic diameter

F_s—Spectacle lens power

Gel—Hydrophilic plastic

GP or HGP or RGP—Hard lens made of gas permeable material

K—Keratometry

KS—Keratitis sicca

LG—Lamellar keratoplasty

OR—Over-refraction (refraction with the contact lens *in situ*)

P—Power in dioptres

PEK—Photoelectric keratometry

Per cent (%), (after a gel material)—Water percentage of the lens;

$$\frac{water}{water + dry\ lens} \times 100$$

PG—Penetrating keratoplasty

PHEMA—Poly (2-hydroxymethylmethacrylate)

PK—Punctate keratitis

PMMA—Polymethylmethacrylate

r_1, r_2, r_3 etc—Radii of succeeding peripheral curves (preceded by the back or front surface of the lens)

RI—Refractive index

RK—Radial keratotomy

r_o—Radius of the base curve

RO—Reduced front optic diameter (or size)—lenticular lens

SF—Shape factor

Si—Silicone lens

SPK—Superficial punctate keratitis

T_c, T_j, T_e—Thickness of the lens respectively at the centre, at the junction of front reduced optic with the front periphery, and at the point 0.5 mm from the true edge

TD—Total lens size

With regard to basic lens design, hard, rigid, gas permeable rigid or hard are synonymous terms. In the few instances where PMMA material is specifically required it will be noted.

1 Lens material

Physical properties

Biocompatibility

Materials used in the manufacture of contact lenses:

- Should be biologically inert.

- Should be non-selective in the absorption of metabolites and toxins, and not take part in enzymatic activity.

- Should not exhibit strong molecular adhesive forces.

- Should not show excessive electrophoretic osmotic properties.

- Should have little friction effect between the surface of the material and the eye tissues.

- Should have a high gas permeability.

- Should be compatible with the surface eye tissue's electrical charges without changing its properties.

- Should not change its properties within the normal biological range of pH (7.6 ± 0.2).

- Should not excite an inflammatory or immune response even when in contact with the eye over a long period of time.

Water absorption

- Water can be held within the material matrix without physico-chemical bonding to the molecular structure (free H_2O), or can be attached by molecular forces (bound H_2O).

- The amount of water held relates to the rigidity and gas transference properties of the final lens.

- The water content of the final lens is not constant and loss can occur from physical pressures and from evaporation after placement on the eye.

Reproducibility of the lens

The accuracy and precision of both measuring and manufacturing methods are important, but many unwanted changes in the physico-chemical properties of contact lenses occur because it is difficult to reproduce the lens' chemistry accurately and precisely every time.

Ageing and radiations

Most polymers degrade over time, especially if subjected to repeated stress, heat and other radiations (for example, UV radiation) and chemicals. Ageing is likely to occur in materials containing impurities (for example, additives, accelerators, fillers, and inhibitors of the polymerization process).

Measurement of properties

Table 1 gives a list of the properties of a material that can be measured and these can be used to standardise lens fitting and wearing behaviour to which new materials must conform. It is preferable to test a new material's properties (or a selected few properties) when a lens has been made.

Table 1. The fitting and wearing behaviour of a lens can be assessed from its:

Specific gravity
Micro-penetration (hardness)
Elasticity
Plasticity
Tensile strength
Water absorption
Surface wettability
Stress and strain
Gas permeability
Gas permeability of lens relative to thickness
Thermal conductivity
Coefficients of size related to $T°$ (linear expansion)
Coefficients of size relative to the material's dry and wet state (linear expansion)
Refractive index
Optical quality
Light transmission %
Material purity
Polymer stability etc.

Surface tension

Surface wettability, contact angle (wetting angle), capillary—all these different terms have a common factor: the surface tension of a solution. The energy between molecules within the bulk of a solution is different from that exhibited at the surface. In the case of films and droplets the tension will be responsible for holding the solution's form. The tension exerted on the sides of a capillary tube by a solution is sufficient to hold a vertical column of the solution in the tube (**1**).

The tear meniscus has a tension which stretches from the lid to the contact lens (see **181**).

The ability of a solution to spread on a contact lens surface depends upon the nature of the lens surface, the pressure of the surrounding atmosphere, the surface tension of the solution and the temperature.

The contact angle or wetting angle of a drop of solution is indirectly related to the ability of a solution to spread on a surface. Tears, for example, have a low angle of contact on glass and a higher one on plastic (see **125**).

Figure **2** shows how the contact angle will change with the effect of gravity; there is a receding and advancing angle. The angle of the average of the receding plus advancing angles should be equal to the contact angle when the solution is not affected by gravity.

Thus, merely to state a wetting angle for a contact lens material *without* other information is of little value to the practitioner.

The surface of the contact lens is one of the most important factors that determines tolerance and tear film adhesion. Many tests have been devised to measure the wetting of lens surfaces by tears; indirect evidence is obtained by using the wettability of water, saline, and contact lens preparations.

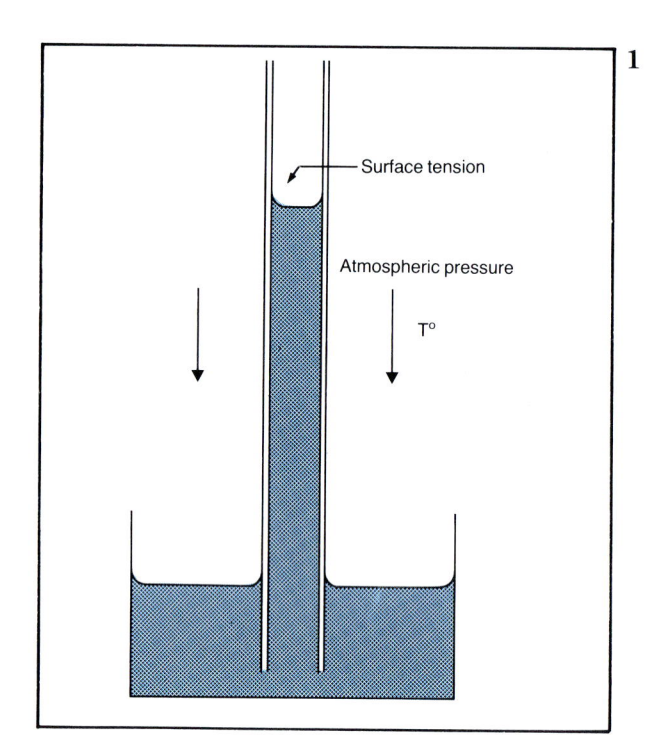

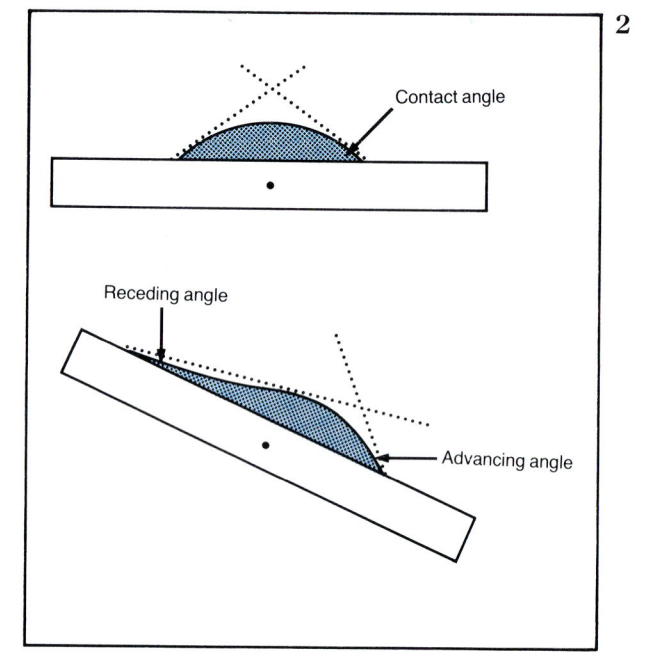

3-6 Using a video camera, one can see that a drop of saline on a dry, cleaned, new lens inserted prior to the blink does not spread, but on subsequent blinks a drop will spread. Thus, the lens coated with tear proteins will permit spreading and normally five good blinks coats the lens. The graph (**6**) shows that *all* materials are coated in the same way. It is more important to measure how adhesive the tear proteins are to a material than how wettable it is. (W.J. Benjamin)

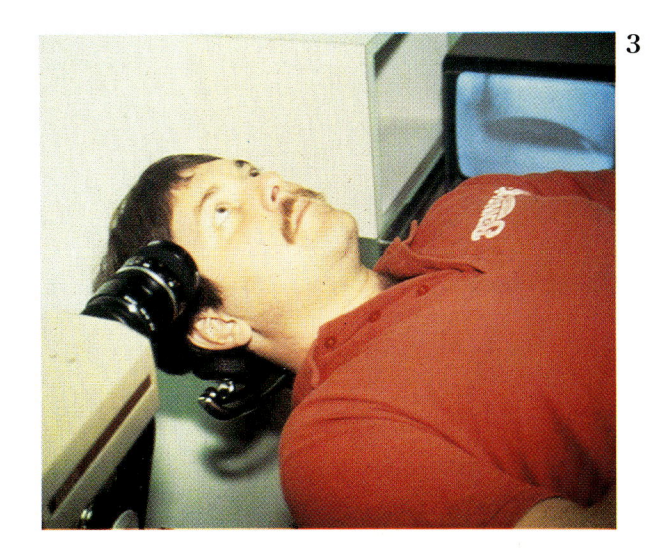

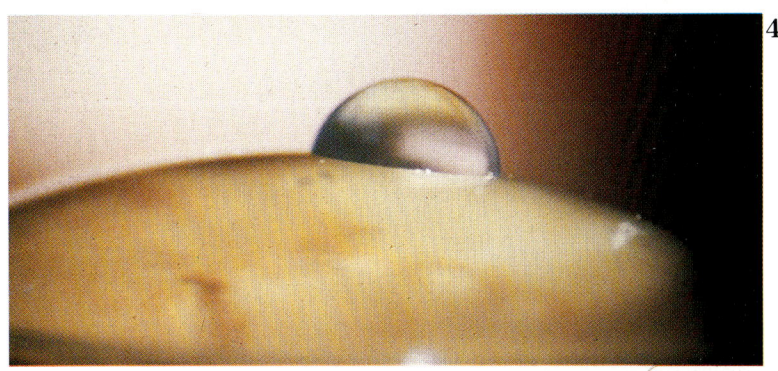

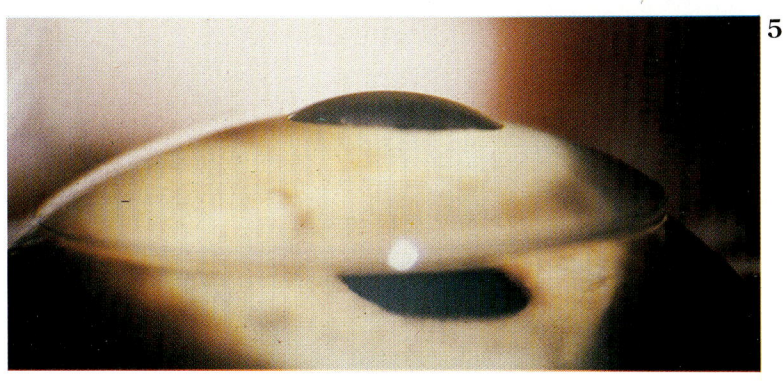

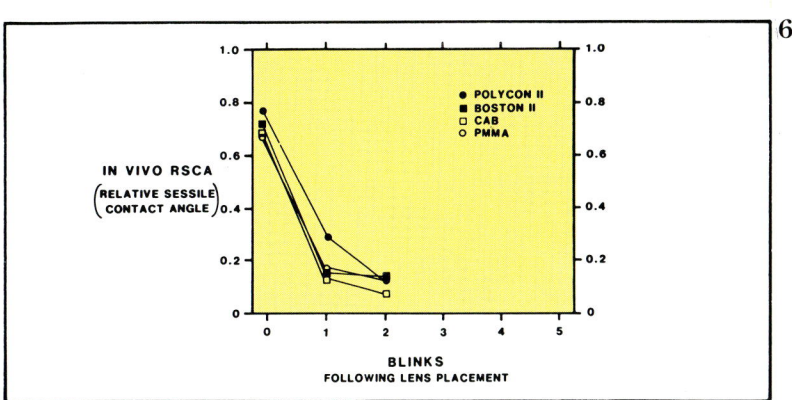

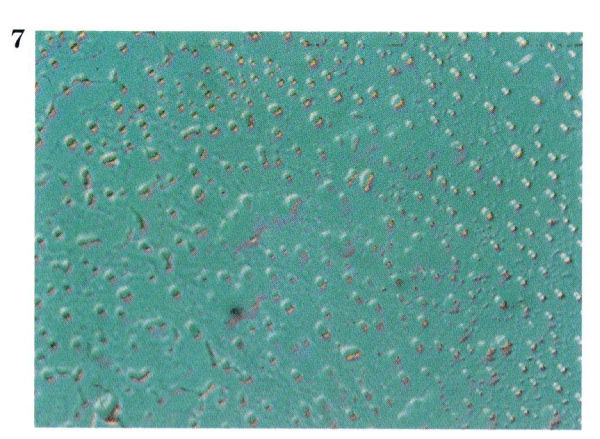

7 Microdroplets of saline on a new gel surface before it is coated by a film of mucin.

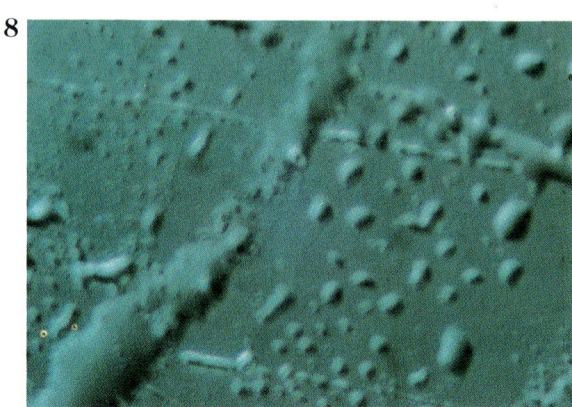

8 Larger, confluent drops of saline on a gel surface.

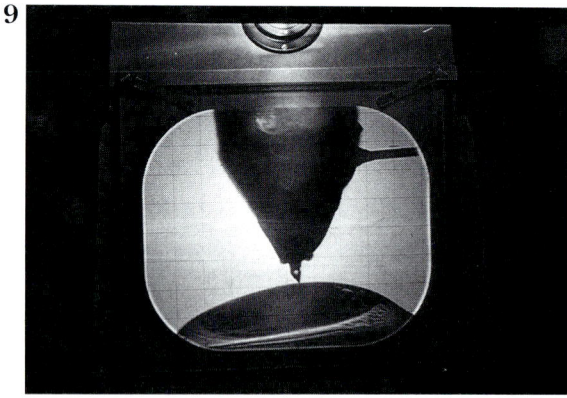

Rigidity of materials

Materials have a wide spectrum of rigidity but they are categorized into two types: soft and hard. However, the definition of a hard or soft lens should describe the behaviour of the lens on the eye and is a combination of the material's properties, the lens design, pressure and other factors (see Chapters 2 & 6).

9 & 10 A lens in a water tank is penetrated with a standard stereo record player sapphire needle. By recording the amount of force it took to penetrate the lens to a certain depth, the relative hardness of the lens was found. Examples of rigidity:
- PMMA is 50 times harder than PHEMA (water content 38 per cent).
- Silicone rubber is 5 times harder than PHEMA.
- The human cornea is 1.5 times harder than vinyl polymer gel (75 per cent water).

Hysteresis

11 Materials subjected to pressure will deform and so will the lens. Pathway (**A**) is taken as stress is applied. Upon release of the pressure the 'memory' of the material should return it to its original shape, as shown by pathway (**B**). But with time and repeated stress, lenses will go out of shape so that when all pressure is removed the slope is not at (**O**) but at (**F**). This is a permanent change in the lens. (See **137**).

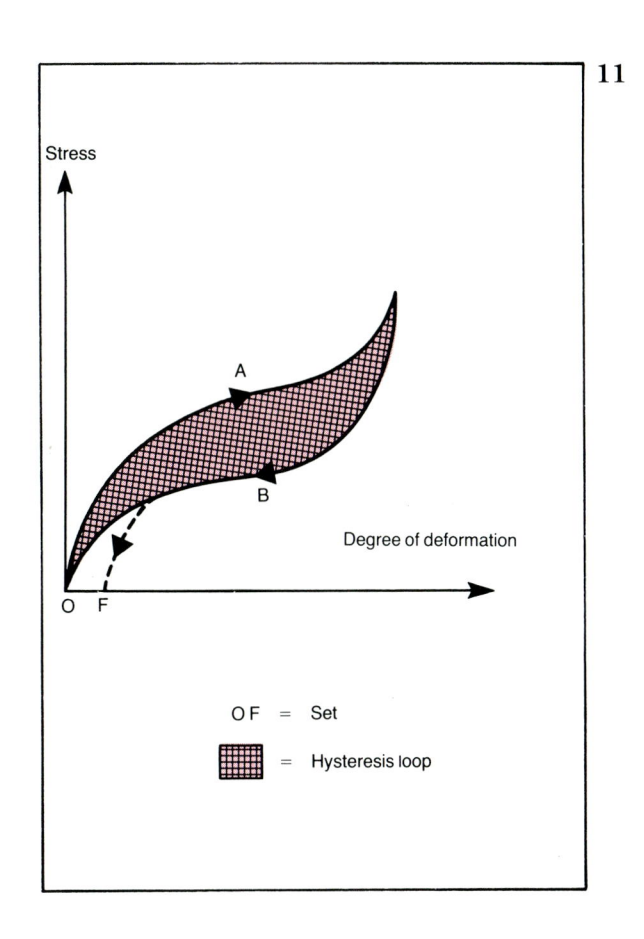

Transparency

For good optical image formation a very high degree of material transparency is required. If dyes (and mordants), which are used to tint the lens, and UV occluders are added incorrectly, they will cause imperfections in the material leading to light diffraction and interference phenomena and image distortion. Polymers that have been incorrectly annealed can show defects in polarized light.

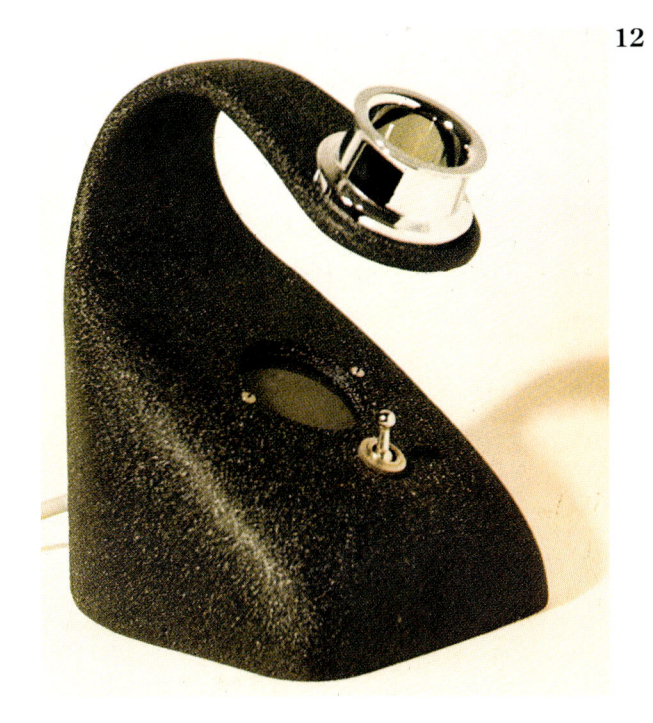

12 A polarizer and analyzer.

13 Two buttons of polymer, the upper one shows internal stress lines.

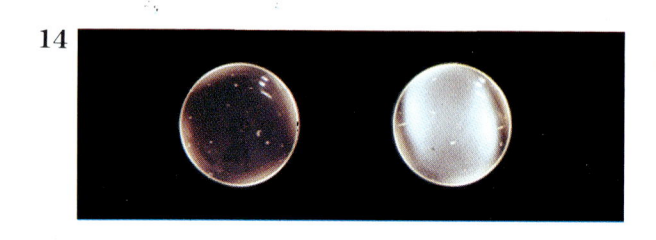

14 Tensile modules formed by pressure on the polymer material during a creep test.

Gas permeability (Dk)

The contact lens forms a variable occlusive gas barrier and a mechanical barrier. The degree depends upon the material size and fit of the lens. A lens can be open or closed when on the eye (see Chapter 6). A lens made of a material that will allow passage of gases is a real advantage to the health of the cornea. The cornea requires 2-5µl $O_2/cm^2/hr$.

Various polarographic techniques attempt to measure this demand after occlusion with contact lenses and also to measure directly the flow of oxygen through the contact lens. The difficulty lies in the standardization of the experimental technology, which limits its usefulness.

Measurement of gas flow

The equipment in 15 & 16 is part of an arrangement that places a contact lens in a dual chamber which passes water—free of gas—on one side and on the other water containing gas of known pressure. The gas diffusing across the contact lens can then be measured, preferably when a steady state is reached for constant conditions of pressures and temperatures. The thickness of the lens has to be known under the experimental conditions. Preferably a standard lens form should be used or a plano disc. Thus:

$$\frac{Dk}{L} = Dk \times 10^{-9} \text{ (cm}^2\text{/s) (ml. } O_2 \times mmHg)$$

or $Dk \times 10^{-9}$ ATVP

(Dk = Diffusion constant; L = Lens thickness; ATVP = Area, T°, Volume, Pressure)

From this $Dk \times 10^{-11}$ (ATVP) is calculated and this is the transmissability of the material. The Dk values are temperature related and should always be stated.

Examples of Dk/L where L=0.1 mm at 37°C:
PHEMA 42%=9   PMMA=0
Vinyl 80%=60   Silicone acrylates=10 to 50+
Silicone rubber=400   Fluorocarbons=60+
(Tolerances are as high as ±5)

NB The gas flux across a material is termed *transmission* (Dk), whereas a specific measurement of flux through a lens of known thickness is termed *permeability* (Dk/L).

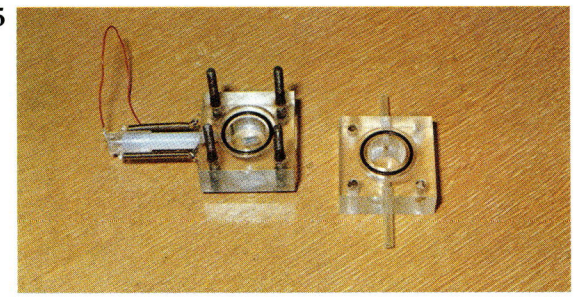

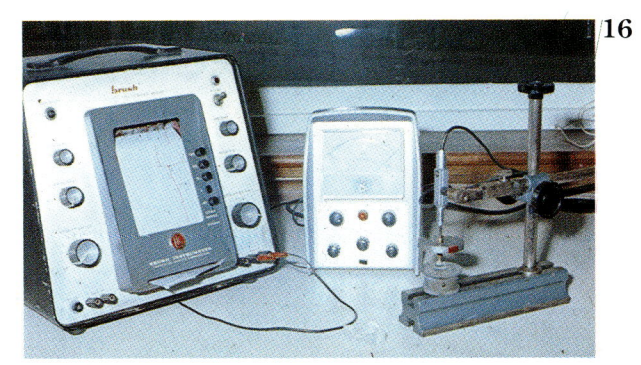

17 Application of the gas (O₂) probe (Clarke type). The polarographic platinum electrode probe (I Fatt) is covered with a polyethylene membrane. A potentiometer records the results over a period of time.

The probe is directly applied to the cornea (**a**). The probe occludes an area of the cornea from O_2, so the readings show a 'drop away' from the atmospheric O_2 pressure of 150 mmHg (at sea level), the slope of the 'drop away' will indicate individual corneal O_2 uptake variations, but also the availability of O_2 from other sources. The shape and size of the probe and the extraneous factors (barrier and edge) shown in (**c**) can affect the reproducibility of the result. The readings can be converted to given corneal O_2 demand.

In (**b**) the readings are given when a contact lens is sandwiched between the probe and the cornea. The results will interpret the Dk/L value (lens oxygen permeability).

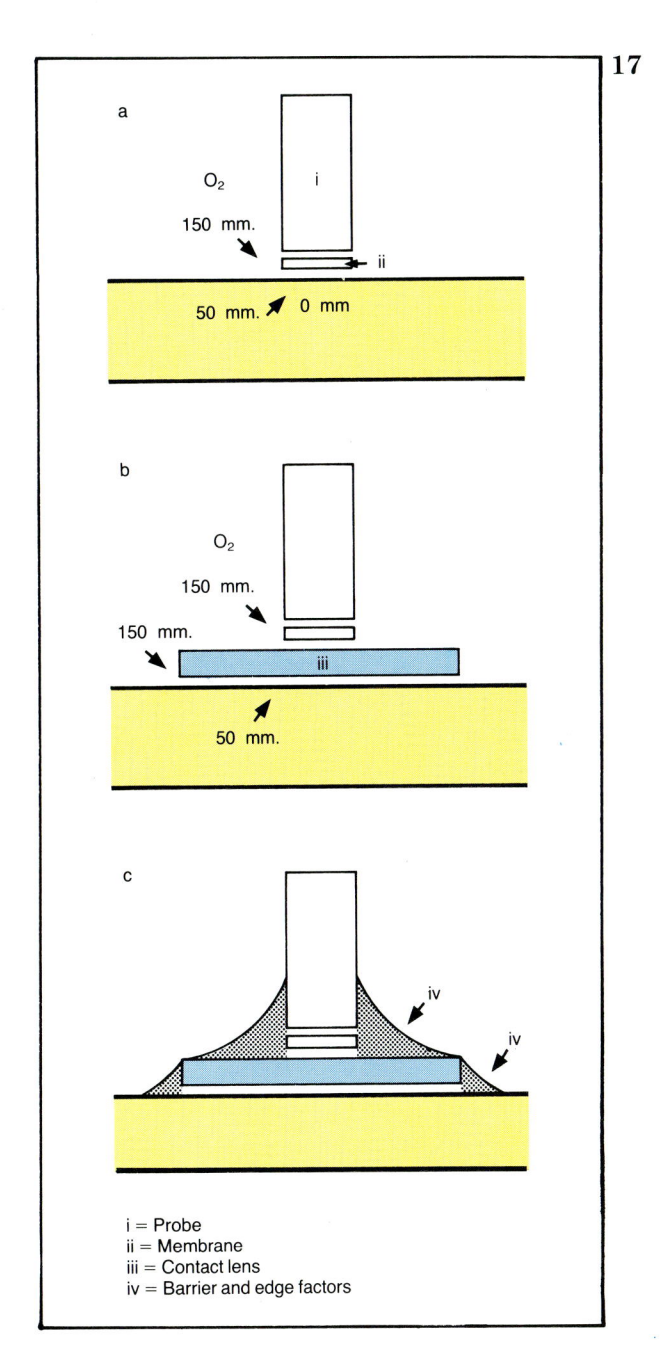

i = Probe
ii = Membrane
iii = Contact lens
iv = Barrier and edge factors

Equivalent oxygen percentage (after R. Hill)

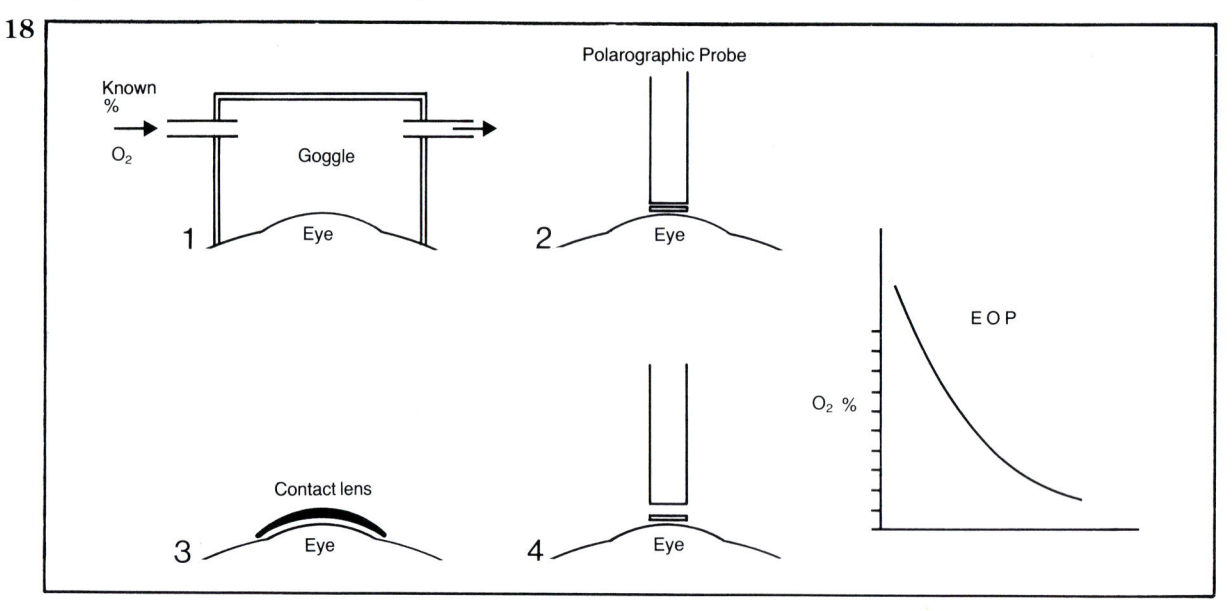

18 Equivalent oxygen percentage. The cornea is exposed to O_2 percentages of different levels by use of a goggle (1). The probe is applied to the cornea and the results are related to O_2 percentage levels (2).

A contact lens is placed on an eye (3) for a finite period and removed; it is then replaced with the probe and the reading is read off as an EOP function (4). Thus a contact lens can produce a state of affairs equivalent to that found under experimental conditions with the goggle.

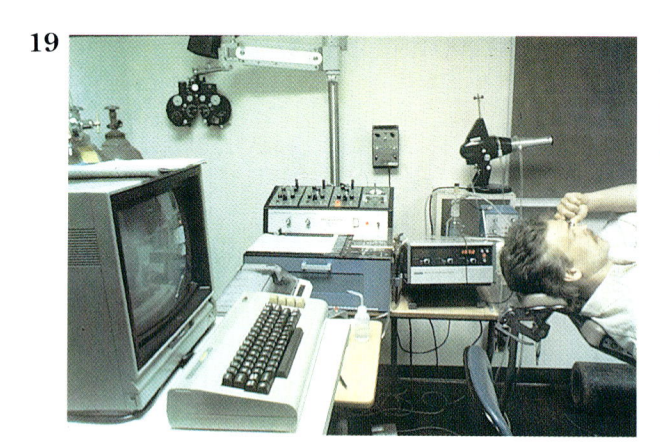

19 Measurement of equivalent oxygen percentage (EOP) (after W.J. Benjamin and R. Hill). The arrangement includes an O_2 sensor, a temperature bath, a blood/gas analyzer, a recording system and compressed gas cylinders for calibration for human subjects.

Chemical formulae
(Formulae of materials by M. Refojo)

20 Poly (methylmethacrylate)(PMMA). Slightly hydrophilic (0.5 to 2 per cent). A material used since the late 1930s. It is inert, with good reproducibility. It can be manufactured by thermolabile and generated techniques, and has almost 100 per cent light transmission. Co-polymers of several types give refractive indices higher than 1.50.

21 Poly (2-hydroxyethylmethacrylate) (PHEMA). Hydrophilic gel. Invented by Wichterle and Lim. It gives a range of materials used chiefly in the water content range of 26 to 42 per cent. Manufactured by spin casting and by lathe generation of the dry material. Using pure monomers the material can be reproduced to high standards. When equilibrated with water, it can be heated to 130°C without the lens losing its form. It will selectively absorb heavy metal and other highly-charged molecules and, as with all other hydrophilic gels, the refractive index varies with the water content.

22 Vinylpyrrolidone (VP). A material which is able to absorb up to 80 per cent water. It can be manufactured into cast and generated contact lenses and has been copolymerized to acrylates. This material has a high gas permeability and its surface is well tolerated by eye tissue.

23 Cellulose acetate butyrate. Several types of this material are possible: the behaviour of impure materials is inconsistent when generated into contact lenses; and water absorption and temperature properties become variable. This is a hard material relative to the gels and is gas permeable. It is used mostly for corneal lens manufacture and to co-link with other polymers.

24 & 25 Silicone rubber—silanes and siloxanes. Methacryloxypropyltris (trimethylsiloxanyl) silane (MOPS), poly(dimethylsiloxane) (**24**); poly (diphenyl-dimethyl-methylvinyl siloxane) (**25**). There now exists a whole range of materials from the pure rubber, which has an extremely high oxygen transmission and is relatively soft, to much harder materials where the gas flow is much less. Rubber itself is lipophilic and ages.

26 Methacryloxypropyltris (trimelthylsiloxany) silane. This copolymer of acrylate and siloxane combines the high gas flow properties of rubber with the hardness of acrylate. From these materials very high Dk values are obtainable. Unfortunately, the high Dk is not always commensurate with a good functioning lens. There are problems of lens deformation, unless the lens is thick, and poor mucous tear adherence. On the other hand, lipid adhesion is rapid.

27 Fluorocarbons—telechelic perfluoropolyether. A hard material that has a high gas flow. It should be noted that polymer mixes, polymer grafts, and copolymers of all these and other materials, makes the chemistry of contact lenses very complicated.

2 Lens design

Basic principles

The basic principles of lens design apply irrespective of the material. The controlling factors of lens design are as follows:

- Back surface fitting shape

- Front surface optic distribution

- Front peripheral shape

- Thickness factors:
  T_c = central thickness
  T_j = junction with optic and periphery
  T_e = edge (0.5 mm from edge)

- Edge where front and back surfaces meet

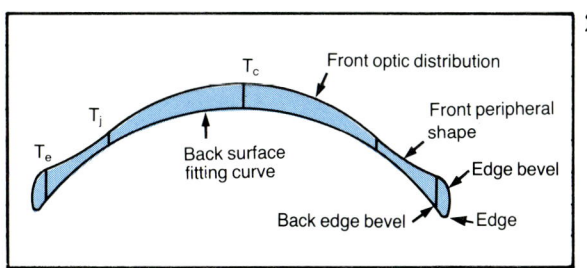

28 Controlling factors of lens design.

- Edge bevels—those portions immediate to the edge

Table 2. Lens specifications by size.		
Types	*Total diameter*	*Stabilizing area*
Corneal	7.0-11.5 mm	Cornea
Corneo–scleral	11.5-16.0 mm	Cornea to sclera
Scleral (haptic)	16-26 mm Usually the vertical dimeter is 1 to 3 mm less than the horizontal diameter. Thus: $\frac{20V}{24H}$ Periphery (haptic) lenses can be moulded to conform to eye shape.	Sclera

Rigidity

- Hard (rigid) lens—essentially a lens which maintains its form when placed on the eye.

- Soft lens—essentially a lens which moulds to the shape of the eye.

- Flexure—a hard lens which bends regularly.

- Warp—a surface which bends irregularly.

(The word 'essentially' is used to advise the reader that there are materials which, when made into lenses, can behave in between the definitions of hard and soft lenses.)

Size

- Corneal lens—a lens which is inter-limbal or less in diameter.

- Corneo-scleral lens—a lens which is 'intermediate' in size.

- Scleral (haptic) lens—a lens with corneal (optic) and scleral (haptic) portions.

Several factors determine the size of the corneal and corneo-scleral lens to be fitted (up to 16 mm in diameter). The important ones are the hardness of the material and the distribution of the thickness, which are complimentary to final lens rigidity. The less rigidity there is in the final lens, the greater the requirement for the lens to be larger for stability of fit.

Table 3 shows a range of materials and the sizes and average thicknesses used in practice. It must be noted that minima thicknesses vary greatly according to the power of the lens and the design. For example, a PHEMA (42 per cent water content) lens can be as thin as 0.03 mm at the centre for a minus lens, whereas a vinyl polymer (60 per cent water) lens of the same power may be as much as 0.08 mm at the centre.

Table 3. Design of lens size and thickness relative to physical properties.

Material	Relative hardness	Water content %	Relative gas (O_2) permeability	Surface wettability angle	Optimal lens size	Average thickness (mm)
PMMA	1.00	1	0	70-50°	7-12	0.12
CAB	0.80	3	3-6	70-50°	9-12	0.12
Siloxane— acrylobutyrates	0.80-0.60	1-3	6-9	30-20°	9-13	0.12
Silicone rubber	0.050	0	100	90-50°	11-13	0.20
PHEMA and copolymers	0.030	26-38	9-25	60°	12-15	0.10
Vinyl hemas	0.020	45-70	25-60	40°	12-15	0.12
Amydo amines	0.015	75	60	40°	13-15	0.20
Vinyls	0.010	80	60+	40°	13-15	0.20

Gas permeability is T° (temperature) and thickness dependent. Wetting angles—regression and advanced angles for hard materials.
N.B. Actual centre and edge thickness is power dependent.

Curves

In general, all preformed lenses have regular geometric shapes that follow the curves produced by taking sections through a cone in different planes. Thus, the section taken parallel to the base describes a circle. All the sections oblique to the base describe aspheric curves which are determined by the angle the section takes to the base. Thus, the curves range from ellipse to parabola to hyperbola (**29** and **30**).

The conic section curves can be described mathematically by using the X and Y coordinates (**31** and **32**) and it can be seen how they are related along the progressively changing curve.

For the purpose of contact lens practice a simplification will be to use the notion of eccentricity (E). A curve can be described by the degree it departs from a circle.

This can best be visualized by looking at Figure 30. The curves within the circle are not normally used in practice; those outside are. Also note that this family of curves is eccentric to one particular radius or curvature of the circle.

Where the curves become practically 'tangential' to the circle, there is a zone of at least 3 to 4 mm where all the lines meet. Over this chord area eccentricity for all practical purposes would be difficult to measure. Practicality *is* important in practice and manufacture. To facilitate the measurement of eccentricity over the range used on the human eye, one uses the shape factor (SF):

$$SF = 1 - E^2 \qquad (1)$$

This is normally just over +0.6 for the cornea.

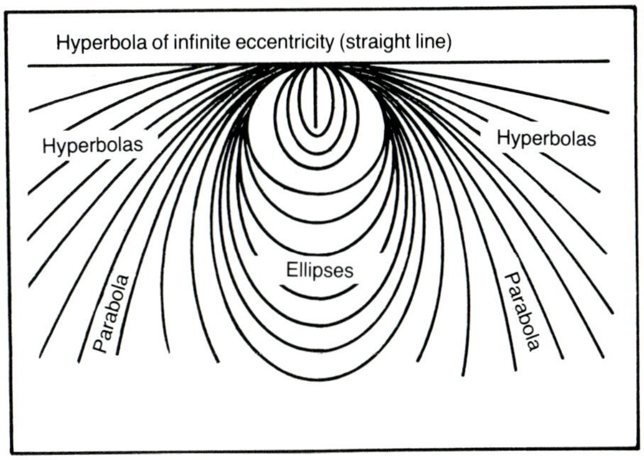

29 & 30 Conic section curves.

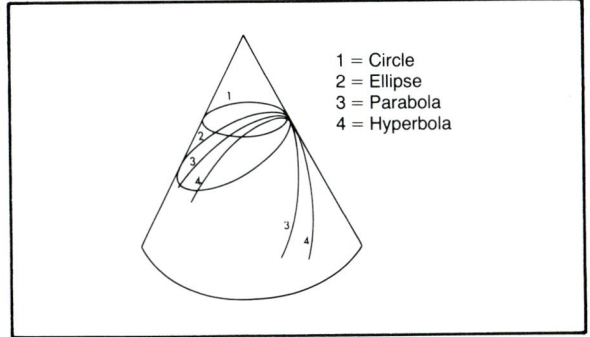

31 Conic section curves and the shape factor.
The diagram shows several conic section curves. They range from very flat hyperbola to the circle passing through the parabolars and the eclipses. The shape factor (SF) for the circle is +1, for the elipse 0 to +1, and the hyperbola has minus quantities.

The diagram is based upon an example for a central base curve of radius 8 mm. The interrupted line describes a fitting curve for an average keratometry reading of 8 mm (fitted on K). The best back fitting lens curve of true conic section has SF = +0.65. The diagram also shows how the co-ordinates X and Y relate to the SF. The formula is given. Even though this drawing is some eight times enlarged from normal size one should note that differences in the curves only become obvious at the diameter 9 mm or more.

$$S.F. = \frac{(2r_0 \times X) - Y^2}{X^2}$$

CL = edge of a 10 mm. contact lens

NOTE: Dotted line is equivalent of a contact lens back curve that would fit the normal eye.

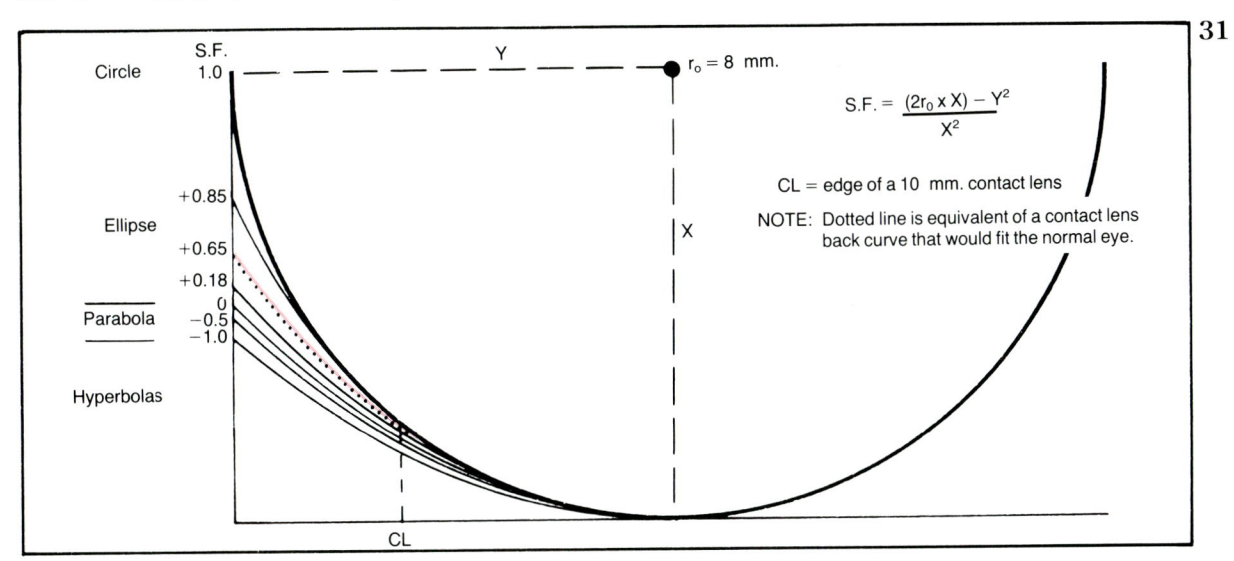

32 Axial edge lift (AEL or Z). The diagram illustrates the AEL measurement given in formula (**3**) and the relationship to eccentricity (E) and the SF see formula (**1**). The continuous curve on the back surface of a contact lens can be related to the AEL required and the back central spherical portion, providing the size of the lens is given and the edge bevel added afterwards. The practitioner, when relating this to keratometry, has to determine the type of fit if trial lenses are not used (see Chapter 6). The use of trial fitting lenses of known AEL or identical AEL helps to access fit and to modify the lens specifications.

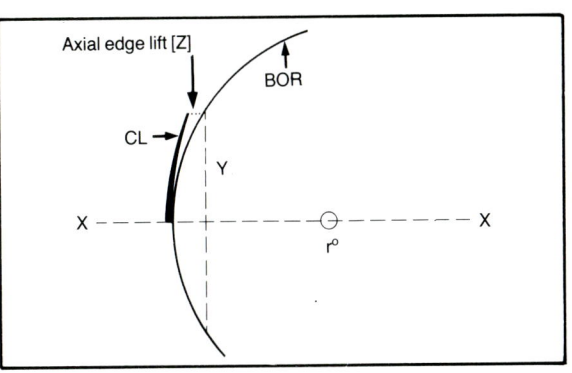

Shape factor

The relationship of the shape factor for a random selection of curves is given in **31**. If one states the central radius and the shape factor the curve will be defined for a given chord (A.G. Bennett).

$$SF = \frac{(2r_o \times X) - Y^2}{X^2} \quad (2)$$

$$E = \frac{1 - 2r_o(X^2 + Z) - Y^2}{(X^2 + Z)^2} \quad (3)$$

The Z factor introduced at this juncture is described as the distance from the edge of the chord (Y) of the circle (r_o) to the eccentric curve and parallel to the axis XX (**32**).

In practice the Z factor is called the axial edge lift (AEL) and is defined as the distance from the edge of the back surface of the lens (before the edge is bevelled) to the back central curve measured parallel to the axis. Note that formulae (**1**), (**2**) and (**3**) are inter-related.

Specification by chord and sagitta

The relationship of a continuous progressively changing curve to the concept of eccentricity has been described. However, most contact lenses use multispherical curves which, when blended, approximate to aspheric curves.

The single curve r_o over chord 2Y (**33a**) can be described by giving the chord and the sagitta (S). Thus:

$$r_o = \frac{Y^2}{2S} + \frac{S}{2}$$

and:

$$S = r_o - \sqrt{r^2 - Y^2}$$

A multispherical curve can be designated by a series of chords and sagitta (**33b**). The use of this method can define a continuous curve in terms of spherical curves.

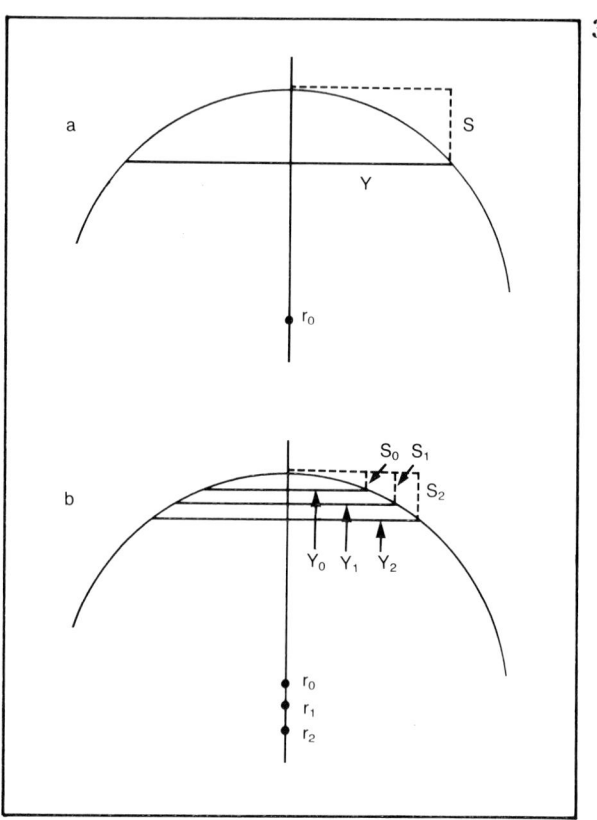

Computerized lens design

The following are soft lens profiles computer-programmed for optimal design and gas flow analysis (prepared by Geoff Cooke, Allergan-Hydron Europe). They have been selected to illustrate various aspects of the professional approach to lens design. Two Dk levels (10 and 50) are taken which for hydrophilic material would be equivalent to 40 and 65 per cent water content of materials respectively. Note that the lens thickness has been magnified relative to its size to show changes in the design.

The data give alternative lens design as determined by front optic size and the relationship to average thickness over the optic and total lens. This then gives the Dk/L readouts for these values.

While they are given as examples of methodology they do not necessarily represent a particular commercial lens.

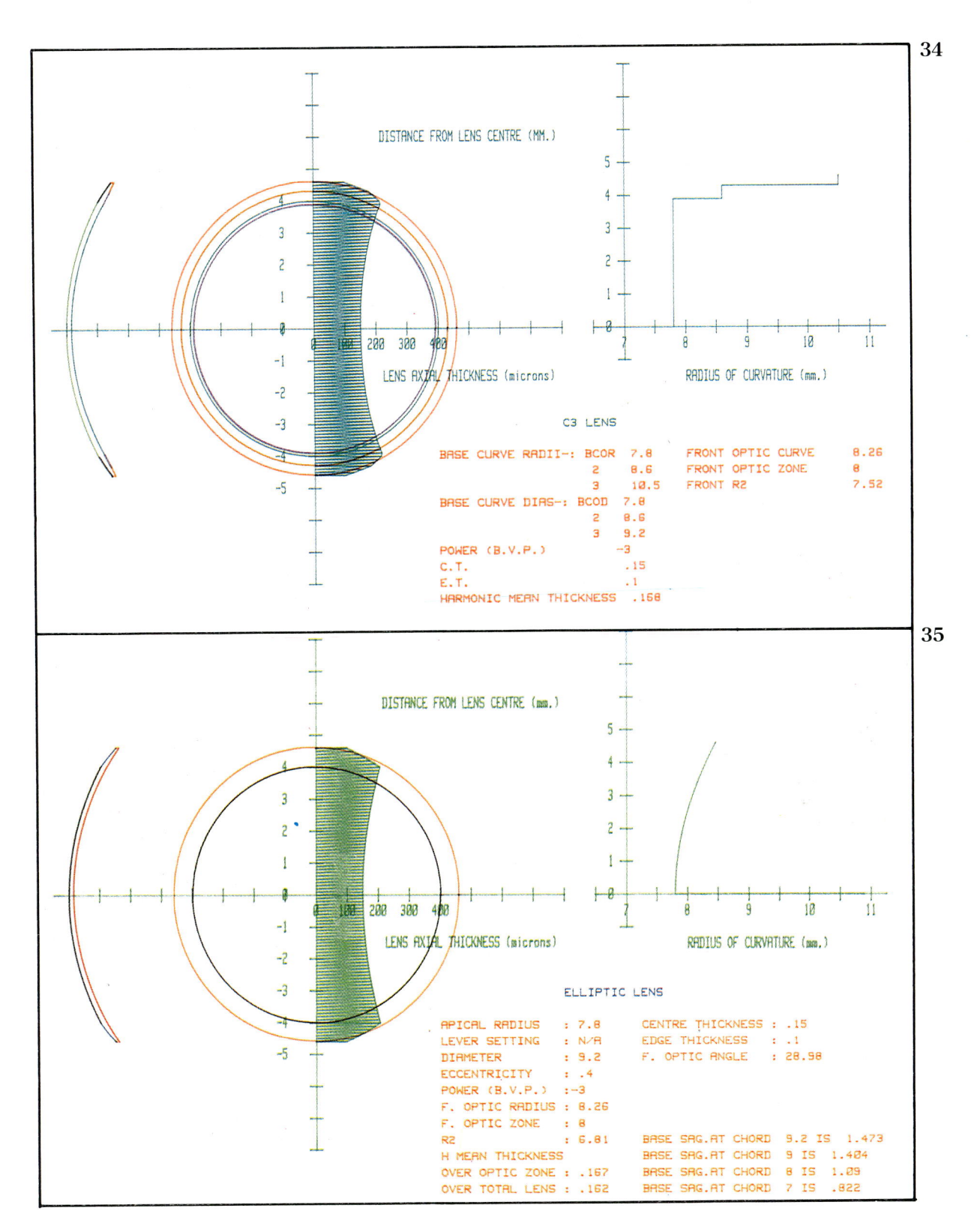

34 & 35 Tri-curved spherical and aspheric lenses. The blue lens should be compared with the green. The back curve of the blue lens is tri-curved spherical while the green is aspheric (E = 0.4 or SF = +0.84). Note that the equivalent central and peripheral radii are 7.8 and 8.6 respectively. Therefore the back curves of both lenses are for practical purposes similar, but can be manufactured by different technology.

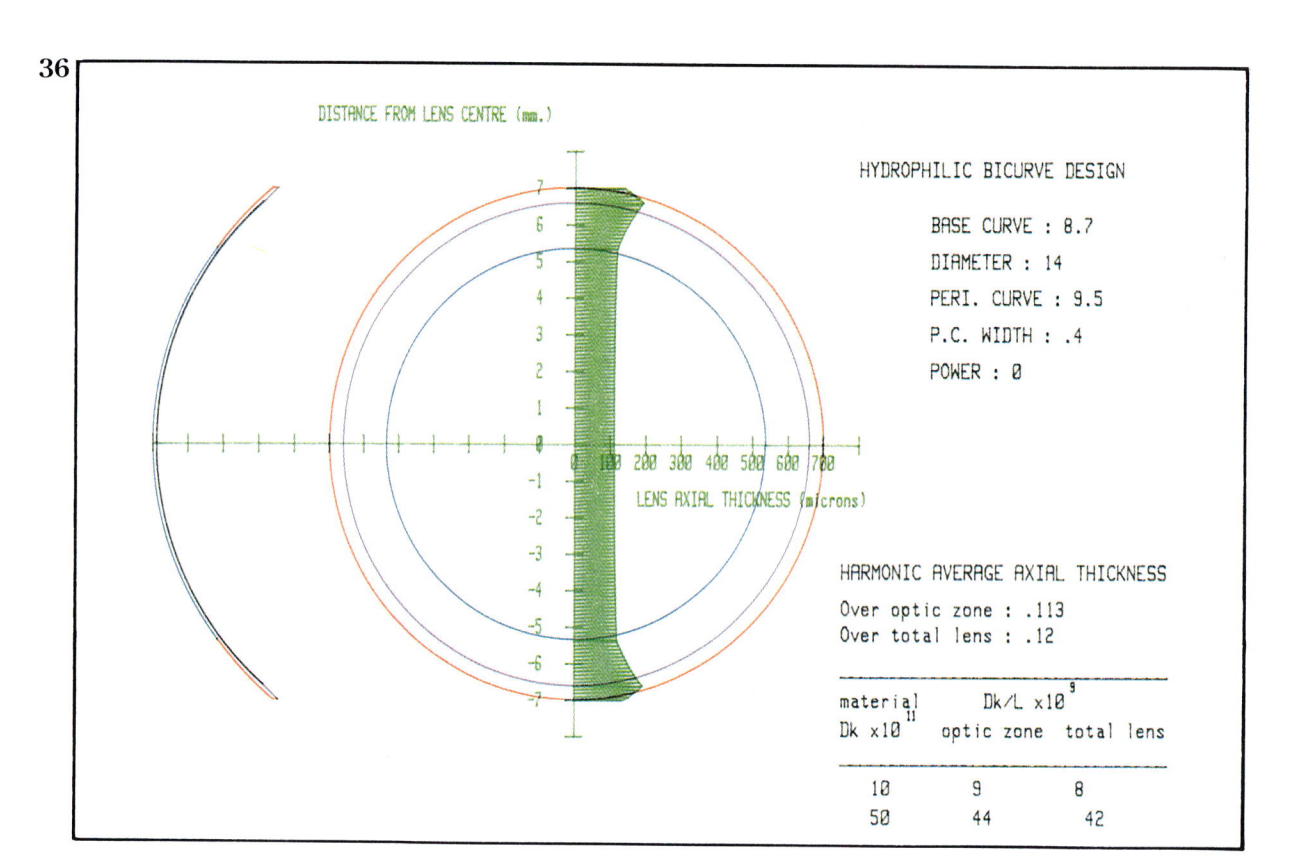

36 Low water content lens. This shows a relatively thick lens if it is made of a low water content material with a low Dk/L value (8×10^{-9} ATVP), which is likely to give hypoxia unless it is fitted loose, whereas the high water content lens gives a satisfactory Dk/L level at the same thickness.

37 & 38 Reduced optic design. These profiles illustrate not only the value of reduced optic design but also higher Dk values. On the other hand very thin low water content lenses should be programmed to give the same Dk/L as the Dk 50 material.

37

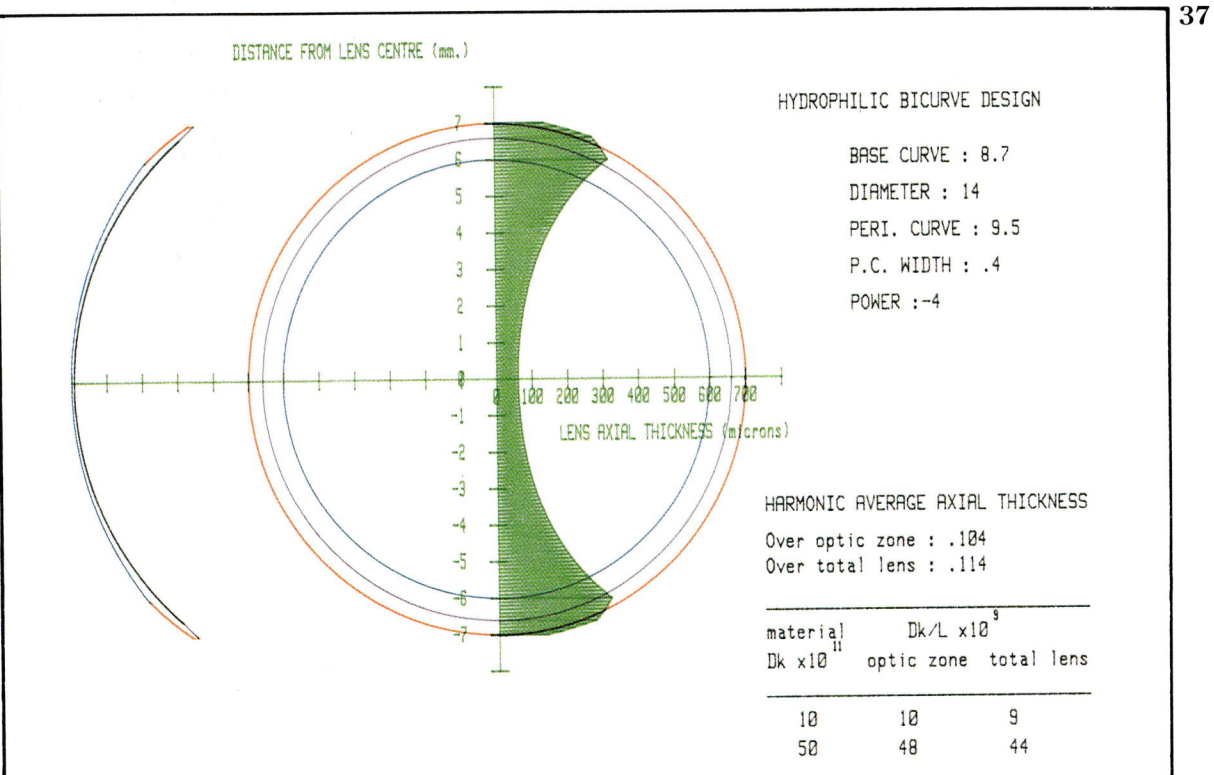

DISTANCE FROM LENS CENTRE (mm.)

LENS AXIAL THICKNESS (microns)

HYDROPHILIC BICURVE DESIGN

BASE CURVE : 8.7
DIAMETER : 14
PERI. CURVE : 9.5
P.C. WIDTH : .4
POWER : -4

HARMONIC AVERAGE AXIAL THICKNESS

Over optic zone : .104
Over total lens : .114

material $Dk \times 10^{11}$	$Dk/L \times 10^9$ optic zone	total lens
10	10	9
50	48	44

38

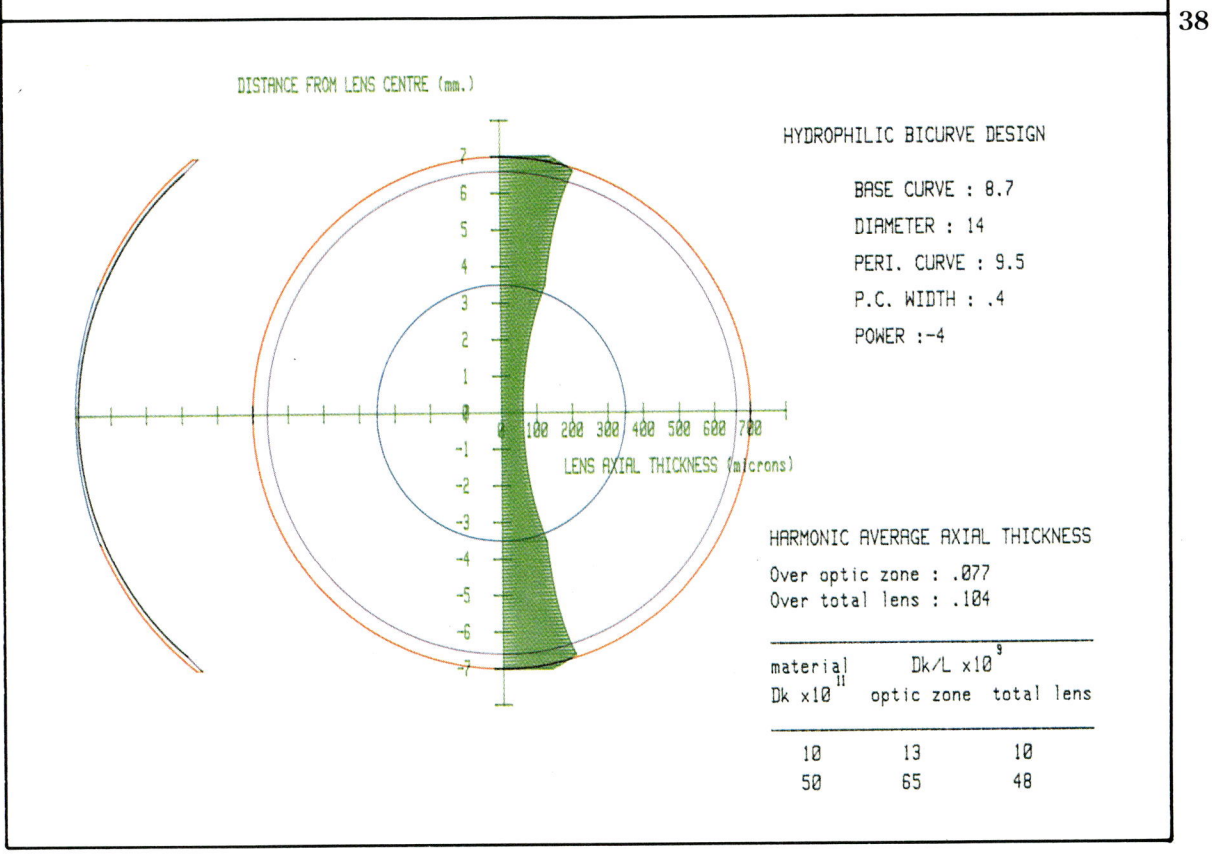

DISTANCE FROM LENS CENTRE (mm.)

LENS AXIAL THICKNESS (microns)

HYDROPHILIC BICURVE DESIGN

BASE CURVE : 8.7
DIAMETER : 14
PERI. CURVE : 9.5
P.C. WIDTH : .4
POWER : -4

HARMONIC AVERAGE AXIAL THICKNESS

Over optic zone : .077
Over total lens : .104

material $Dk \times 10^{11}$	$Dk/L \times 10^9$ optic zone	total lens
10	13	10
50	65	48

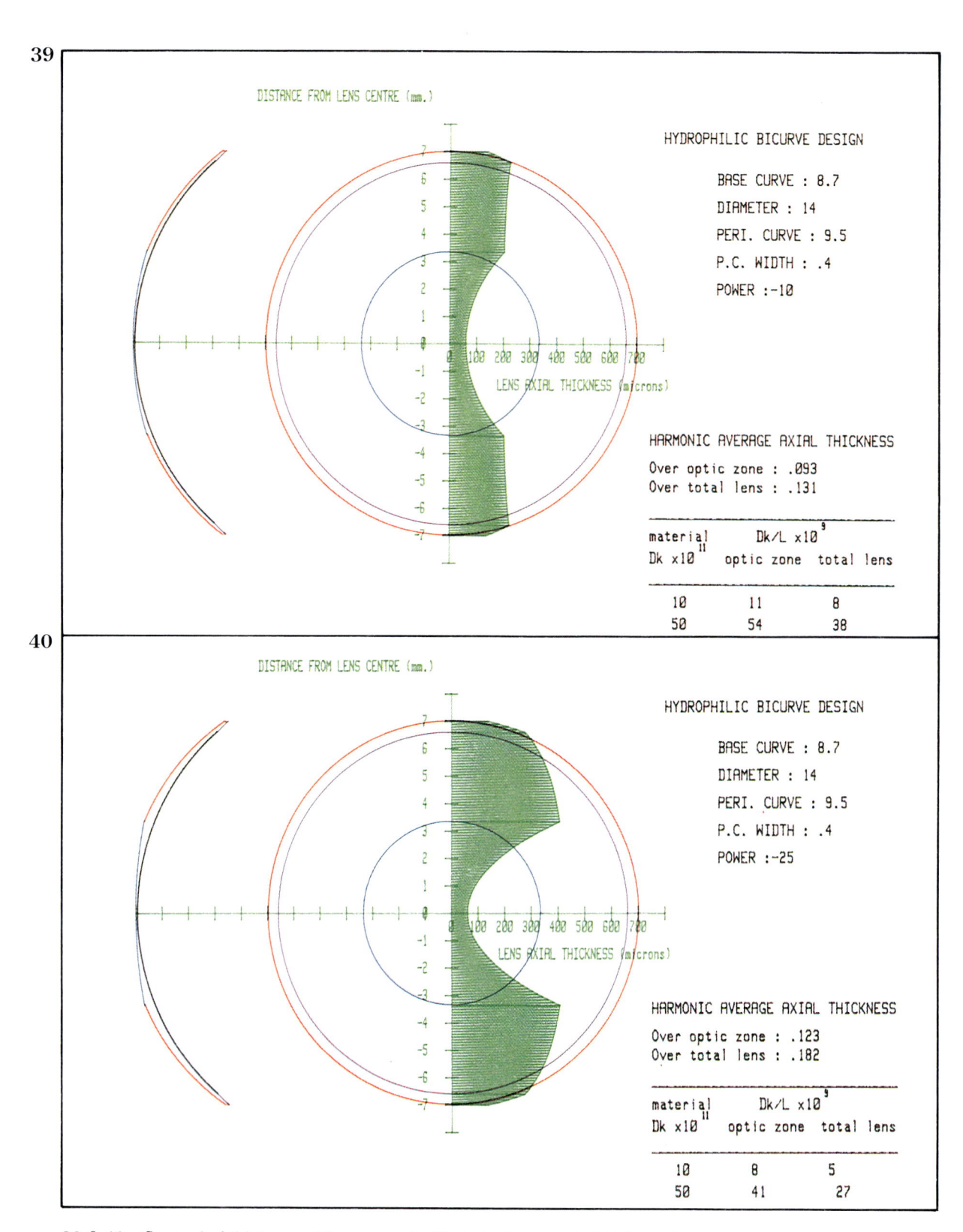

39 & 40 Control of thickness. These examples illustrate the control of thickness for high minus powers using reduced optics.

41

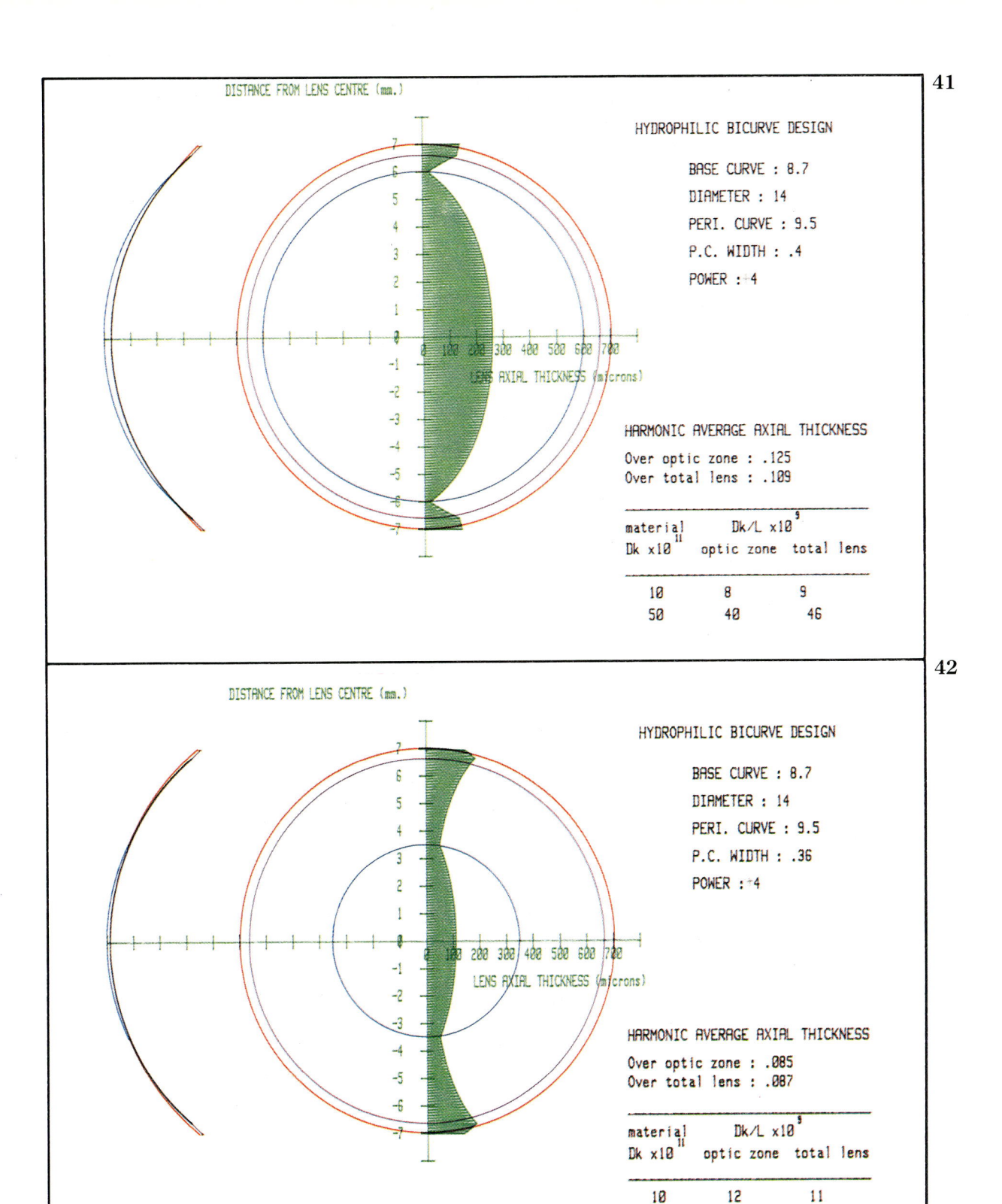

HYDROPHILIC BICURVE DESIGN

BASE CURVE : 8.7
DIAMETER : 14
PERI. CURVE : 9.5
P.C. WIDTH : .4
POWER : +4

HARMONIC AVERAGE AXIAL THICKNESS
Over optic zone : .125
Over total lens : .109

material $Dk \times 10^{11}$	$Dk/L \times 10^9$ optic zone	total lens
10	8	9
50	40	46

42

HYDROPHILIC BICURVE DESIGN

BASE CURVE : 8.7
DIAMETER : 14
PERI. CURVE : 9.5
P.C. WIDTH : .36
POWER : +4

HARMONIC AVERAGE AXIAL THICKNESS
Over optic zone : .085
Over total lens : .087

material $Dk \times 10^{11}$	$Dk/L \times 10^9$ optic zone	total lens
10	12	11
50	59	57

41-44 Negative peripheral carrier design. All these lenses are plus lenses and the use of a negative peripheral carrier design is obvious as well as their reduced optics. Even with high water content lenses the total Dk/L is within the hypoxia levels. Thus a new design could be programmed for, say, an optic of 6 mm instead of almost 7 mm as here.

43

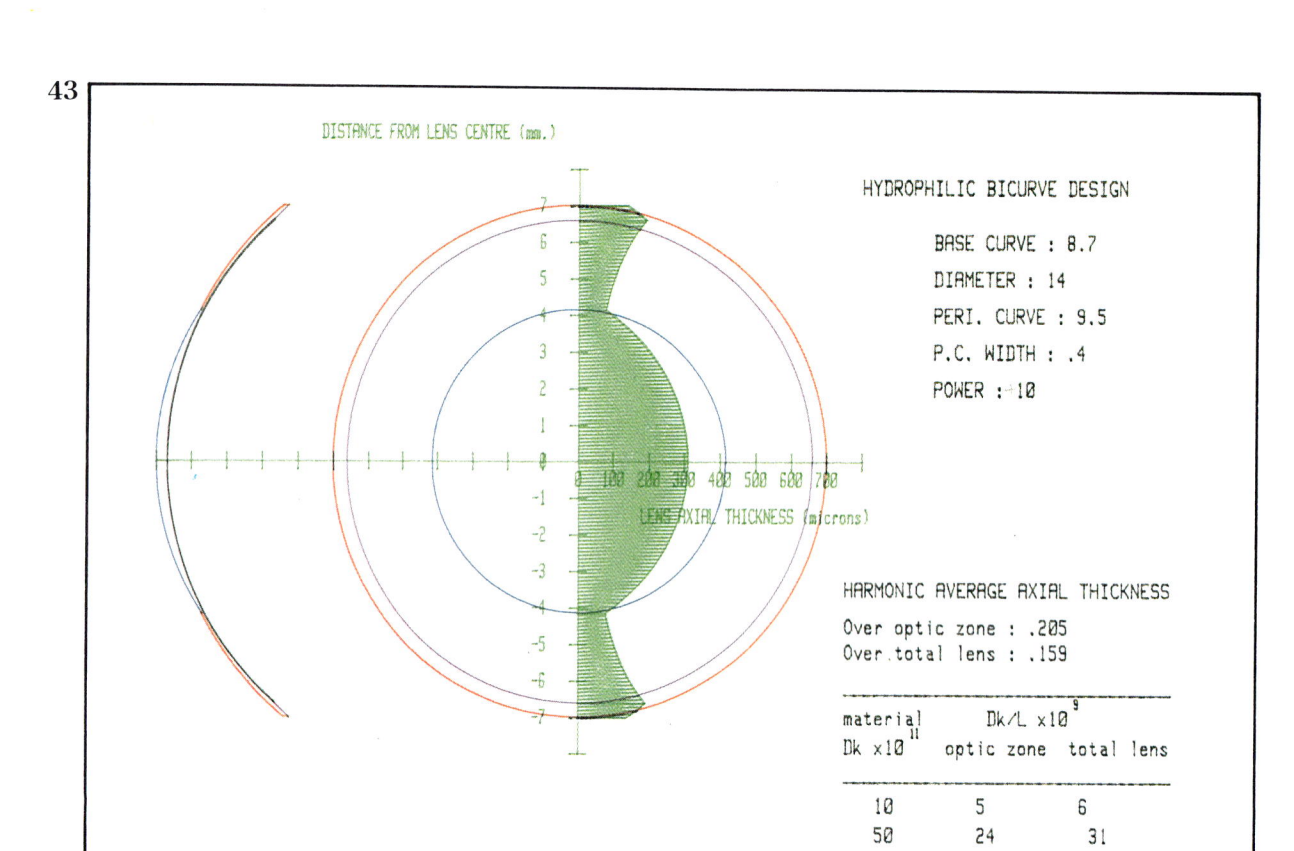

HYDROPHILIC BICURVE DESIGN

BASE CURVE : 8.7
DIAMETER : 14
PERI. CURVE : 9.5
P.C. WIDTH : .4
POWER : +10

HARMONIC AVERAGE AXIAL THICKNESS

Over optic zone : .205
Over total lens : .159

material $Dk \times 10^{11}$	$Dk/L \times 10^9$ optic zone	total lens
10	5	6
50	24	31

44

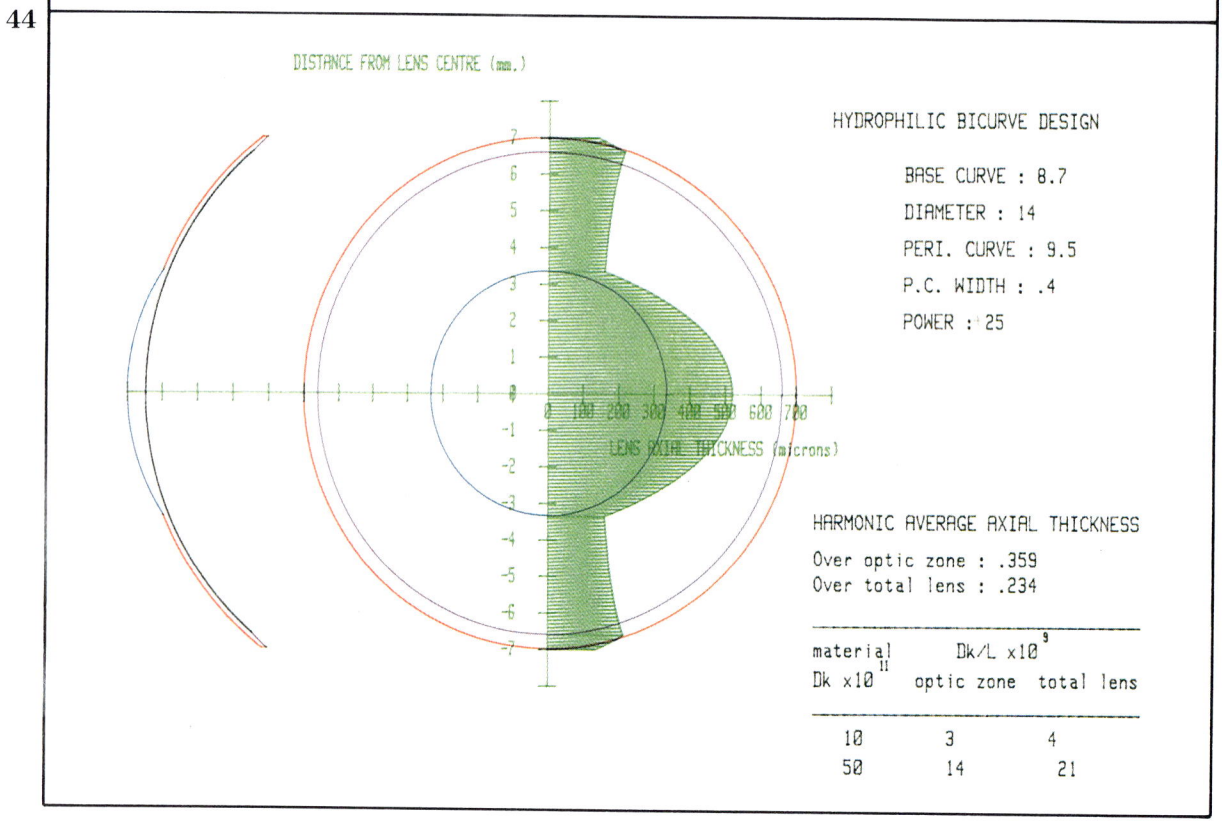

HYDROPHILIC BICURVE DESIGN

BASE CURVE : 8.7
DIAMETER : 14
PERI. CURVE : 9.5
P.C. WIDTH : .4
POWER : +25

HARMONIC AVERAGE AXIAL THICKNESS

Over optic zone : .359
Over total lens : .234

material $Dk \times 10^{11}$	$Dk/L \times 10^9$ optic zone	total lens
10	3	4
50	14	21

Lens thickness distribution and gas flow

45 Lens form and gas flow. Given the Dk of the material and the lens thickness profile the gas flow can be calculated for any part of the lens. In the example, the negative powered lens is of a very high power (-30.d.). Two different designs are shown. The left-hand design has a thick junction zone that will not permit good gas flow whereas the right hand design permits good gas flow.

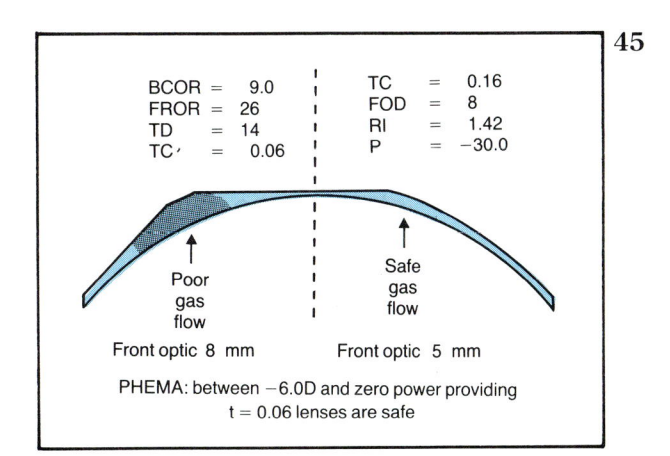

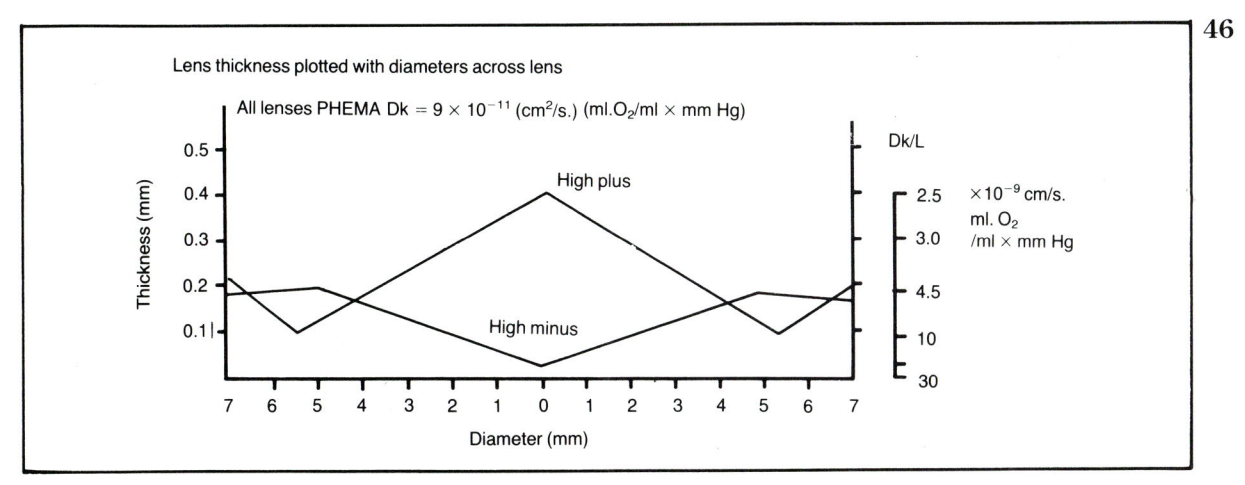

46 Two PHEMA lenses are plotted to show their thickness distribution and the related Dk/L. If a Dk/L of 30 were to be considered safe for the normal cornea, then most of these lenses would fall outside these limits. In the case of the negative lens only the central zone appears safe. It must be stated that there are other factors besides thickness that clinically permit the wearing of such lenses.

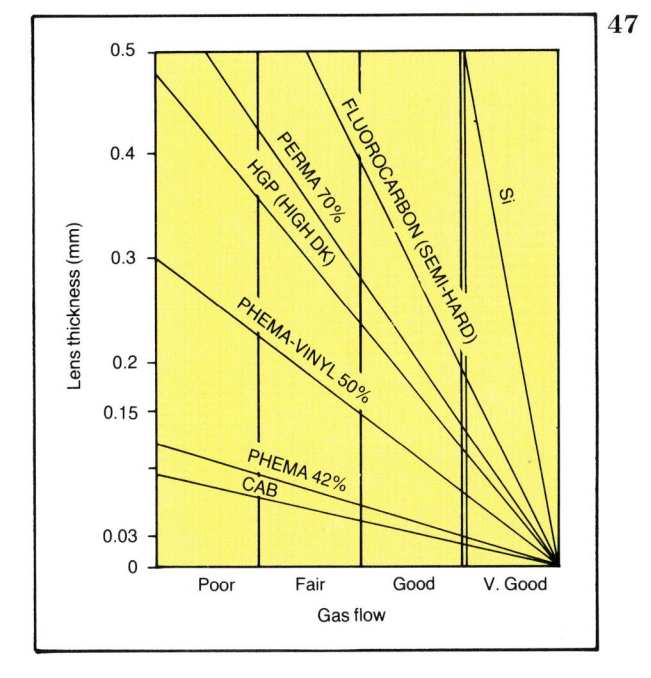

47 Several materials are now compared as to thickness and gas flow. It must again be emphasized that thickness is not the sole criterion for physiological tolerance.

27

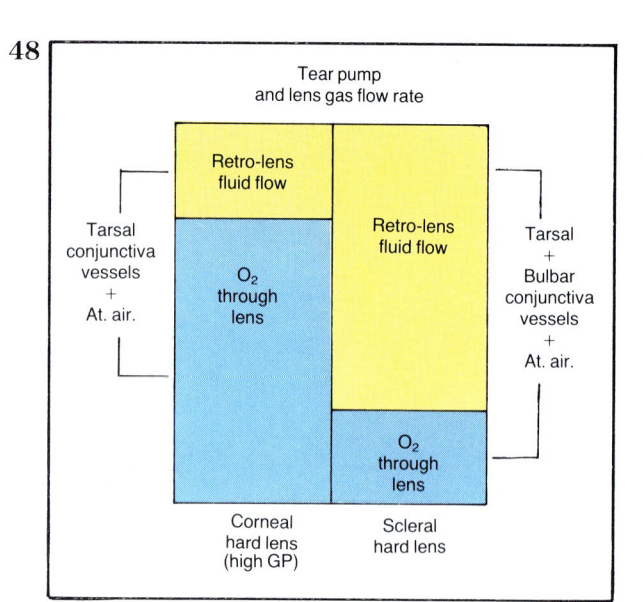

Tear pump retro-lens and gas flow

48 Lens design and the tear pump mechanism. O_2 can diffuse to the cornea via the tear fluid, and for a gas permeable corneal lens the relative amounts passing through the lens as compared with the tears under the lens may be 25-50 per cent, depending upon lens size and fit.

A large scleral lens made of the same material may even obtain its O_2 from the area of conjunctiva under the haptic.

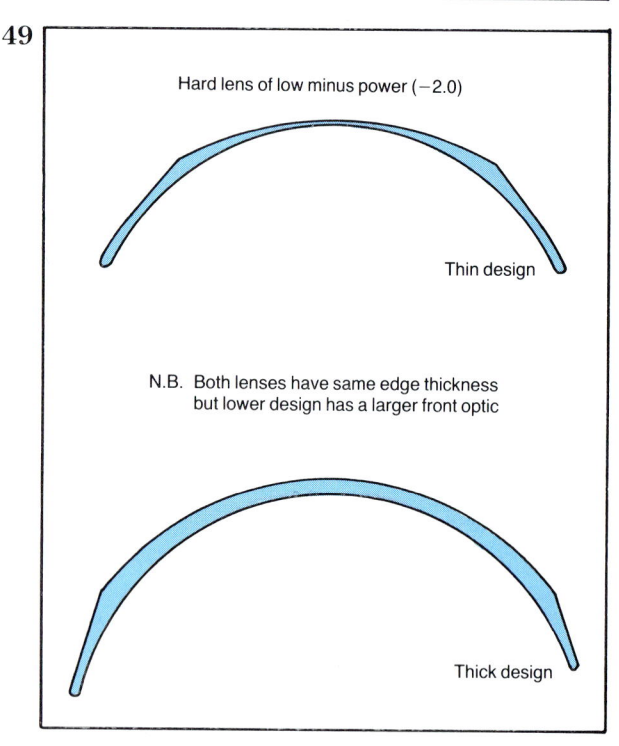

Low power design and thickness control

49 There are some points of improvement for low power lenses. The top design has a very thin centre and reduced optic with a conventional edge thickness. However, often, because it is a low power, a single front curve is used with the result that the lens is unncessarily thick at the centre. The edge thickness is the same in the two lenses.

Reduced front optics

50 Front peripheral offset curves. Front peripheral curves will add thickness to the lens carrier portion and are of use in plus reduced optic lens design.

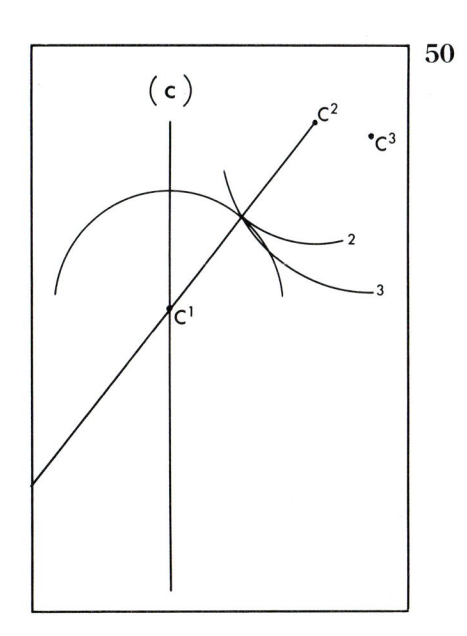

51 To reduce the bulk of both plus and negative power lenses and to distribute the thicknesses more evenly, the diameter of the front optic can be reduced to as small as 5 mm. (Alternatively, an aspheric design can be used.) In the case of the plus power lens a negative front surface is used at the periphery.

The negative power lens when reduced (to **b**), still has a thick edge design. A further reduction (to **c**) permits an offset negative carrier.

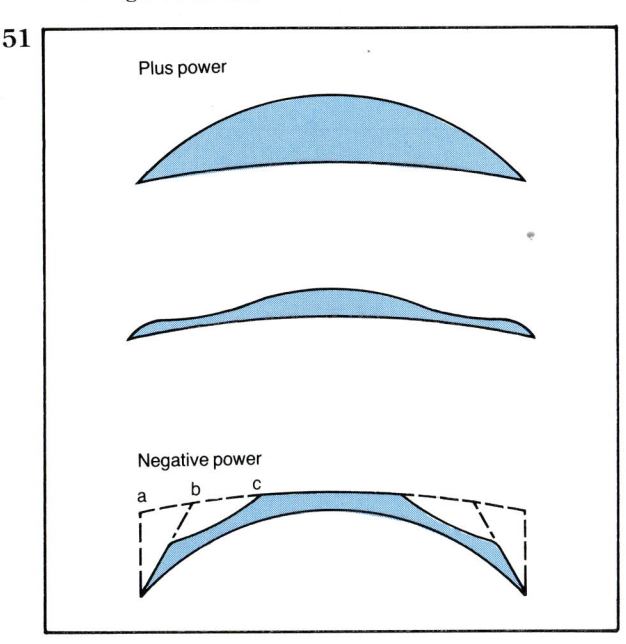

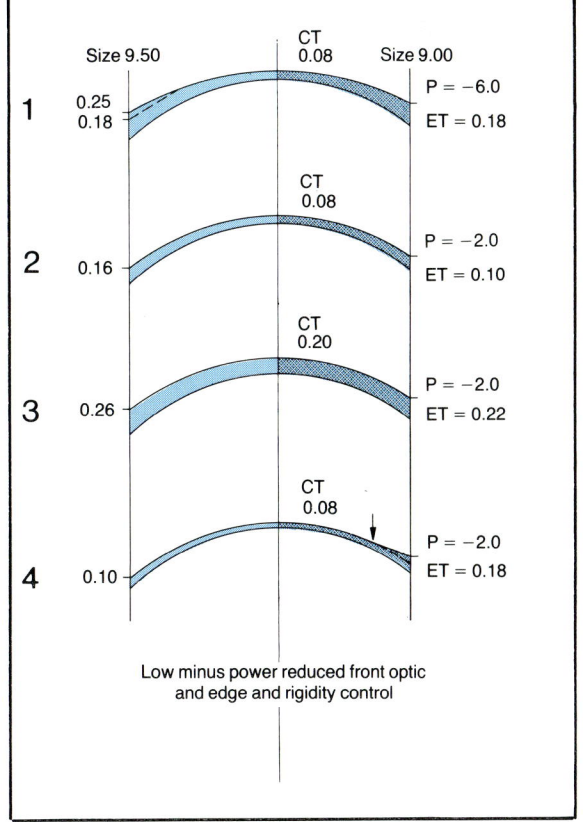

52 Thickness and rigidity of low power lenses. The scale drawings (edge designs omitted) are of −2d. and −6d. lenses. They show the effect of thin lens design on front optic and edge thicknesses—problems that particularly affect low rigidity materials such as silico-acrylate co-polymers:

1. −6d. lenses with a single front curve for the 9 mm size, but for the 9.5 mm size it has a reduced front optic to allow a thinner edge.

2. −2d. lenses of the same centre thickness as in (1), but now the periphery of the small lens is too thin and is likely to result in lens deformation. The 9.5 mm size results in a thicker periphery and greater rigidity.

3. −2d. lenses with single front curves to show the resulting excessive peripheral thickness.

4. −2d. lenses with the same thin centre as in (2), but now, by using peripheral front offset curves, substantial thickness to the edge can be given to the lenses increasing their rigidity and using the gas transmission properties of the material to its best advantage.

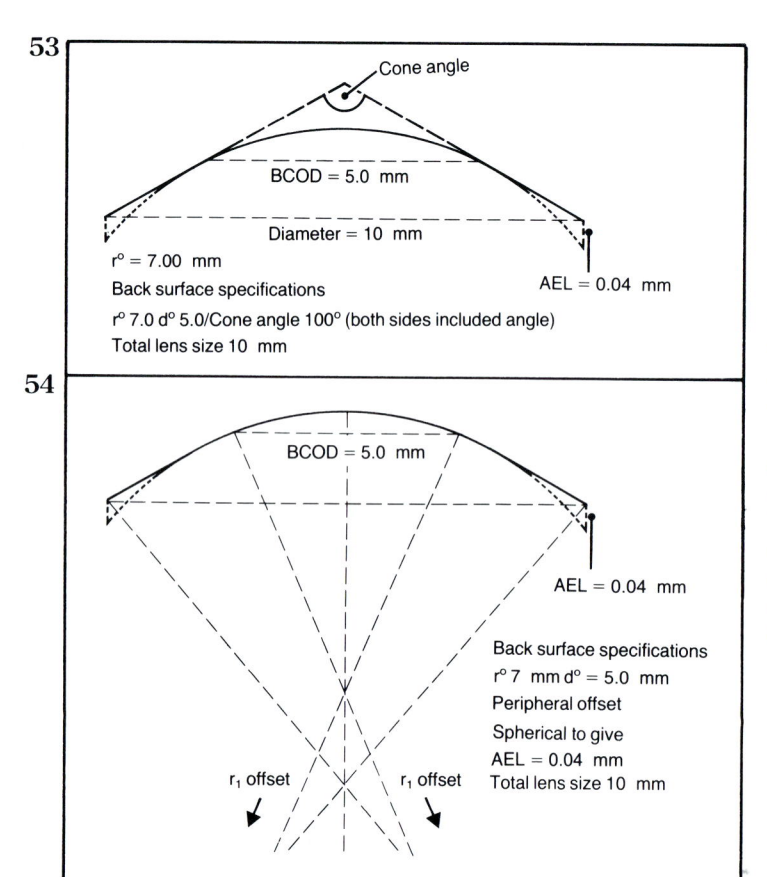

Pseudo-conic surfaces

The use of several spherical curves to simulate a true aspherical surface has been described. The simple way to simulate a true aspherical surface is to use the central spherical curve and an additional peripheral curve that is either a tangential-peripheral cone (**53**), or a peripheral curve that is spherical with its centre offset from the central axis (**54**).

In both these instances, in order to provide an axial edge lift useful for the size of the lens it is necessary to have a smaller than conventional central back zone. In these instances the central fit is always steeper than the keratometry. Such lens designs are of use in keratoconus and keratoplasty.

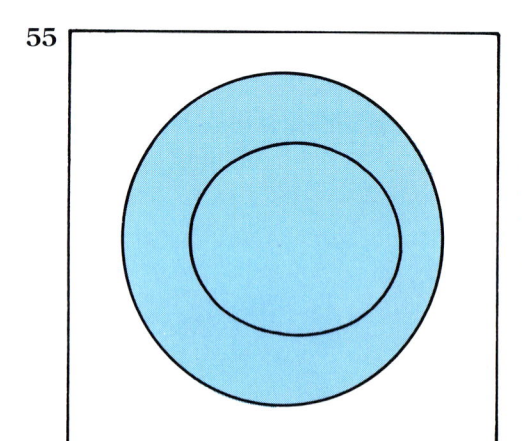

53 Cone angle; BCOD = 5.0 mm; Diameter = 10 mm; r^o = 7.00 mm; AEL = 0.04 mm
Back surface specifications
r^o 7.0 d^o 5.0/Cone angle 100° (both sides included angle)
Total lens size 10 mm

54 BCOD = 5.0 mm; AEL = 0.04 mm
Back surface specifications
r^o 7 mm d^o = 5.0 mm
Peripheral offset
Spherical to give
AEL = 0.04 mm
Total lens size 10 mm
r_1 offset r_1 offset

Toric back surface junction

55 Toric back surfaces can be limited to the peripheral curves, the central back curve being spherical, or the whole of the back curves can be toroidal. Where a spherical surface joins a toroidal surface an oval junction occurs, as in the diagram.

Best (optimal) lens forms

56 The spectacle lens can be designed using front and back surfaces to give the best image formation. This is especially important in the case of steep surfaces. Lens A is an example of a plus power lens in which the peripheral curves have been designed to reduce aberrations in the form of interrupted lines. For the contact lens this could be best done by use of a front aspheric curve.

A negative power contact lens, as shown in B, could reduce its aberrations by steepening the back peripheral curve. However, this is inconsistent with a good fit.

57 Effect of gas transmission upon lens design. Gas (O_2) flux through a contact lens is in direct relationship to its thickness. Thus a material such as PHEMA, 40 per cent water at 0.03 mm thick, may give a Dk/L equal to 30 (ATVP), whereas vinyl, 80 per cent water and able only to be made 0.1 mm thick, gives a Dk/L equal to 50. The respective Dk's are 9 and 62 x 10^{-11} (ATVP). Thus, a high Dk is not in itself sufficient information as to lens gas flux.

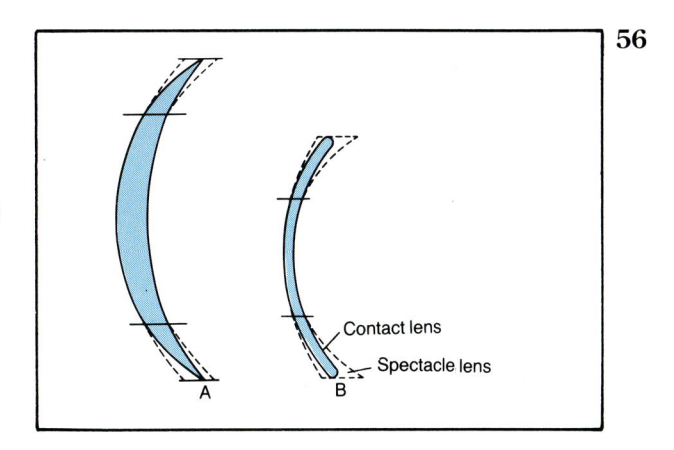

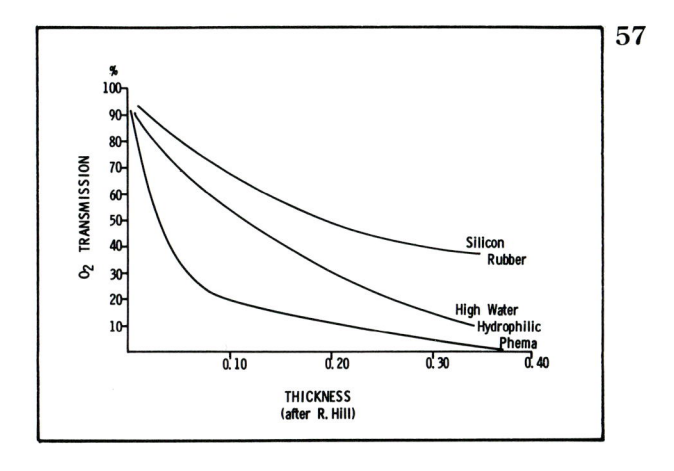

3 Manufacture of lenses

There are two levels of lens manufacture: the laboratory that makes single lenses to practitioners' prescriptions, and the commercial manufacturers who are chiefly concerned with defined, mass-produced product lines. It is the latter that has a responsibility to research and development, often working with institutions. The details of manufacture are sometimes protected by patents so only an outline of the procedure for making a lens is given here.

Lathe cutting

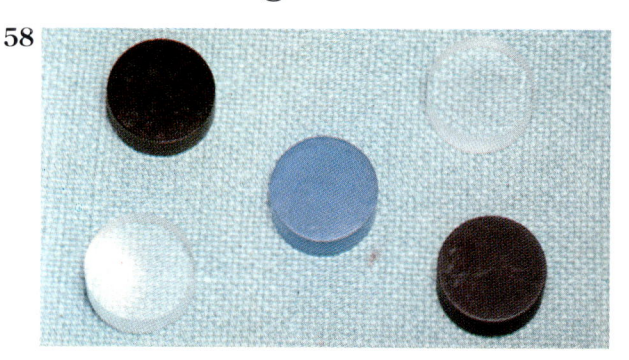

58 Hard, dry plastic buttons. The cutting tool is usually a specially cut diamond. Laser cutting is a more refined technique.

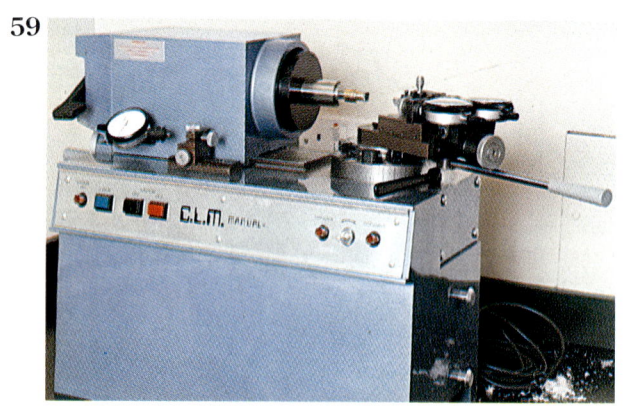

59 & 60 A manual lathe is shown cutting the front of the plastic to give a spherical surface. In practice the back surface is cut first with as many different back curves as required, including the edge back curve.

Lathes can be automatic and computer controlled; they can also have a template inserted that guides the cutting tool to give a continuous aspheric or pseudo-aspheric curve, for example.

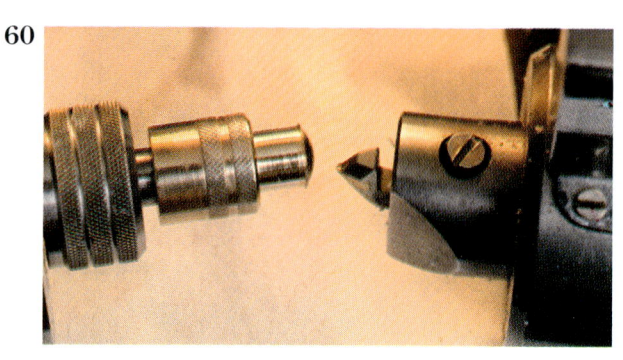

61 This shows the surface immediately after the lathe has cut the plastic (x 10). Using a fine diamond tool and/or a laser, the grooves can be almost indiscernible to the naked eye. Back and front surfaces are generated in this way and the thickness controlled to tolerances of ±0.01 mm.

Many hydrophilic and nonhydrophilic lenses commence in this way. The hydrophilic lens will eventually be equiliberated with saline and therefore the cut dimensions have to make accurate allowance for the material's linear expansion factor.

62 The grooves are polished out as much as possible by automatic machines using tools with conforming surfaces and polishing medium.

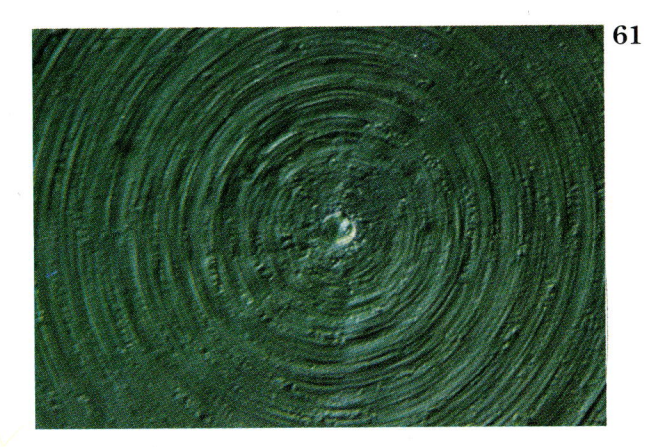

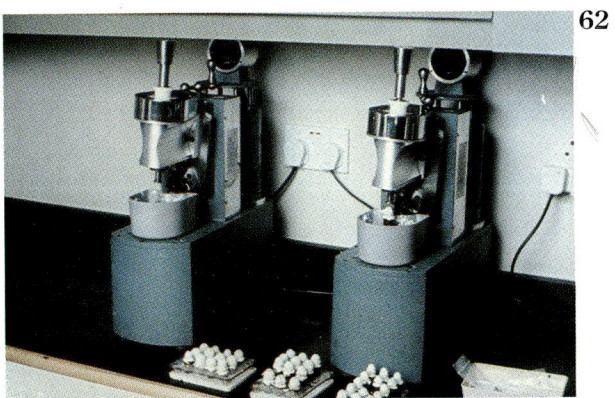

Lens edging

63 & 64 Edging of lenses may be just a hand polishing process if the lathe has cut both the front and back edge surfaces. There are edging machines which not only form the edge but control the lens size.

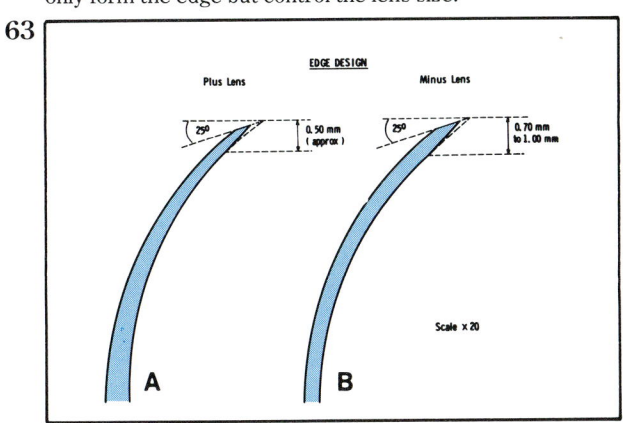

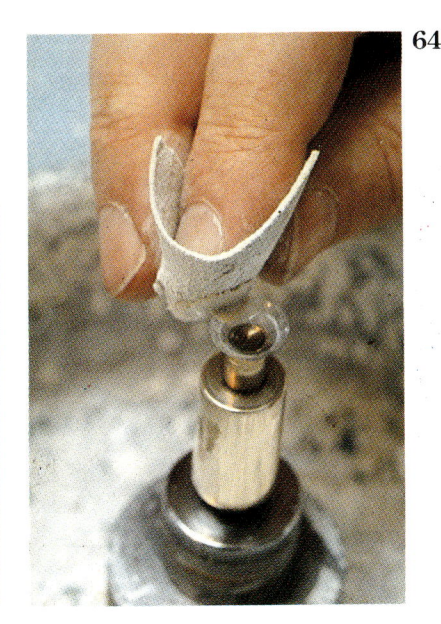

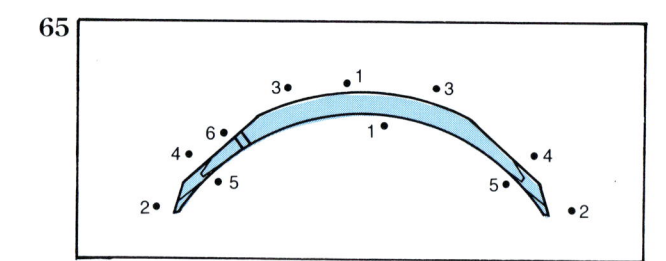

Lens modification

65 After the lathe cut hard lens has been manufactured and worn, a limited number of alterations can be carried out:

1. The surface and edge can be repolished.
2. Thickness permitting, the edge and form of the bevel can be refashioned.
3. The power can be altered by lapping ±0.75d. (not always over the whole surface).
4. The size of the lens can be reduced.
5. The peripheral surface and sometimes the intermediate surface can be flattened and the surfaces at the junctions reblended.
6. The lens can be fenestrated (by drilling).

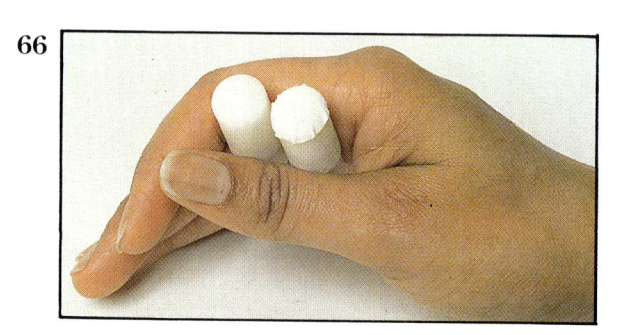

Pressure grinding

66 & 67 Diamond-bonded tools (66) are used to grind out surfaces (a lapidary process), and when covered with a suitable material and polishing medium, they will polish and blend junctions between surfaces, forming a smooth transition (**67**).

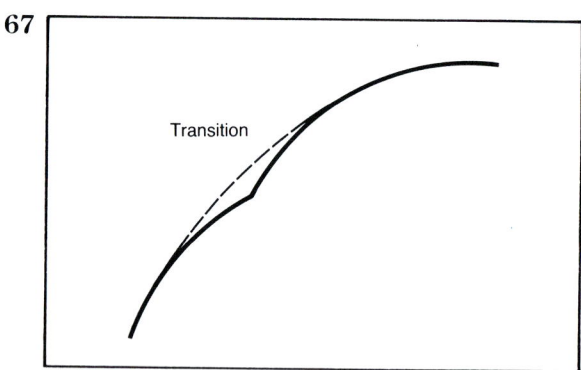

Moulding

Spin moulding

68 A process patented by Wichterle uses the polymer mix in the fluid state, which is placed into a mould. The front surface of the lens is formed by the mould. As the cast spins the mix polymerizes and sets hard. The speed of the mould rotation, the viscosity and the amount of polymer determine the aspheric shape of the back surface of the lens. Thus, many different size and thickness variations are possible, but the final lens design is constrained by the method. Bausch & Lomb are the chief exponents of this type of lens. The lenses have an excellent surface finish.

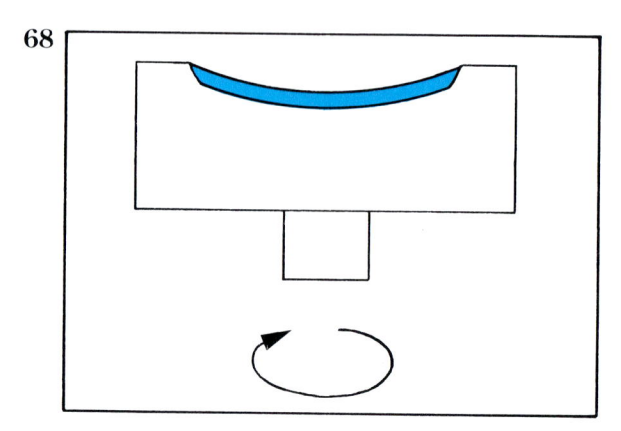

Injection moulding

69 Injection moulding using metal dyes. This technique was used for scleral lens manufacture in the 1940s and 1950s. It has been suggested recently (Pullum, 1987) that this method is now applicable to silicone-acrylate co-polymer and thus to a moulded gas permeable scleral lens. The figure shows the male and female dyes of the lens shape made from an eye model.

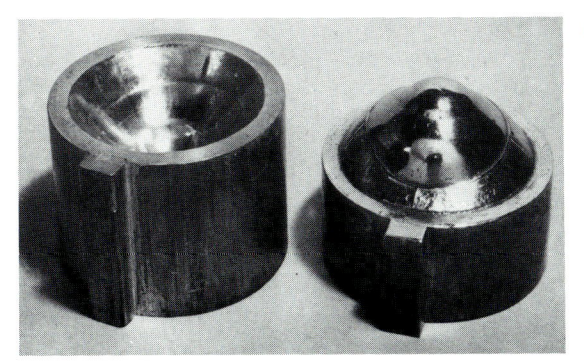

Metal dyes have now been replaced by plastic dyes, which can produce several hundred corneal lenses an hour. (Figures **70-72** are courtesy of Cooper Vision.)

70 Purpose-built precision machinery on the laboratory floor.

71 The individual male and female components of the mould are specially-designed to produce an edge without flash (overflow of polymer).

72 Multi-moulds of plastic material to take the precise amount of injected liquid polymer.

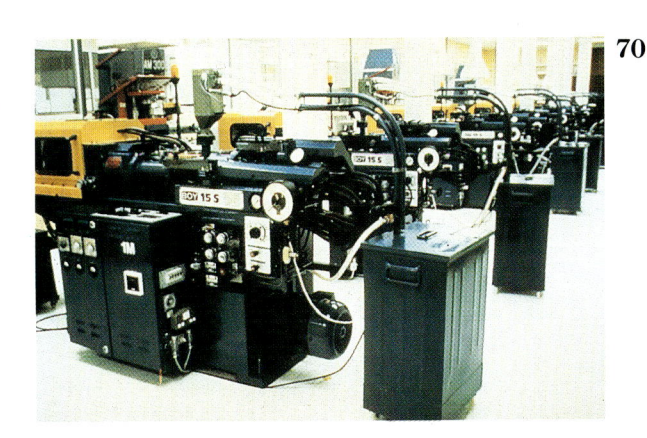

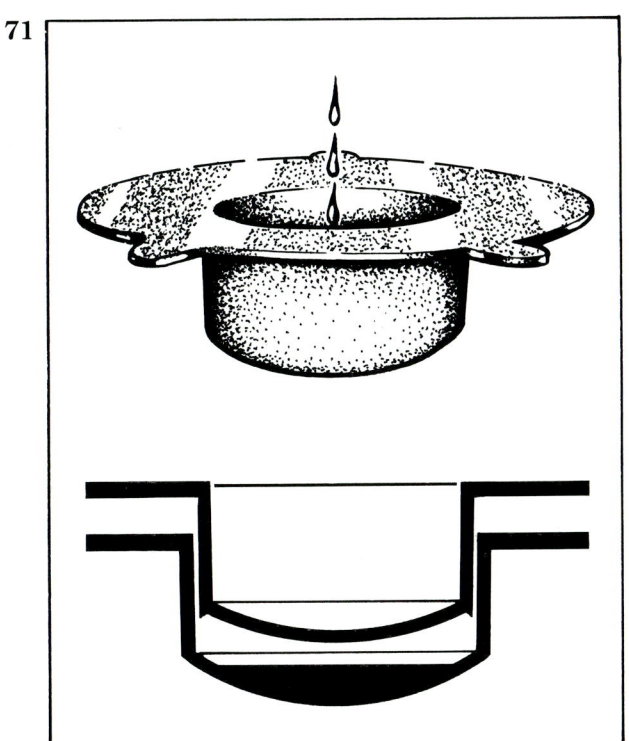

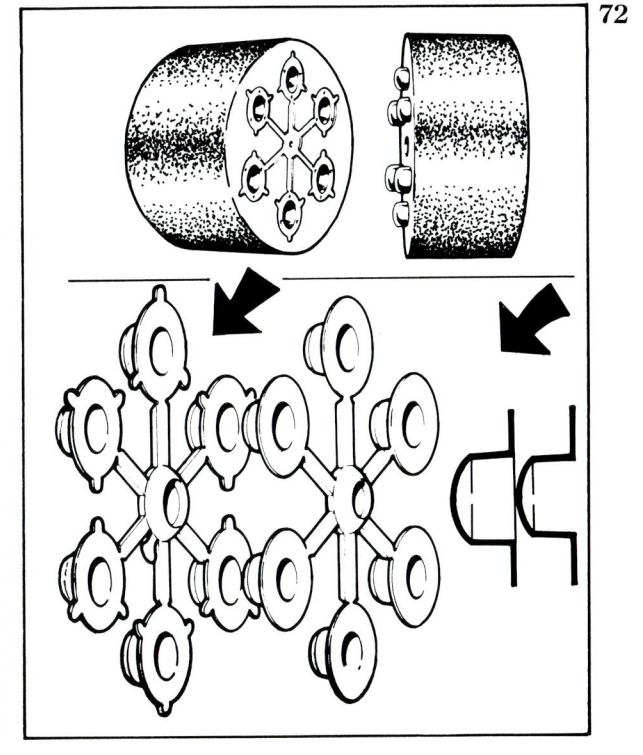

Scleral lens manufacture

Although the making of a scleral lens and its fitting cannot be separated, the basic technical procedure is given here and the clinical aspects in Chapters 6 & 7.

The scleral lens plays a particular role in the treatment of various eye diseases and is the foundation of prosthetic practice.

Methods:
- Lathe cutting from a solid button of plastic—the final lens is referred to as a 'preformed geometric scleral lens'.
- Moulding—using heated sheets of thermolabile plastic pressed on to plaster models of the eye or injecting liquid or crystal polymer between dyes (polymerization is by heat and pressure).

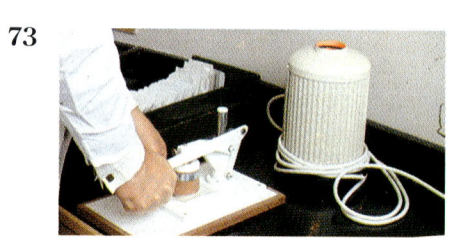

73 Heated PMMA (or other thermolabile plastic) 0.6 mm thick is inserted between the plaster model and a conforming pad or curved heat-resistant surface. Pressure is then applied evenly with the aid of a hand press.

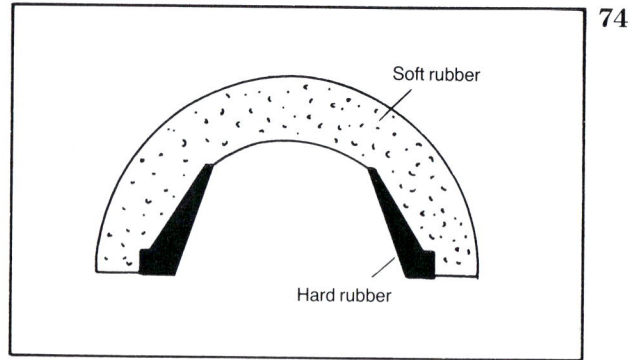

74 Cross-section through the curved, heat-resistant pad which clamps down on to the hot plastic.

75 & 76 The shape is cut out of the plastic sheet.

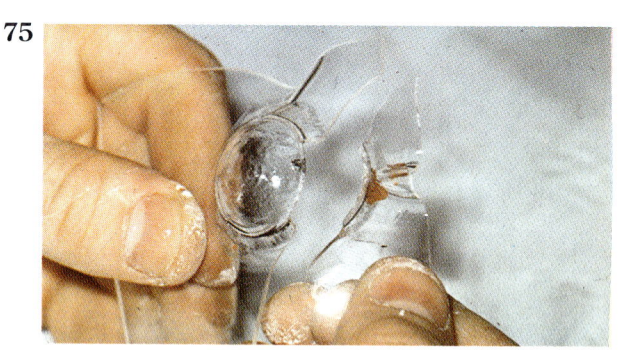

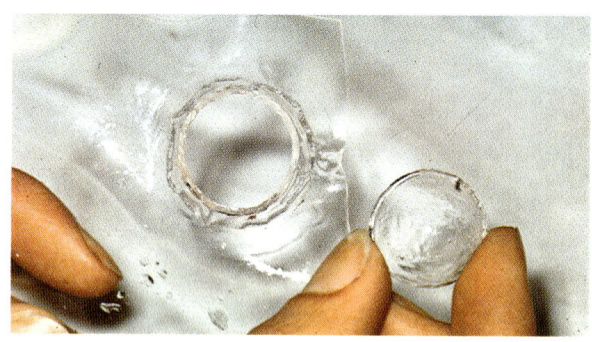

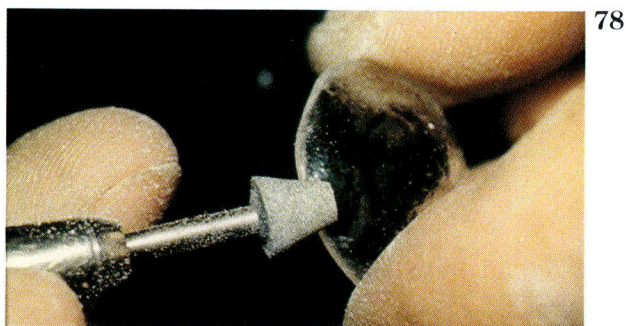

77 & 78 The edge is ground and polished.

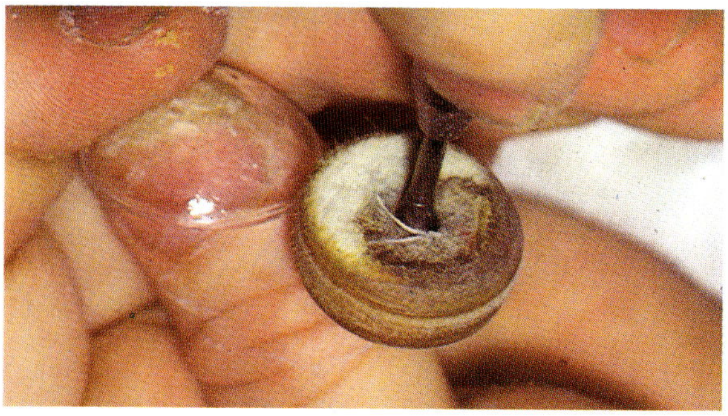

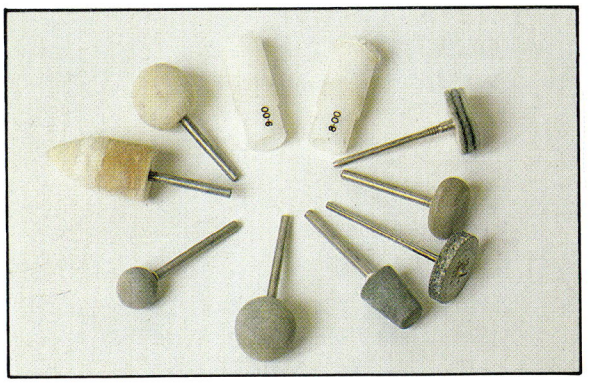

79 & 80 Diamond-bonded tools and hand-held rotating drive equipment are used to form smooth transitions and give essential clearance areas.

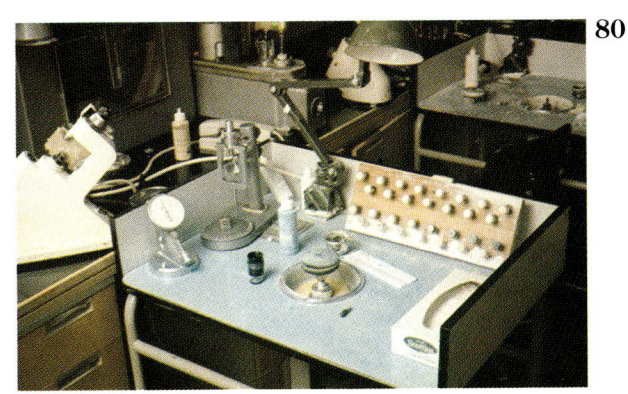

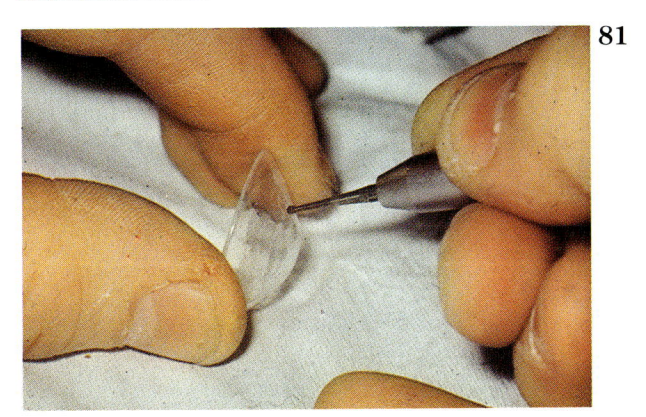

81 A fenestration is drilled at the junction of the optic with the haptic.

Lathe generation method

82 & 83 Scleral lenses can also be manufactured to geometric curves using the lathe generation method. This method is of value using hydrophilic plastics to make scleral lenses and also gas permeable nonhydrophilic materials which are not thermolabile. The diagrams give the optic and haptic diameters. If using gas permeable material, the distribution of thickness should ensure thin zones over the limbal transition (**82**).

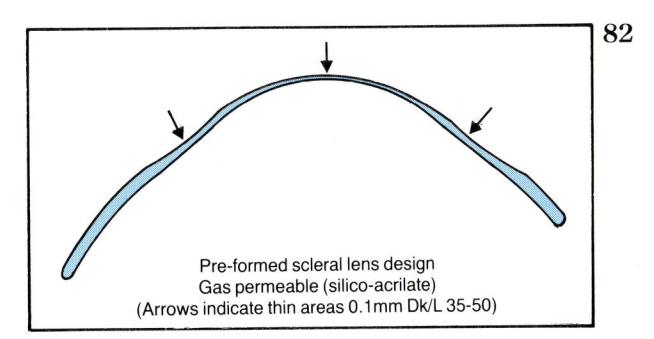

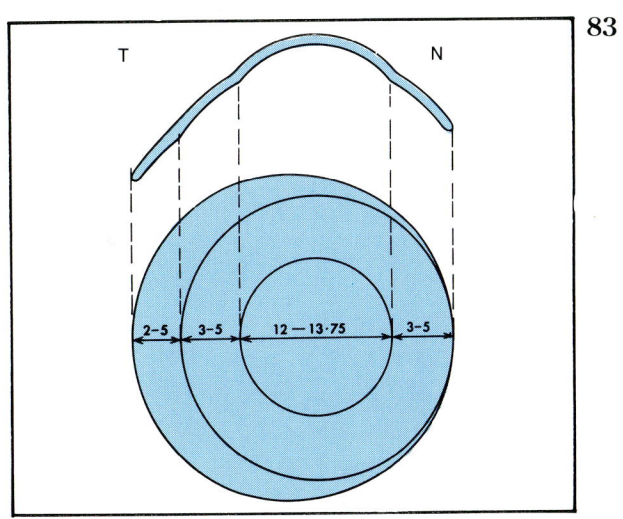

Pre-formed scleral lens design
Gas permeable (silico-acrilate)
(Arrows indicate thin areas 0.1mm Dk/L 35-50)

37

4 Checking of lenses

Standards

Standards are necessary for all health products: this includes the lens and the preparations used for its care and to improve the patient's tolerance. Standards state the tolerances that can be accepted in the purity of the ingredients, in the finished product, its packaging, labelling, safety, and for the measurements of the lens. *Standards do not necessarily control the proof of the function of the lens.*

The lens is measured by the manufacturer and the practitioner, but there are many limitations since the accuracy and precision of the instruments used and the conditions under which the tests are done are rarely stated. There are some simple measurements that the practitioner can make on all contact lenses and, providing the tolerances are known, these can be useful.

It is axiomatic that the instruments used should be more precise than the tolerances allowed in the manufacturing process, otherwise a design drawing of a lens to be manufactured to an accuracy of 5 per cent error may eventually be measured by an instrument with a 10 per cent error.

Magnifyers and microscopes

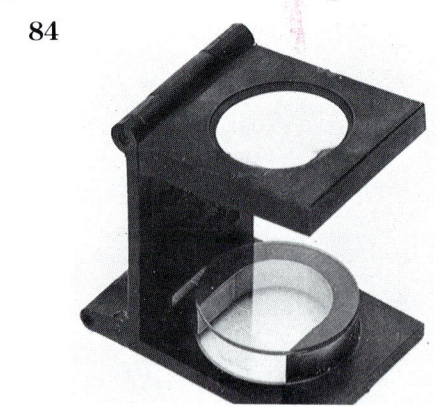

84 **Simple magnifier** with a tank and a graticule—for measuring the size of a lens (± 0.1 mm tolerance).

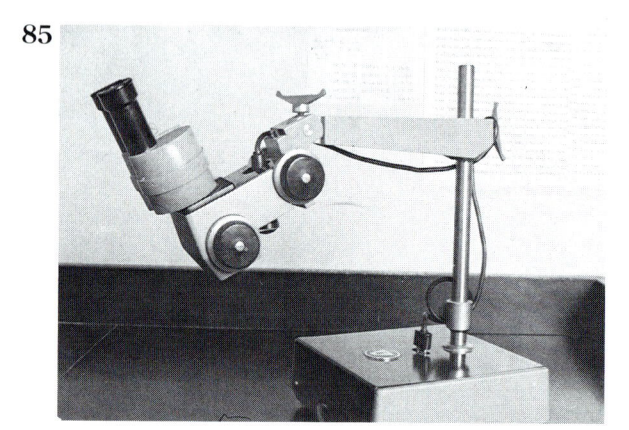

85 **Microscope** with a working distance objective $M = \times 20$. Self-illumination oblique beam. A very useful instrument for examining contamination of solutions, lens contamination, and all surface and edge defects.

In research and manufacturers' quality control, conventional light and scanning microscopy (even TEM) have been used.

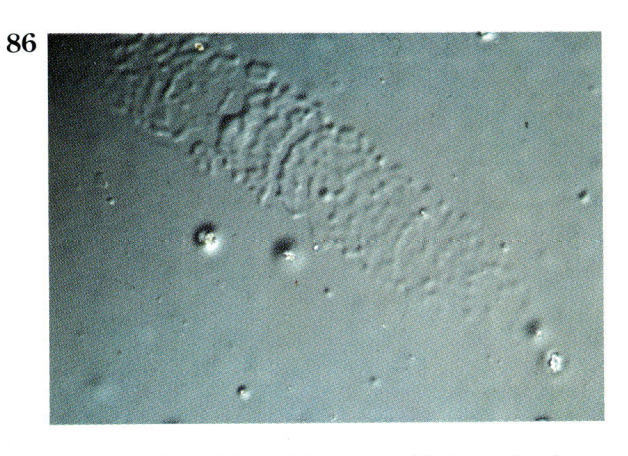

86 & 87 Blemishes. Injection moulded lens showing surface polymer blemishes.

88 Stress lines in the polymer of a new hydrophilic lens.

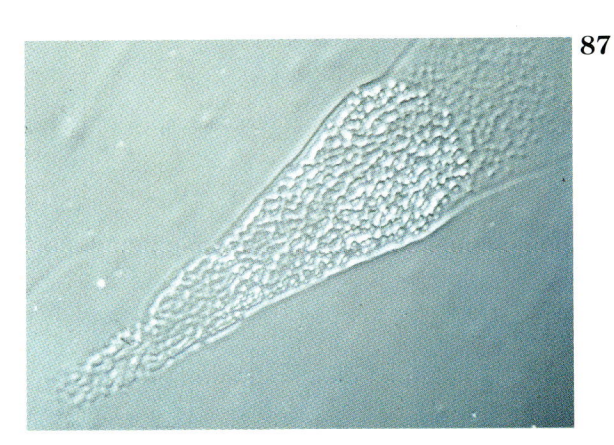

89 Cracked edge of a gel lens.

90 Rough edge of a gel lens.

Shadowgraphs

91

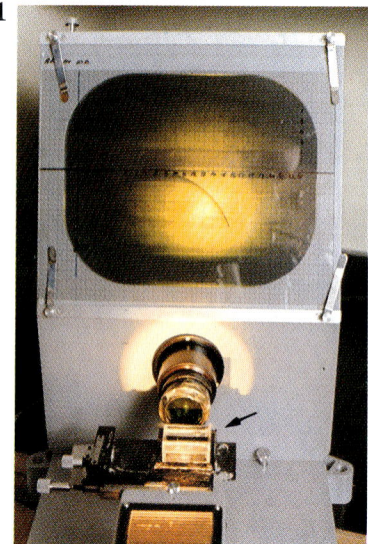

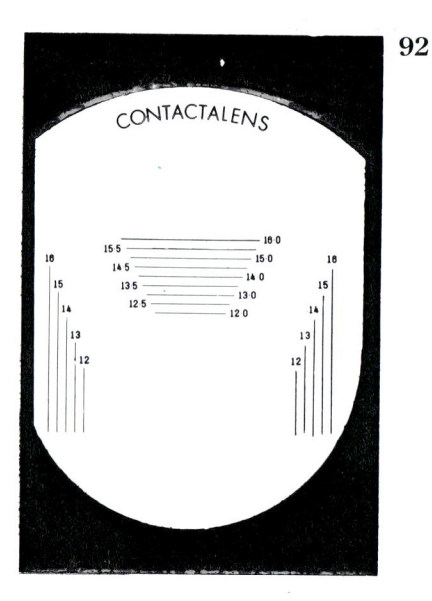

92

93

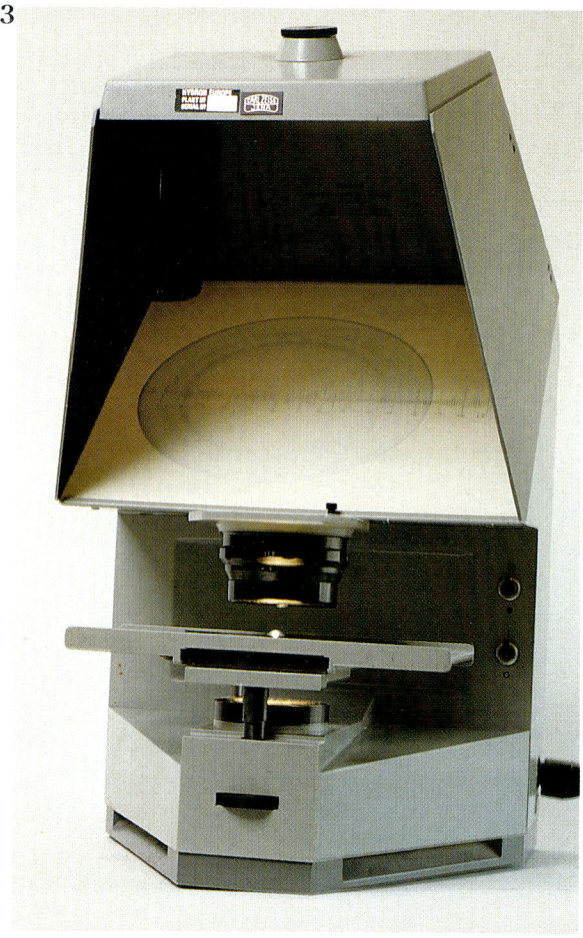

91-93 The stage on which the lens is placed can be rotated and moved until a section shadow of the lens is in focus. The screen can be marked to give direct readings of the size thicknesses sagitta over chords and even matched to curves drawn on the screen. Tolerances for such equipment depend on the quality of the instrument. The small, low-magnification instruments used by practitioners have linear tolerances of ±0.1 mm over measurements greater than 5 mm. The instrument is most useful to show splits and tears in soft lenses and all types of spoilage. Soft hydrophilic lenses are examined by placing them in a saline tank (**91**, arrow). In figure **93**, a coloured hard lens (9 mm) is on the stage.

Lens curvature

94 & 95 Radiuscope (Drysdale's principle). In its simplest form it can be used to read the central and peripheral radii, plus and minus curves and lens thickness. Figure **95** shows the binocular instrument fitted with a digital readout.

Using a light booster or image intensifyer system it is possible to obtain readings from soft lenses in water tanks.

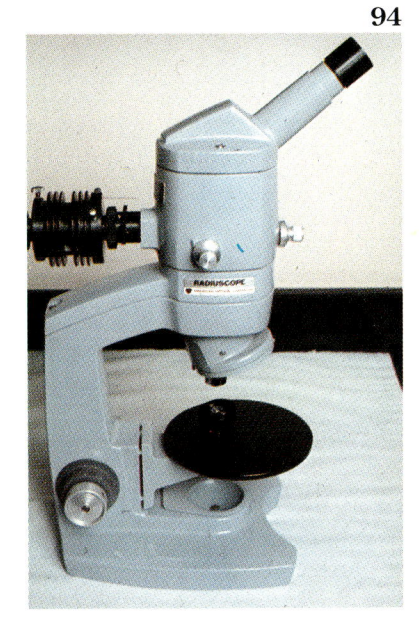

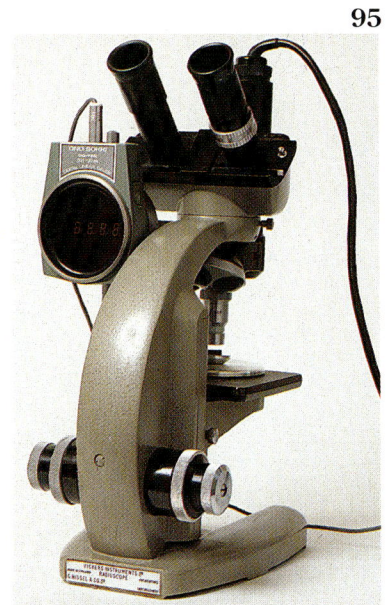

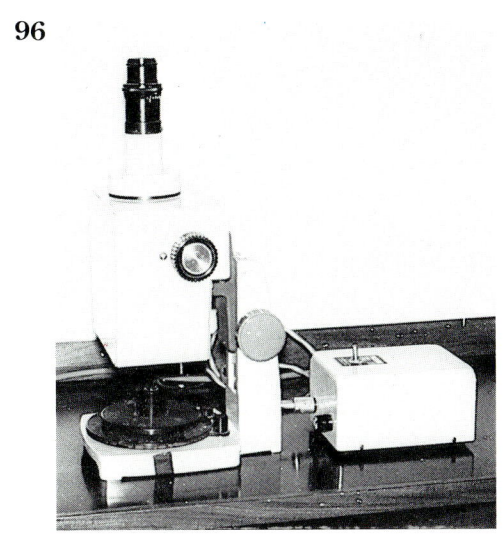

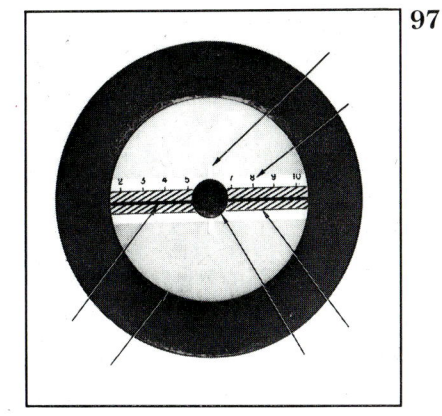

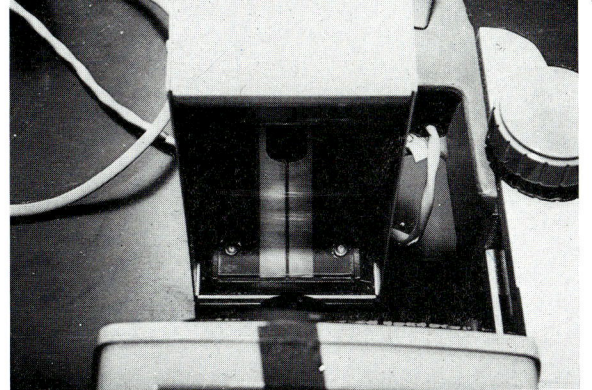

96-98 Toposcope. Using interferometry patterns (Moire fringes), the whole surface of a lens can be scanned to give a notion of the change in curvature (**97**).

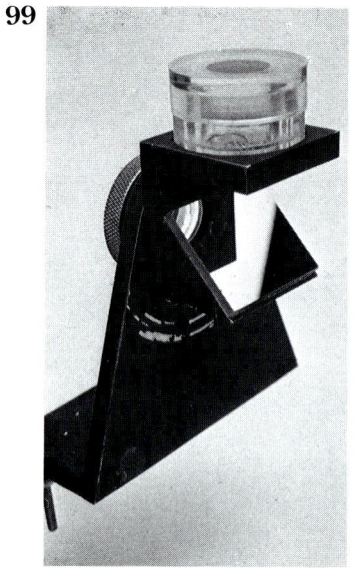

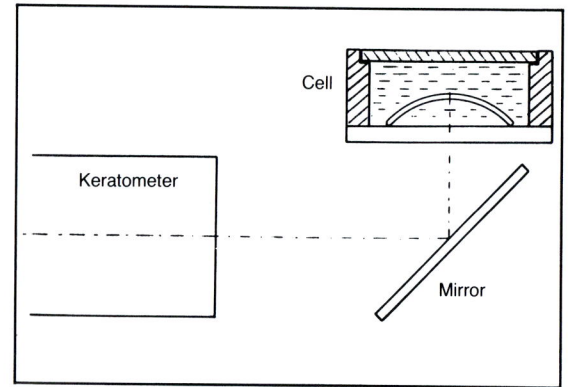

99 & 100   This tank/mirror device (Chaston) is attached to the keratometer to allow readings to be taken of soft lenses providing the illumination system is sufficiently bright. A similar system (Wesley-Jesson) is possible for hard lenses.

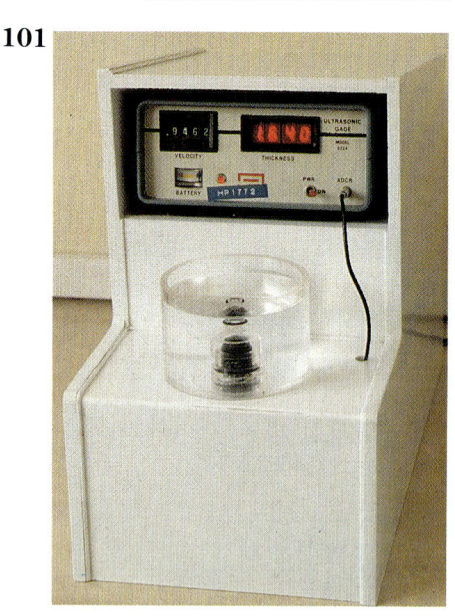

101   Ultrasound sagittometer (US)—Panametrics. This instrument is particularly suited for soft lenses. A readout of the sagitta is obtained and converted into radii.

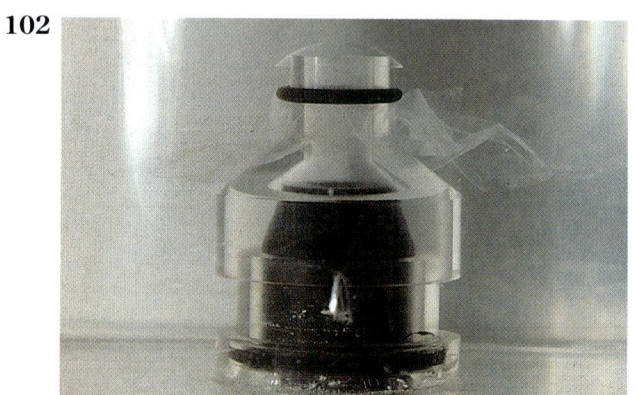

102   A close-up of the tank and the support for the lens over the short US emission scource.

Thickness gauges

Several types are available and are indispensable for hard lens practice.

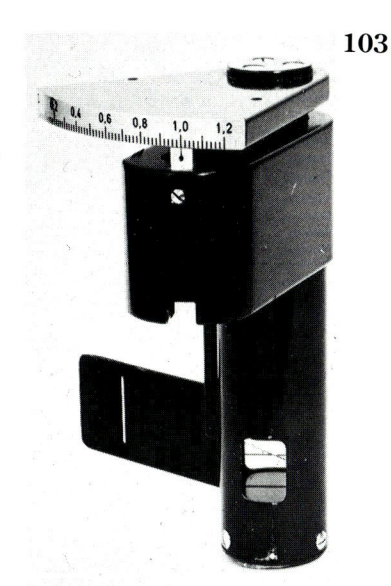

103 Pachometer. This instrument is attached to a slit beam microscope. It is used for the measurement of corneal thickness and is therefore a diagnostic tool for the early detection of oedema. Its can also be used to measure the thickness of a contact lens *in situ*.

104 & 105 For hydrophilic lenses, a type of gauge has been used where anvil contact with the lens and plunger completes a circuit and records the thickness (to ±0.01 mm).

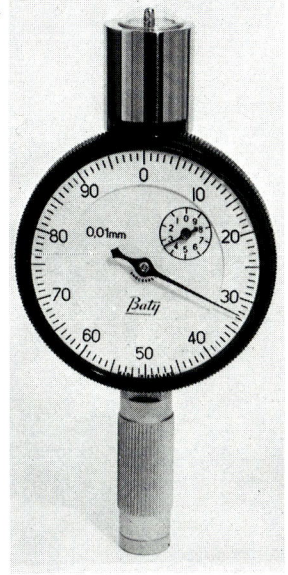

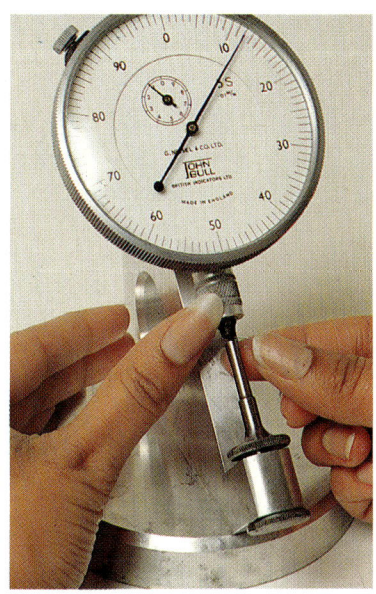

Power

106 Focimeter. The lens is placed over the instrument's aperature and a reading is taken. In the instance of hydrophilic lenses the water is blotted off the surfaces before taking a reading. Note that the back vertex power is used so the concave surface of the lens is as near as possible to the aperture.

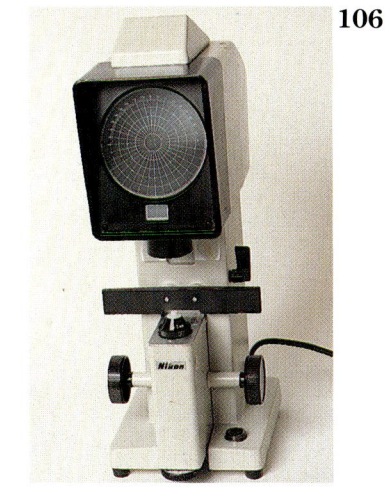

Size of hard lenses

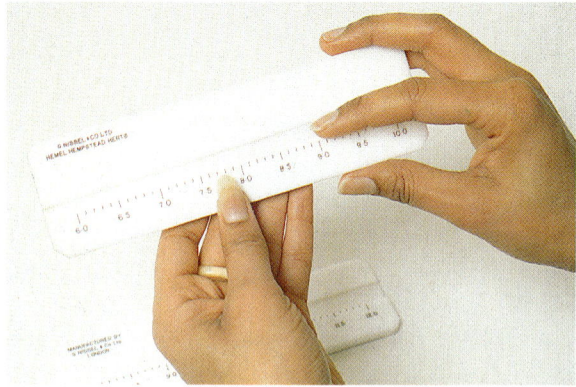

107 The 'V' slot gauge is used to measure the diameter of hard contact lenses. The specialist contact lens practitioner can verify lenses by confirming their diameter, power, back curve, thicknesses, quality, edge finish, and contamination.

Table 4. Acceptable tolerances in lens measurement		
	Hard	**Soft**
Total diameter	±0.02 mm	±0.03 mm
Centre back optic—radius	±0.01 mm	±0.02 mm
Power	±0.12 0 to 10d ±0.25 over 12d	±0.25 0 to 12d ±0.37 over 12d ±0.50 over 20d
Thickness Edge (0.50 mm in) Optic-periphery junction Centre	±0.01 mm	±0.01 0 to 12d ±0.02 over 6d ±0.03 over 20d

Requirements for a new lens in its container from the manufacturer
- No clouding or haze in the solution
- No deposits on the lens or as sediment in the solution
- The lens should be clean

(As viewed against a white, well-illuminated background × 2 magnification.)

Water content of soft hydrophilic lenses

The water content is related to the refractive index and also to the gas transmission properties of the lens.

It is often necessary to find out what the water content of a lens is in order to help identify the material and monitor the effects of evaporation during wear.

108 & 109 A soft contact lens refractometer and it's optics (N. Efron and Noel Brennan). The instrument is calibrated with saturated salt solution (S20°C) and then the hydrophilic lens is placed in the container and a reading taken.

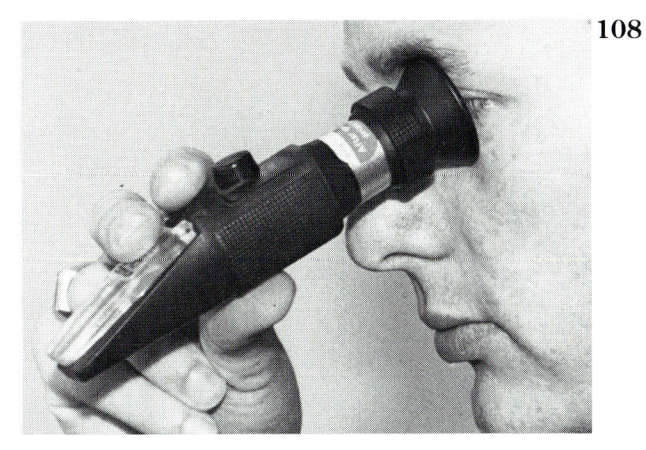

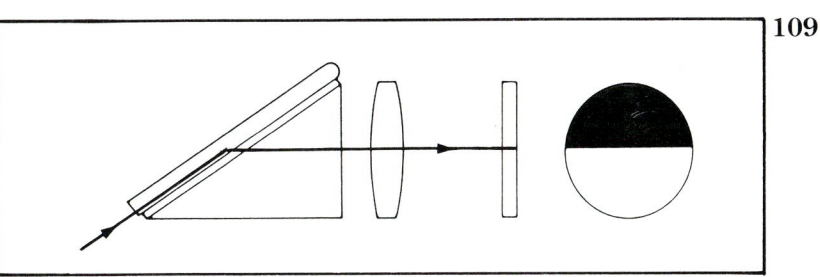

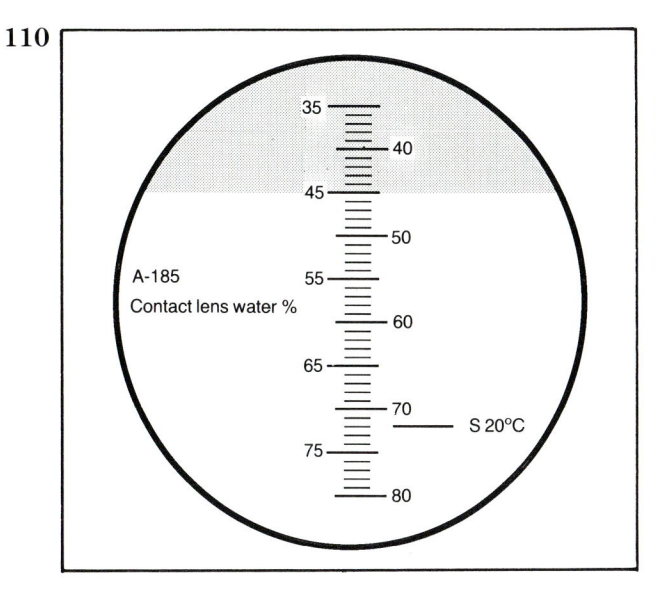

110 In this reading the lens shows a 45 per cent water content.

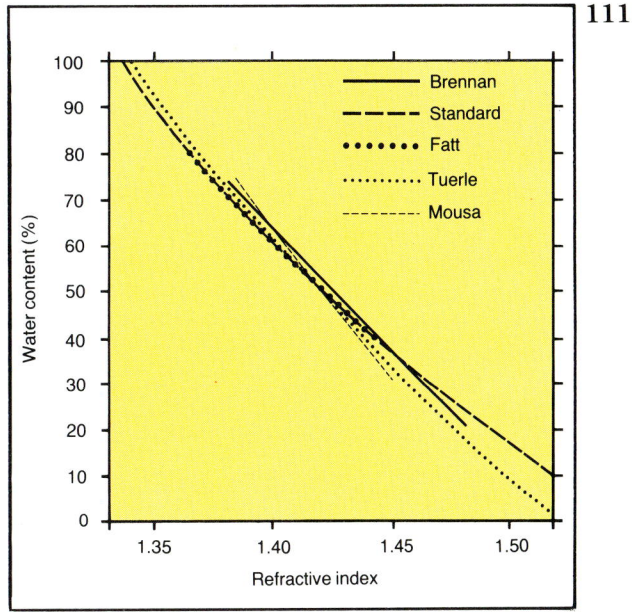

111 The graph can be used to find the relative refractive index of the material.

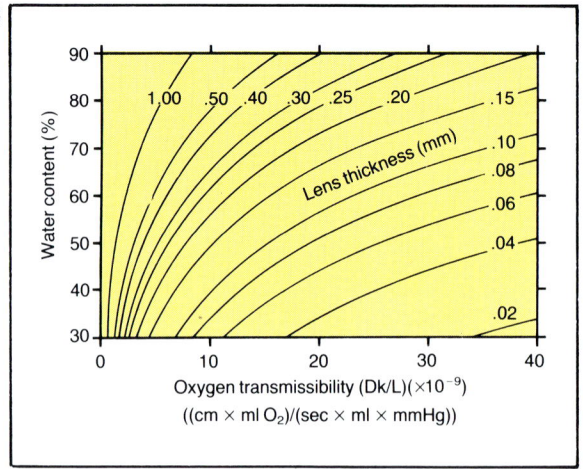

112 **Knowing the water content,** the oxygen transmission can be calculated. The graph gives the readings in Dk/L x 10^{-9} (N. Efron and Noel Brennan, *Optician* 10.2.87, p.29-41). The lens thickness *in situ* can be estimated from the pachometer reading (see page 43), or from the manufacturer's data supplied with the instrument. The results are useful to determine possible corneal zones of hypoxia.

Specific gravity of HGP lenses

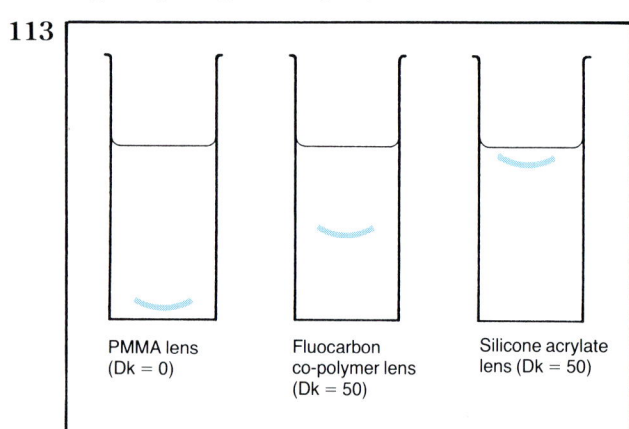

The flotation method of determining the specific gravity (SG) of the lens material (M. Refojo) uses 20 tubes containing progressive concentrations of CaCl solution to give SG readings between 1 and 1.2. Thus the increments are of the order of 0.01. For example, one could distinguish between two lenses of identical Dk if one lens had an SG of 1.1 (e.g. fluocarbon co-polymer) and the other an SG of 1.07 (e.g. silicone acrylate).

113 The diagram simulates equiflotation for a lens of SG 1.1 (centre), while in the same solution a PMMA lens of SG 1.2 sinks to the bottom and a silicone acrylate lens of high silicone content floats to the top.

Table 4a. Identification of the contact lens, material, and specification

- Lens size: by 'V' slot guage (for hard lenses) or magnifyer measure or shadowgraph
- Lens power: by focimeter
- Lens curvature: by radiuscope and/or ultrasound sagittometers (other methods are available)
- Lens thickness: by thickness gauges (for hard lenses) and shadowgram or pachometer (for soft lenses)
- Water content of hydrophilic lenses: by refractometers
- By thick lens formula[*] to find the refractive index if given the power, thickness and curvatures of a lens
- Specific gravity: by using the flotation method chiefly to find a lens of fluorocarbon content and high Dk (high SG as compared with a high Dk lens of silicone acrylate which has a low SG)

Depending upon the physico-chemical properties of the plastic, changes in lens form can occur when the lens is soaked in solutions or stored at extremes of temperature. Such changes are particularly relevant to cellulose acetyl butyrates and co-polymers. A manufactured lens may change the radius of curvature by 0.25 mm (in high powered lenses) after prolonged periods of storage.

[*] Thick lens formula:

$$F^1_v = \frac{F_1}{1 - {}^t/_n \times F_1} + F_2$$

5 Care and spoilage

Contamination of the lens

A large industry has evolved concerned with the care of the contact lens. In those instances where care systems fail or the patients' own protective systems are inadequate, infection can be a serious complication.

In the first instance, the inert contact lens can become coated with a biofilm, and then with precipitations and cell debris plus added contaminants of the environment and those accidentally introduced by the patient (for example cosmetics). Teeth are often coated with plaque, and contact lenses suffer in a similar way unless satisfactorily cleaned by tear flow and lid action. Where these fail adequately to clean the lens then preparations have to be used.

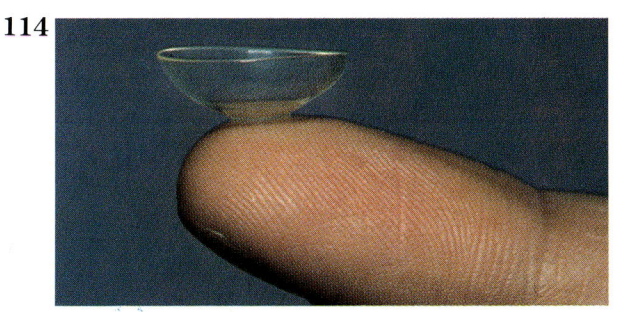

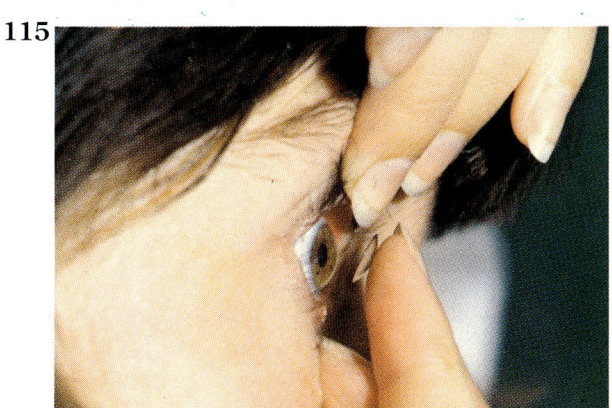

114 & 115 Insertion of lens. All lenses have to be placed into the eye by the hand, therefore, irrespective of the techniques used to clean, sterilize, disinfect, rinse or wet the lens, the ultimate procedure can be a source of contamination. Clean hands free of soap films and contaminants such as oils and greases are important to avoid contamination.

- Sterilization is a process to kill all micro-organisms: while this is used by the manufacturer for any preparation or lens that has water as a constituent, it is not the method used by the patient. Disinfection is the process that makes a lens safe from infection. Most of the methods advised to the patient are those of disinfection.

Heat disinfection

116

Heat disinfection is used for hydrophilic soft lenses, and mainly low water content gel lenses (below 40 per cent). High water content contact lenses show premature ageing with repetitive heat disinfection. At 80°C, the minimal effective time is 20 minutes.

116 & 117 Electrical disinfection using a dry heat case with lenses in a saline case. This method ensures a rapid rise in temperature to almost 100°C, and then a slow decline which exposes the lens to over 80°C for a period of 40 minutes. This is effective against most bacterial contaminants but not fungal spores.

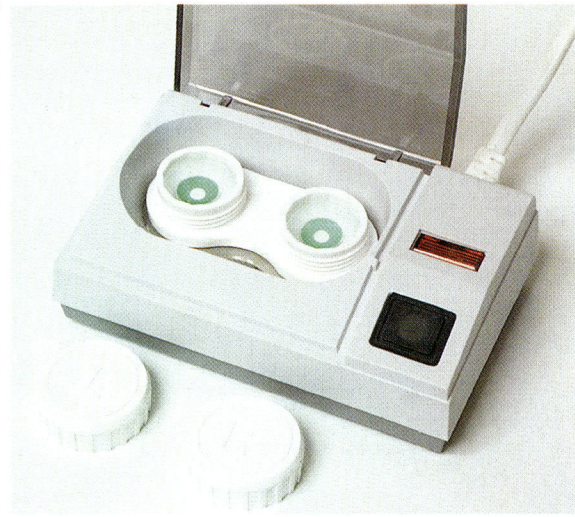

117

118

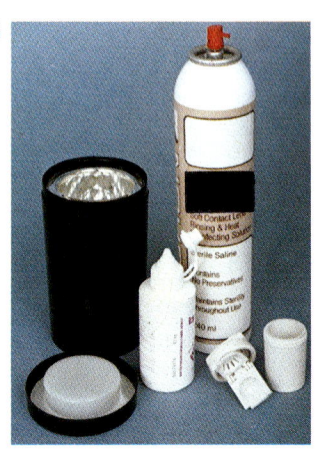

118 Thermos flask. The cleaned lens is placed into its case with fresh saline and then into a thermos containing boiling water. A slow decay of heat, from a peak of 90°C, takes place over a period of several hours. This is a safe and inexpensive method of disinfection.

Chemical disinfection

Several chemicals are commonly used to disinfect contact lenses—chlorhexidine, thiomersal (mercury salts), hypochlorites, quaternary ammonia compounds, hydrogen peroxide, benzalkonium chloride (nonhydrophilic only), and sorbic acid, for example. The concentration has to be such that a rapid kill time of micro-organisms can be proven, especially of the viruses—adenovirus and HIVs for example. The final solution must not be toxic to eye tissues. In most instances a neutralizing process or saline rinsing is required. Processes avoiding chemicals that selectively bind with the plastic of the case or lens are preferable. For example, chlorine is an effective disinfectant at 4 to 8 parts per million. With the lens wet, microwave techniques do not damage the lens but if the lens is dry, this method will seriously damage the lens surface.

Chemical elution

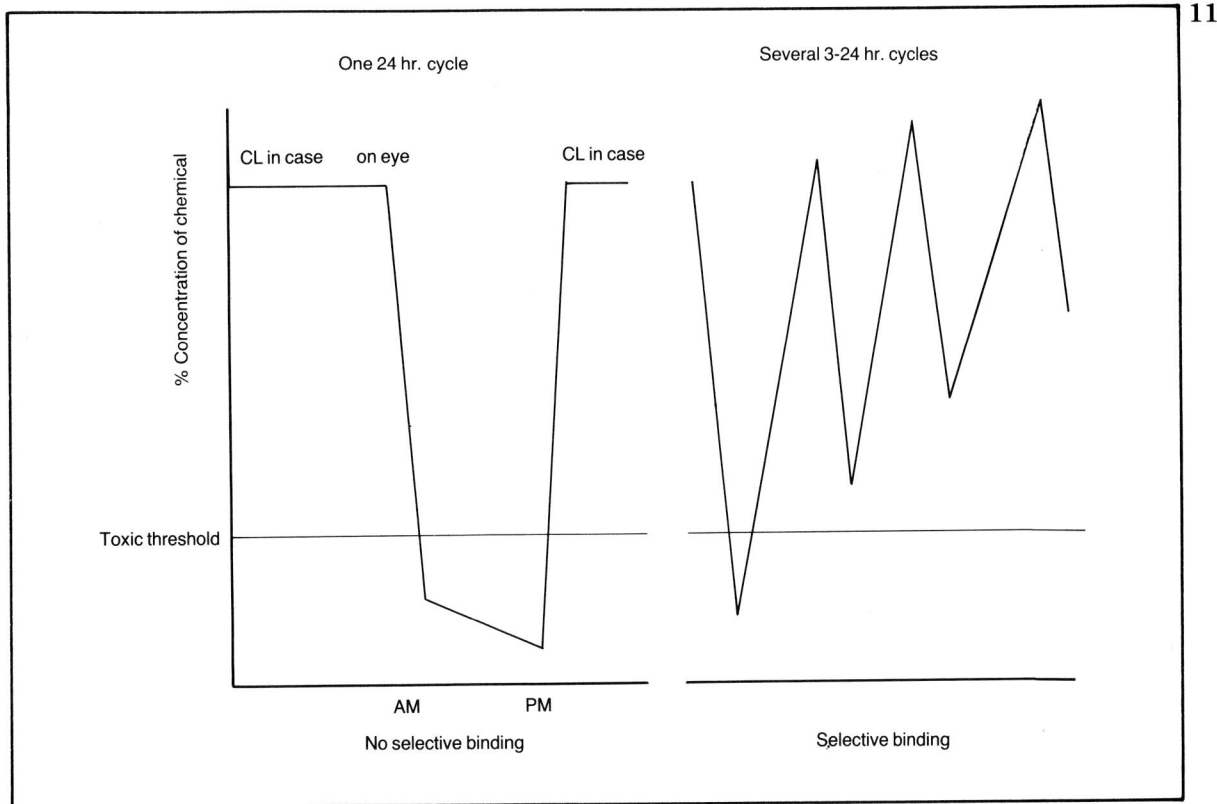

119 Elution rates of disinfectant chemicals. The lens can take up chemicals which bind selectively to the polymer. On the other hand, some large molecule preservatives only attach themselves to the lens surface. These imaginary schemas show two different types of preservative.

On the left, a toxic (to the eye) concentration is present in the lens case. Almost immediately after rinsing and placing in the eye this falls to a nontoxic level and by the end of the daily wear period is almost completely eluted. Replacement in the lens case in the evening again brings the concentration to a toxic level.

On the right is a chemical disinfectant (for example, chlorhexidene). After the first soak it is at a toxic level and during wear on the first day drops to a nontoxic level. However, it never sufficiently elutes on the subsequent cycles of wear and there results finally a lens that is increasingly tending to toxic concentrations.

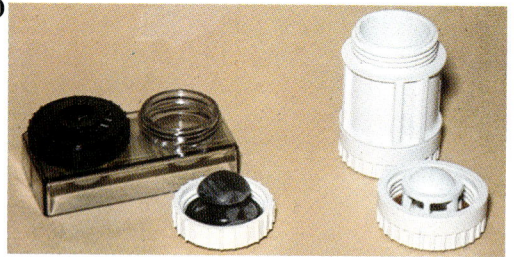

120 Case for lens storage. This design is not ideal because the lens could adhere to the dome of the holder and not be exposed to the chemical.

Biocalyx can enclose bacteria in the case and lead to their survival. A new case is therefore advised periodically.

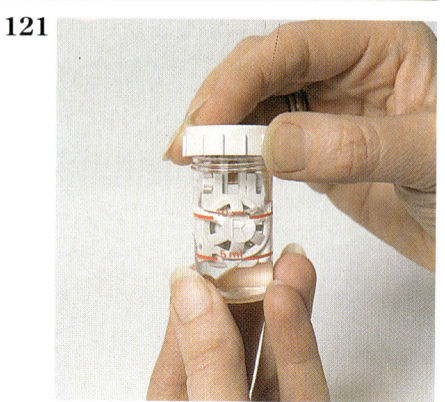

121 Peroxide method. The neutralization of the peroxide is usually from alkaline-buffered saline solutions, and reductases such as pyruvates, or catalytic reactors. The photograph shows a case into which accurate quantities of the disinfectant and then the neutralizing solution can be placed.

Cleaners

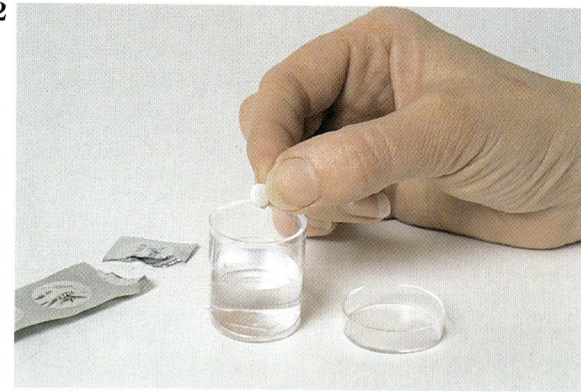

Several cleaners are available for both hard and soft lenses. Chemical degraders of proteins and lipids such as borates (lipofrin) activated by heat are specifically reserved for the practitioner. Mild abrasives and detergents are available for patient use; solvents such as alcohols are also used. They must all be rinsed off the lens and the manufacturers' instructions rigidly complied with.

122 Lipase and protease preparations are for removing protein film from the lens (used for both hard and soft lenses). Several rinses with saline are necessary after the lenses have soaked in the solution.

123 Practitioner method of cleaning lenses combining controlled heating with vibration and a solution.

124 Ultrasound tank. A method that has to be used with the correct solvents to effectively clean lens surfaces. Ultrasound methods can cause the lens to go opaque. Phillips suggests that 15 to 16 k Hz for 5 to 45 minutes is safe.

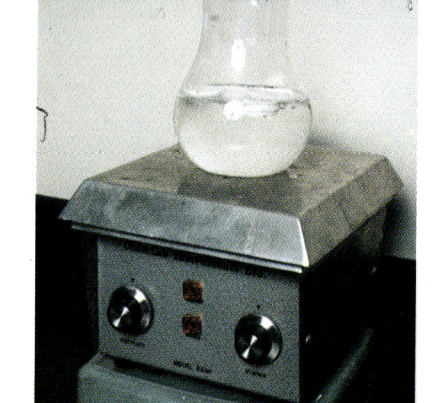

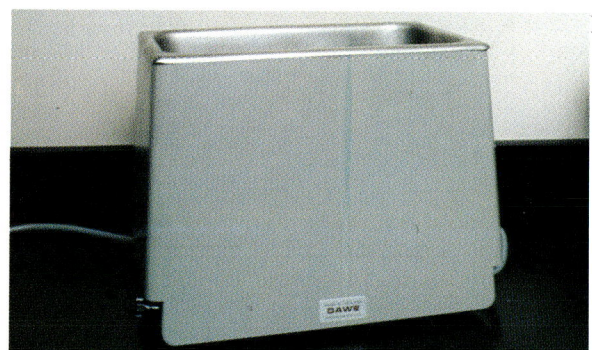

Lubricant drops

One of the most common problems encountered is the drying of the lens surface and eye during wear. Instilling supplementary artificial tear drops of varying viscosity is the usual way of reducing the problem effectively. However, there comes a 'watershed' situation when the drying is more rapid than the rate of drop instillation, which leads to the covering of the lens surface with the solutes of the tears and artificial tears. All contact lens preparations entering the eye should simulate tears with regard to pH, osmolarity and wetting properties.

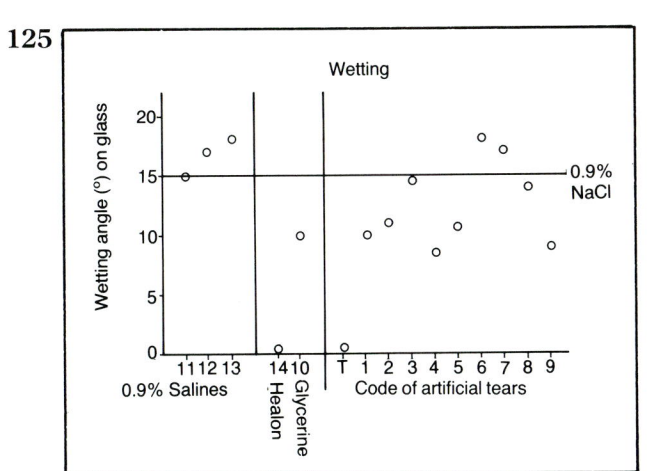

125-127 These data for wetting, pH and osmolarity compare several commercial preparations (1-9) with human tears (T) and also with three salines (11-13). Healon and glycerine 2 per cent solutions are also compared (Ruben and Hopkins). The conclusions are:

- Wetting: Healon is as good as tears.
- pH: most of the preparations are within tear range.
- Osmolarity: most of the preparations are within tear range.

There is still room to improve the wettability of contact lens surfaces.

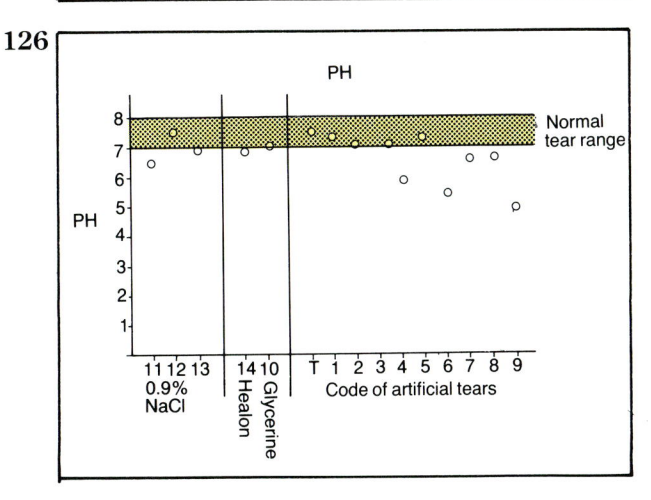

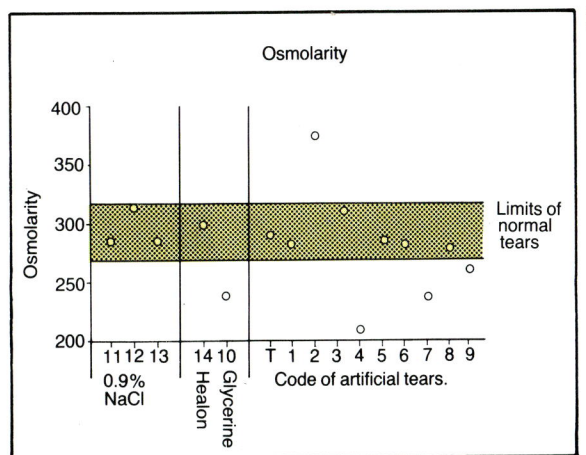

Lens spoilage

Contact lens spoilage may be due to:

- Ageing—breakage of molecular linkages resulting in: loss of transparency; change in water absorption; surface adhesion loss; surface break-up; colour changes (to yellow).
- Loss of lens shape, e.g. deformation resulting from silicone rubber shrinkage.
- Colour change from: absorption of metal ions from water; metabolism derivatives, e.g. dopamine adrenaline cycle; amino acids, e.g. tyramine, tryptophan; domestic dyes and cosmetic colourants; accidental contact with fluoresceine; drugs secreted into the tears; foreign bodies, e.g. iron pigments.
- Surface and subsurface deposits: calcium salts (PO_4 and CO_3); mucolipid calcium conglomerates.
- Infection of the lens from fungus and bacterial colonies.

Damage to the ultrastructure

Damage to polymer plastic can result from:

- The manufacturing process—surface damage from friction or the pressure of high-velocity micromissiles, for example.
- Polymer-chemical anomalies resulting in polymerization blemishes in a surface and cavitation of material.
- Physical-chemical action in the form of: chemical corrosives, which break up polymer linkages; UV radiation; weathering and ageing, resulting in polymer degradation; heat, e.g. from a disinfection process; biological action, e.g. from body enzymes, infection, and fungus growth into the polymer.

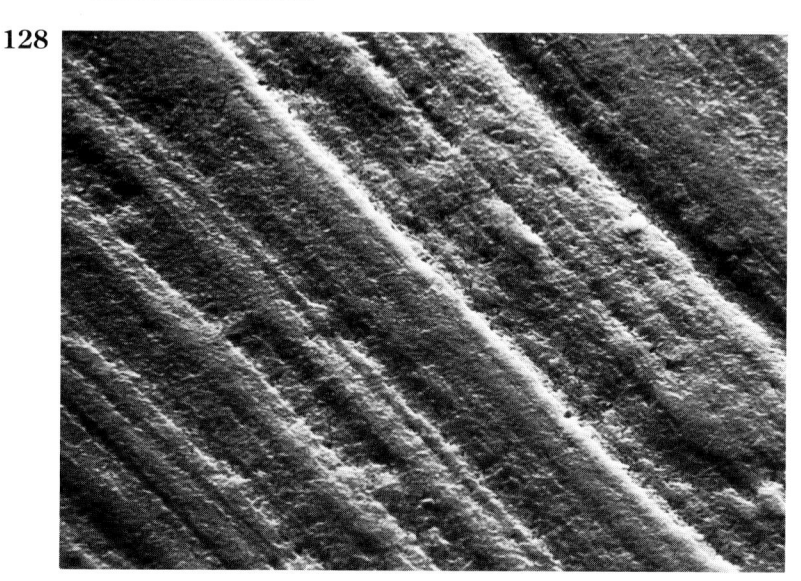

(Figures **128-133** are from *An Atlas of Polymer Damage* by Lother Engel, Hermann Klingele, Gottfried W. Ehrenstein and Helmut Schaper (Wolfe Publishing, 1978).

128 & 129 Surface of a gas permeable polymer. Note the grooves and intervening lattice stretch patterns. The cavities shown in **129** are most likely due to amorphus crystalline transformation, This is due to heat produced at the surface by the cutting procedure. ($\times$ 500 & $\times$ 10,000)

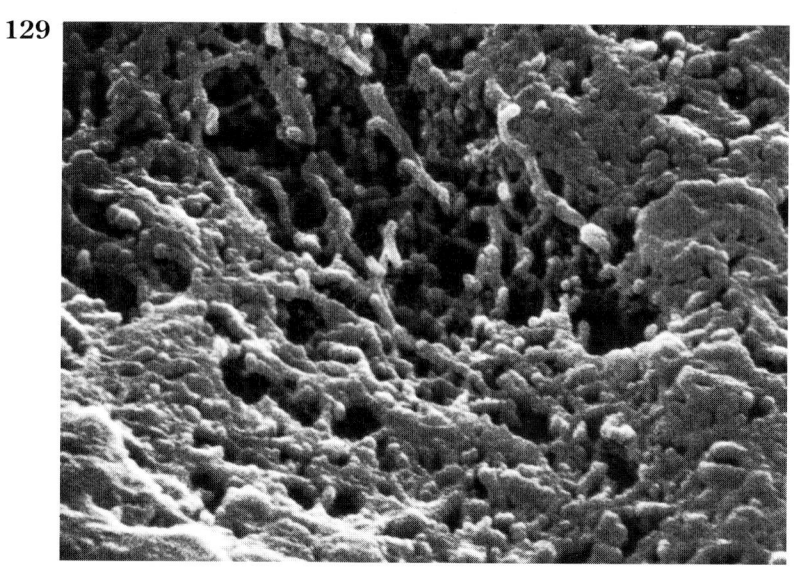

130 Brittle polymer. Some polymers are brittle and friction will cause wear to the surface. The illustration shows particles less than 1µm agglomerated to form deposits. (× 2200)

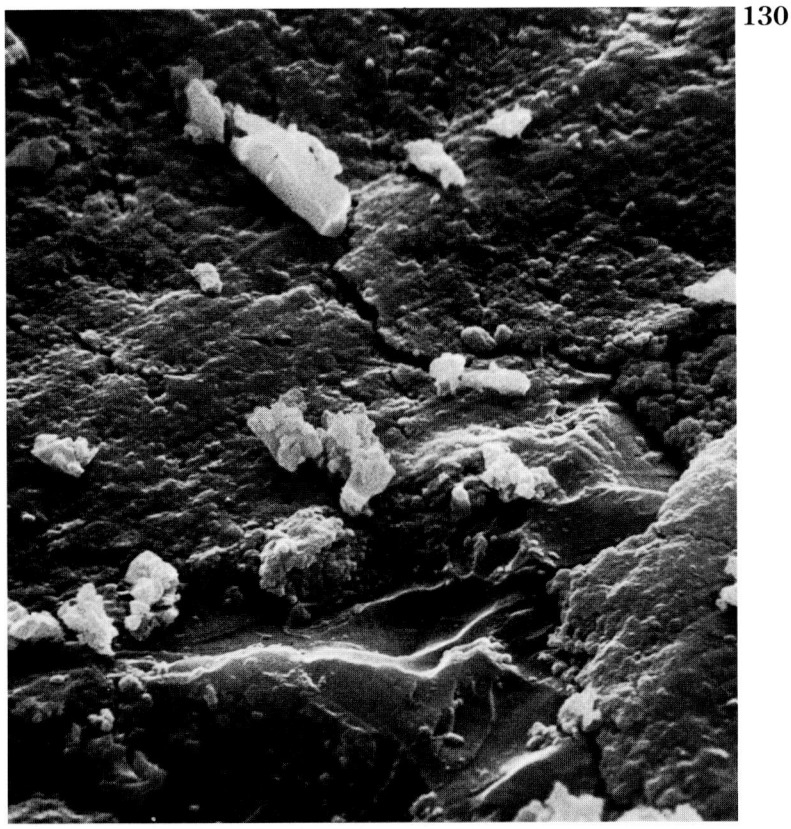

131 Elastic polymer. Hard, solid microparticles, if rubbed into an elastic (as opposed to brittle) polymer, will tear the surface forming loops, which give a fishnet appearance. (× 220)

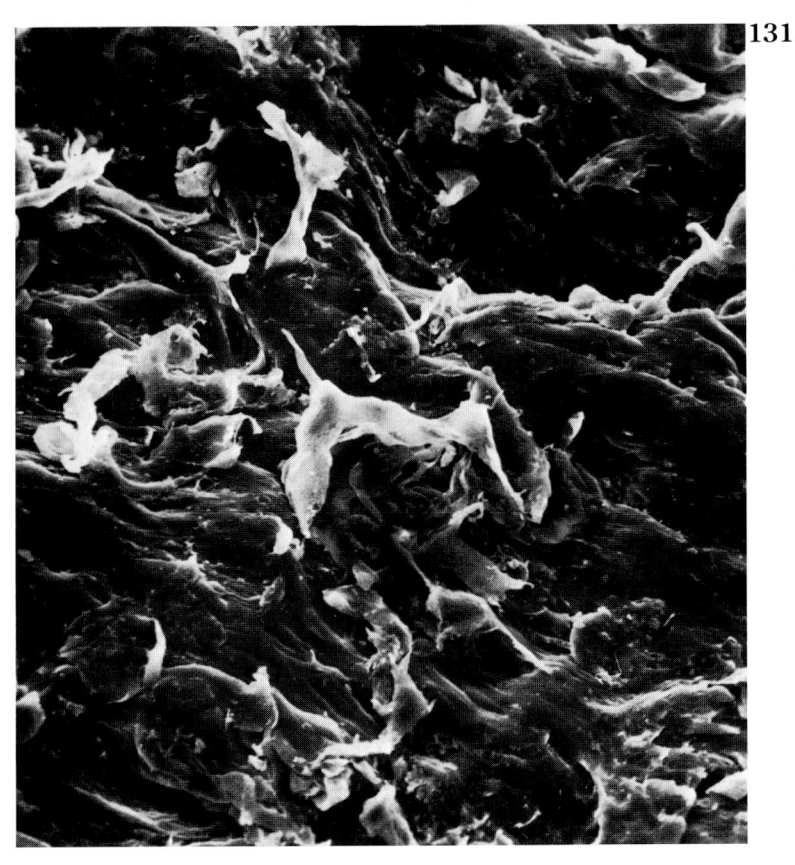

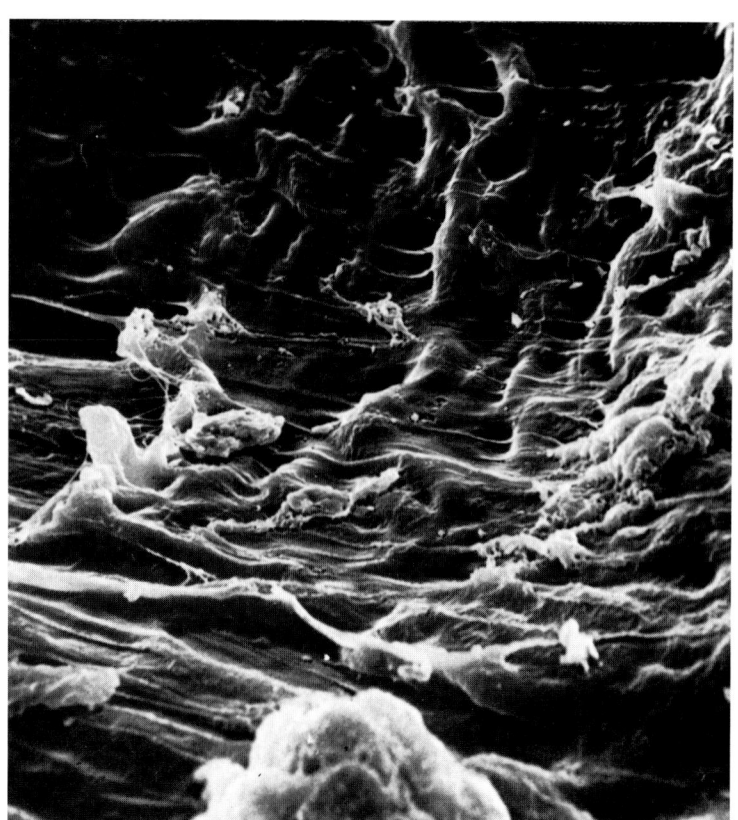

132 Erosion of the surface with torn and stretched polymer fibrils. (× 1200)

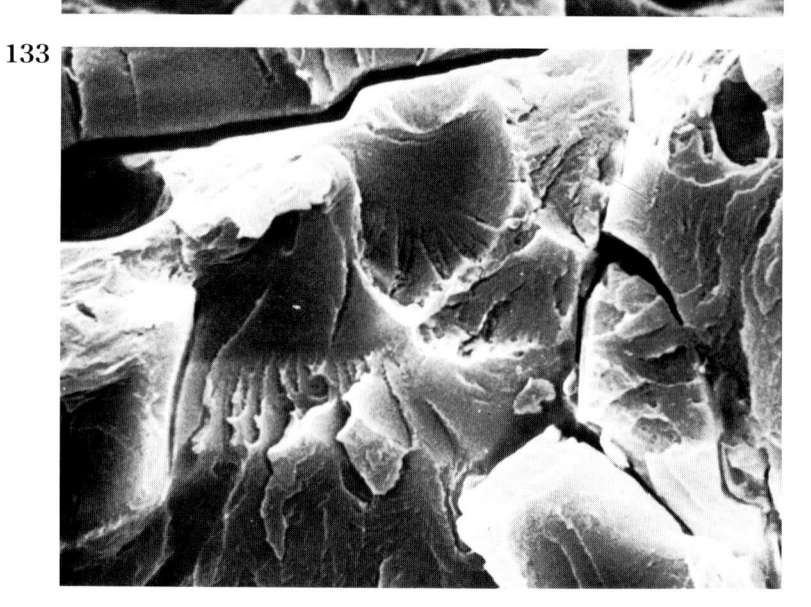

133 High-velocity water droplets. The impact of high velocity (400m/s) water droplets (1.2 mm diameter) on PMMA will result in fractures and splinters because of the brittleness of the material. (× 1800)

Polymer damage

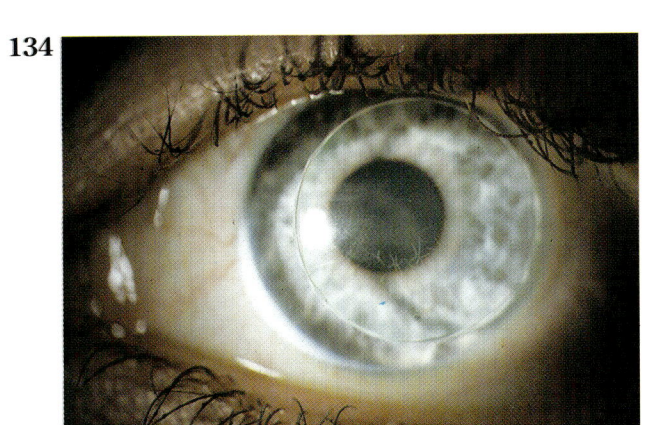

134 Gas permeable hard lens on the eye, showing crazing of the lens surface. (Graeme Young)

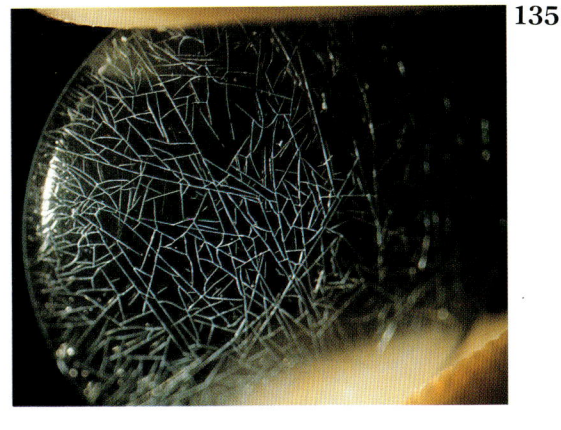

135 Gas permeable hard lens, showing gross crazing of the material. (Graeme Young)

Surface crazing can be of two types: the break up of a surface film; and cracks in the surface of the lens substance—due to changes in the stress patterns between the surface and deep molecules.

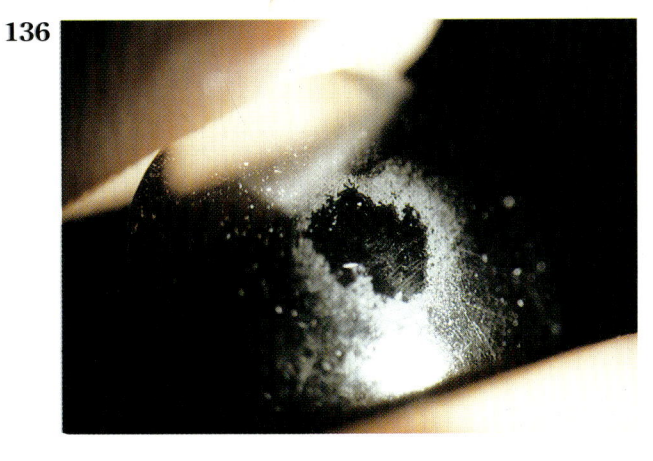

136 Surface deposits of mucoprotein on a gas permeable hard lens. (Graeme Young)

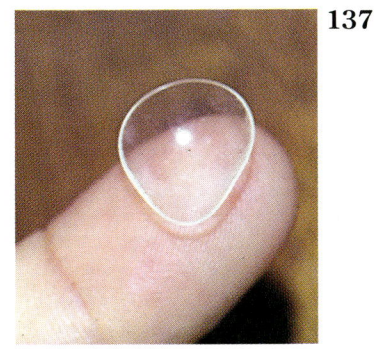

137 A gel lens (55 per cent water) has warped after several months of wear.

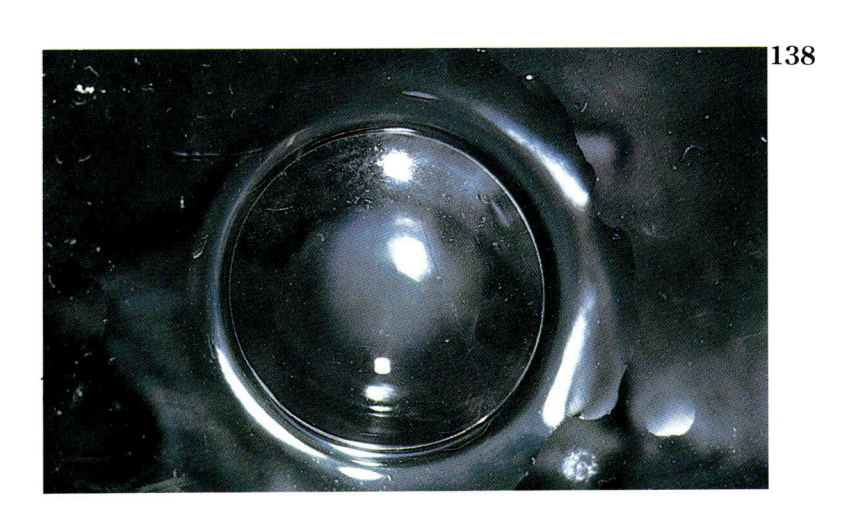

138 Polymer degeneration and increased absorption of water has caused the amorphous white discolouration.

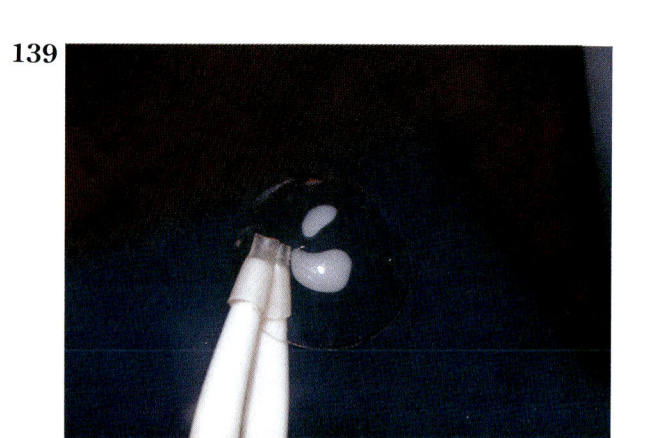

139 White or grey discolouration caused by polymer degeneration and increased absorption of water.

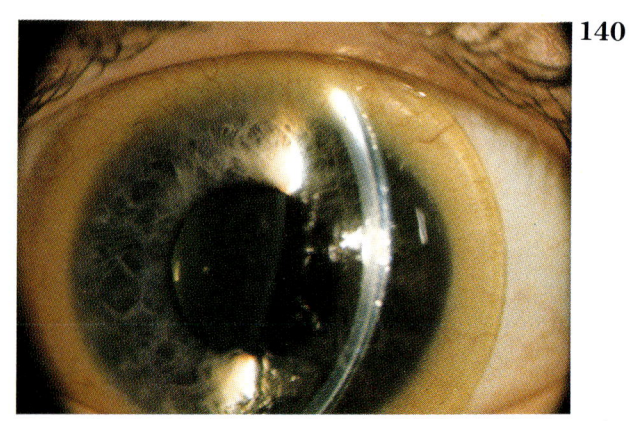

140 Brown discolouration (unicular), thought to be due to heavy tobacco smoking.

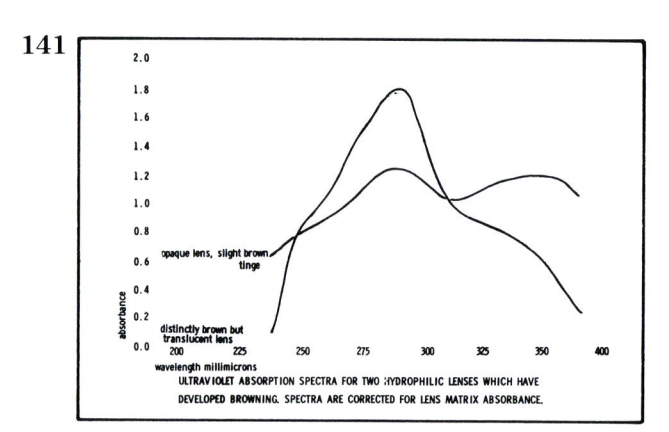

141 UV spectrophotometry of a coloured lens which gave high peaks at 280. Possibly metabolic in aetiology and involving an amino acid. (A. Winder.)

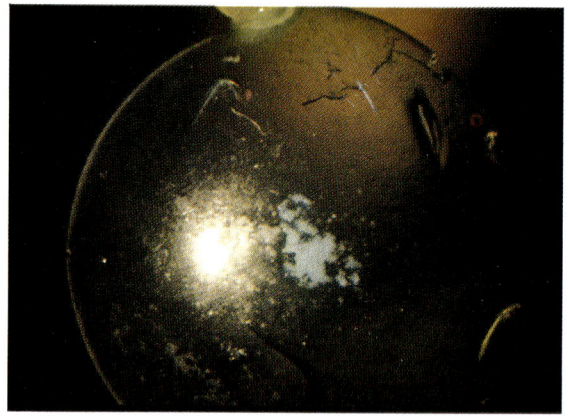

142 Dry eye patient. Note the haze over the lens and the milky-white deposit.

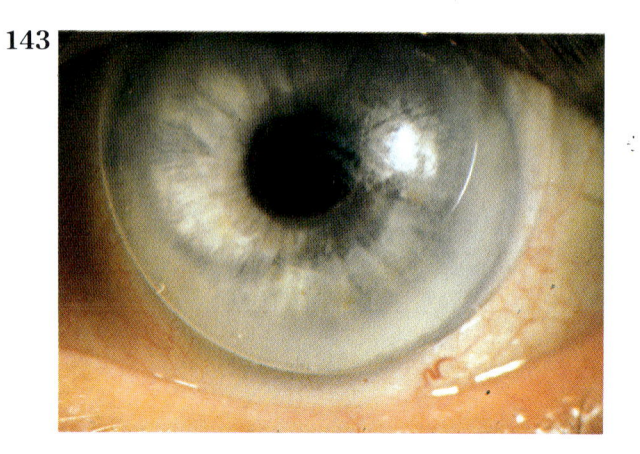

143 Lipid haze on a silicone rubber lens.

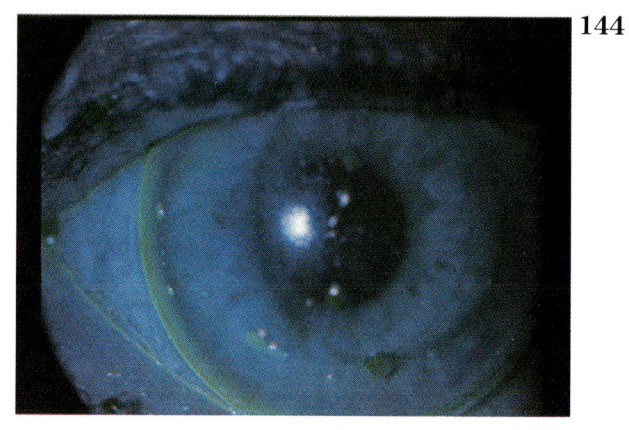

144 Lipid haze, with mucoprotein deposits, on a silicone rubber lens.

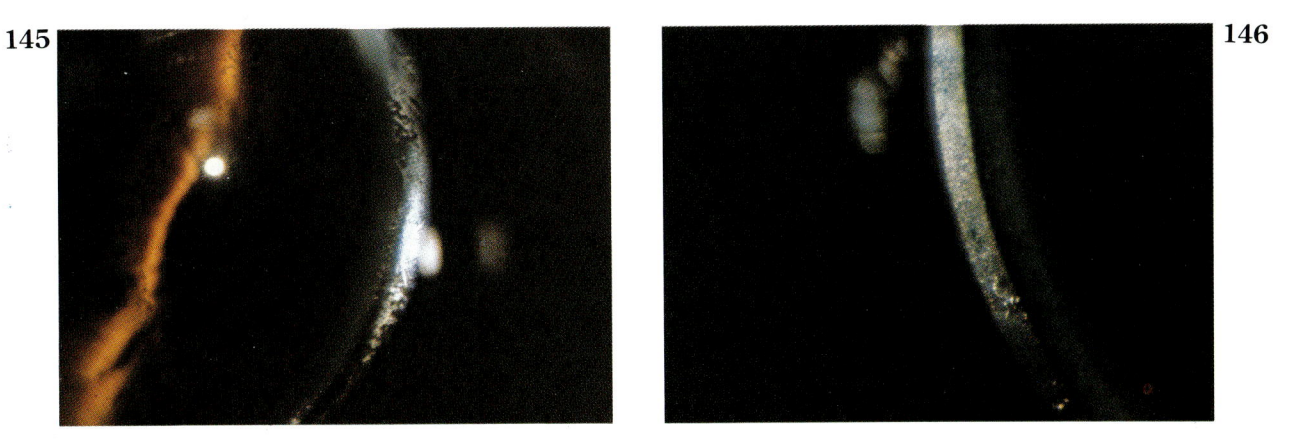

145 & 146 Crazed dry surface and lipid haze, with mucoprotein deposits on silicone rubber lenses. (Note a similar effect on the gas permeable hard lenses in **134-136**.)

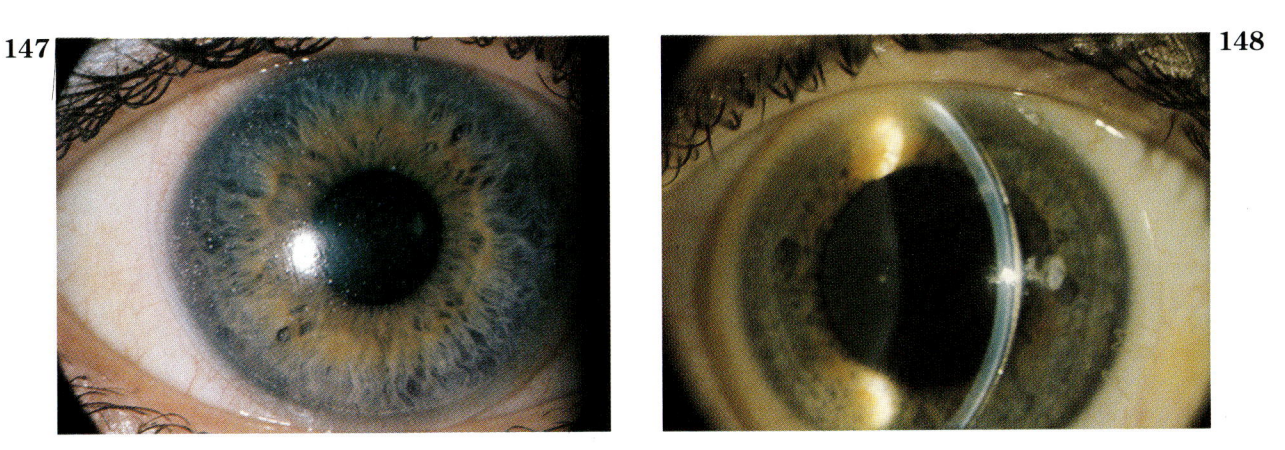

147-149 Calcium. Discrete white calcium salt deposits. (These can be removed by soaking in EDTA 1 per cent.)

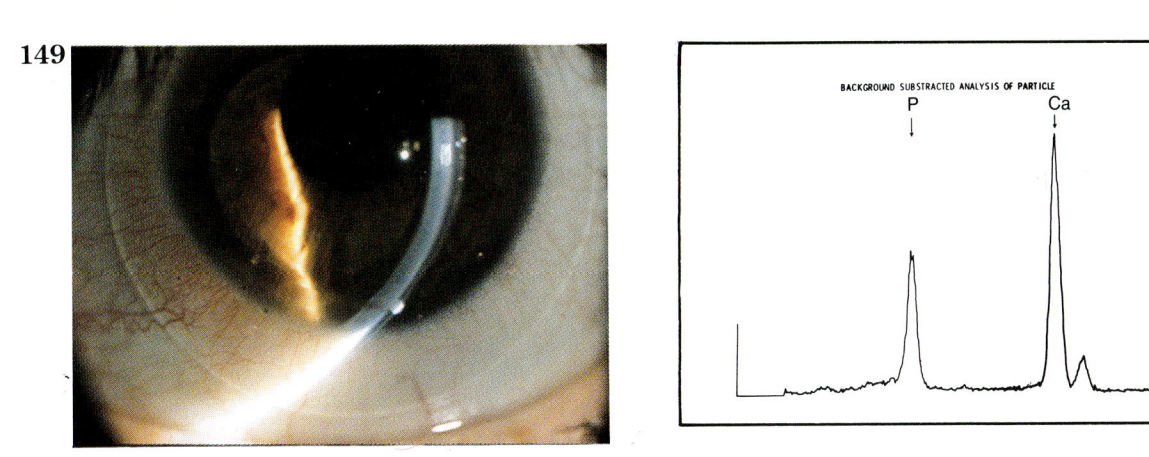

150 Microatomic probe readout showing calcium present in a spoilt lens.

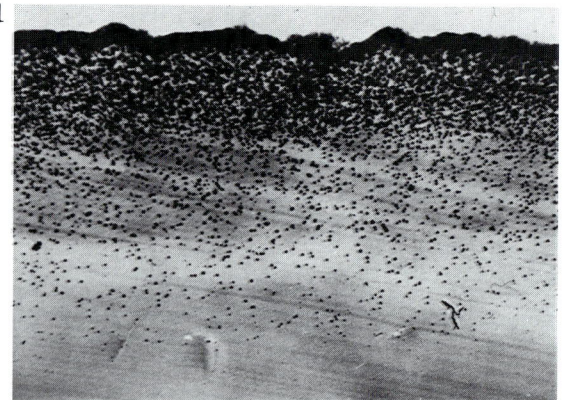

151 Calcium penetration. Light microscopy and selective calcium staining of the lens in **150**, showing the depth of calcium penetration.

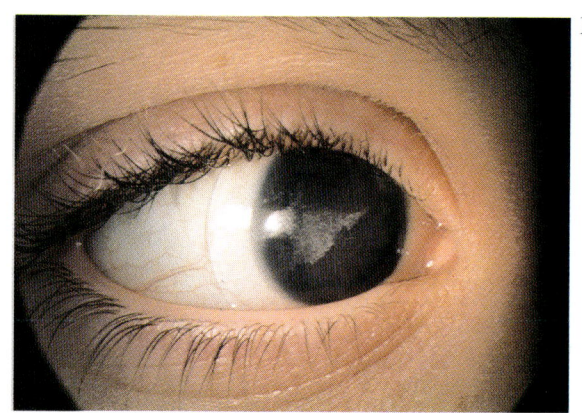

152 Discrete grey-white deposits and polymer degradation.

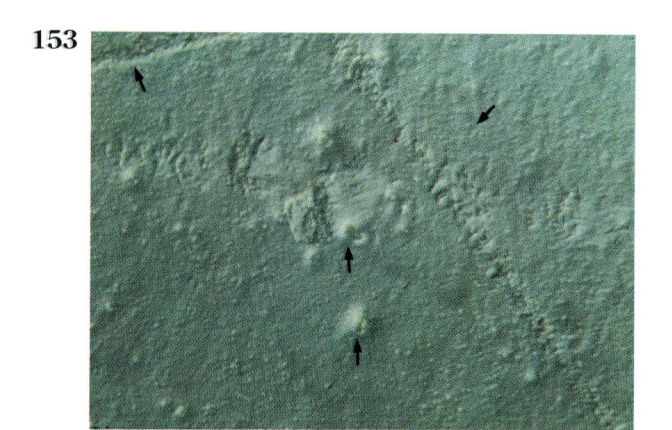

153 Phase-contrast microscopy (× 50) of a PHEMA lens surface. Note the granular appearance, craters, lathe-cut grooves and polish tracks.

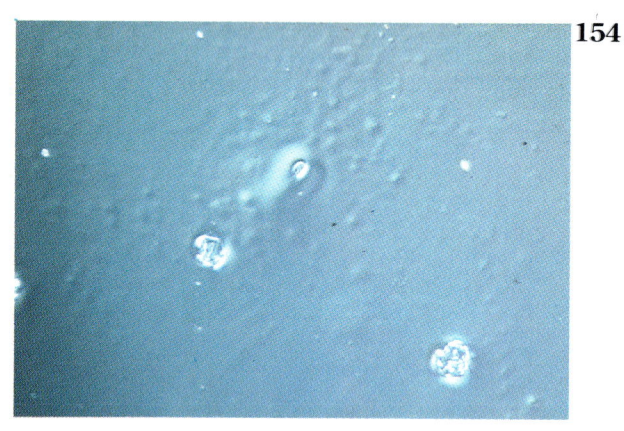

154 Craters in the surface of a gel lens. Some are open and are the result of surface granules breaking up.

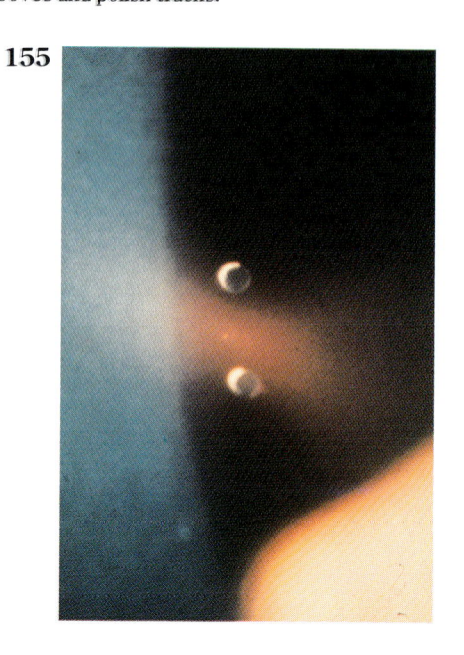

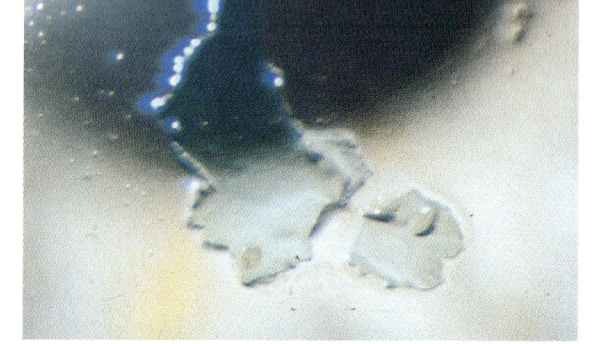

155 Cystic degeneration of a high water content gel lens. (× 30)

156 Surface polymer break-up.

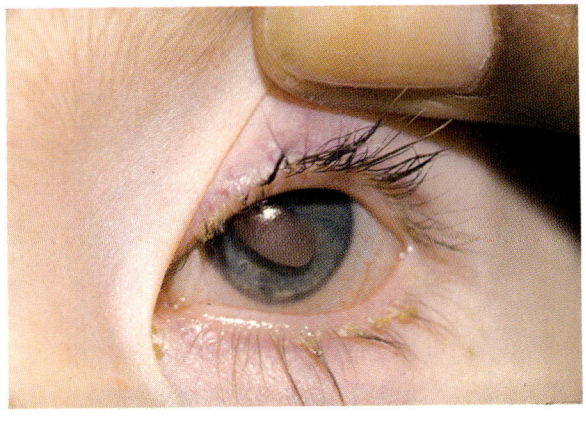

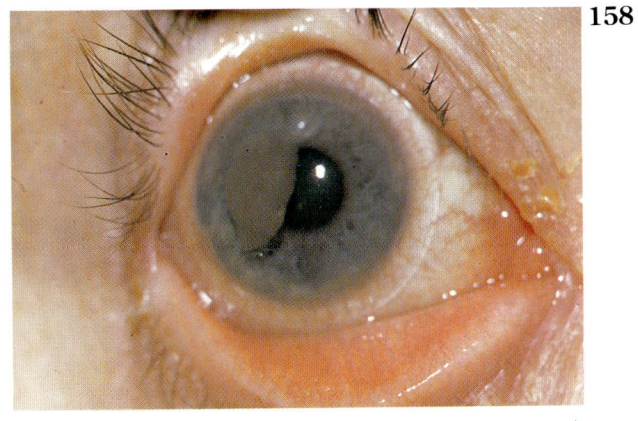

157 Polymer degeneration. The degenerate polymer has imbibed water and appears a translucent grey colour.

158 Polymer degeneration (as in **157**) in a soft lens worn by a rheumatoid arthritis patient.

159 Iron foreign body deposit on a PHEMA lens surface.

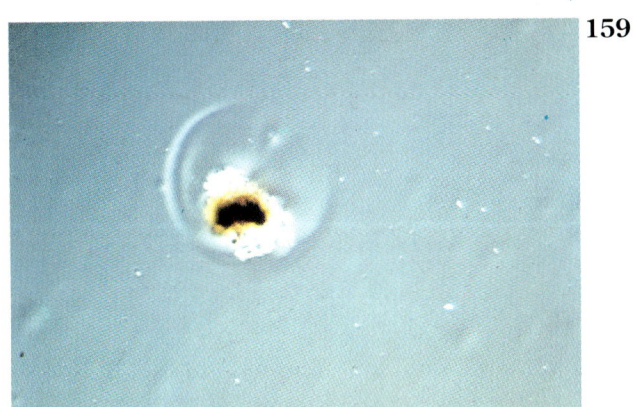

Microscopy of lens surface degeneration

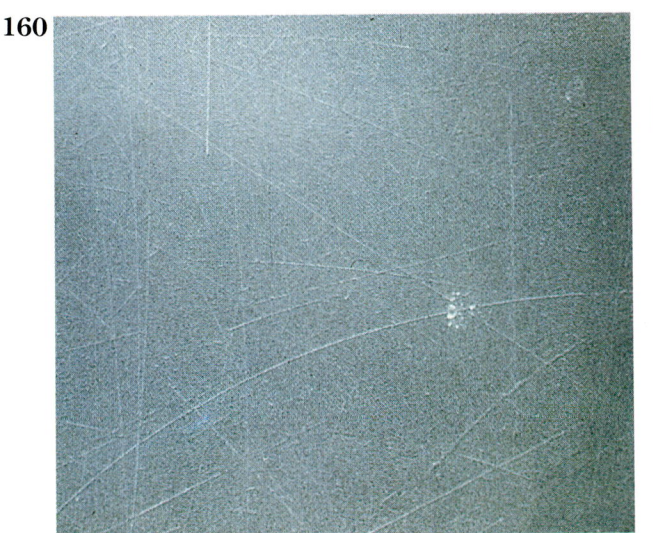

160 Clean surface. A clean (not worn) hydrophilic lens surface. Note the fine pitting and the polishing scratch marks. (M. Piccolo and R. Boltz)

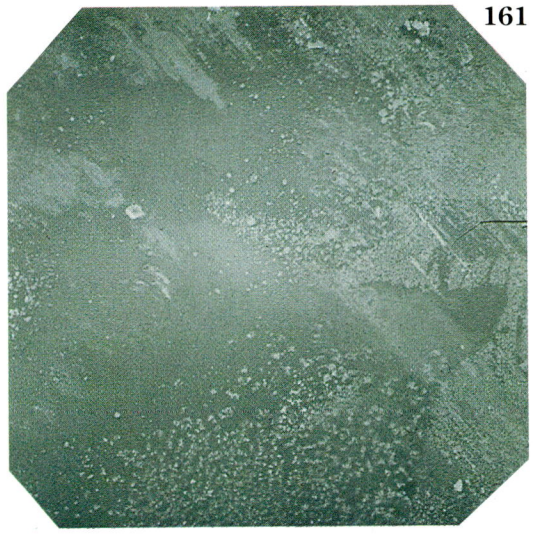

161 Protein coating. The surface shows typical protein coating. This lens has been worn for several weeks. (M. Piccolo and R. Boltz)

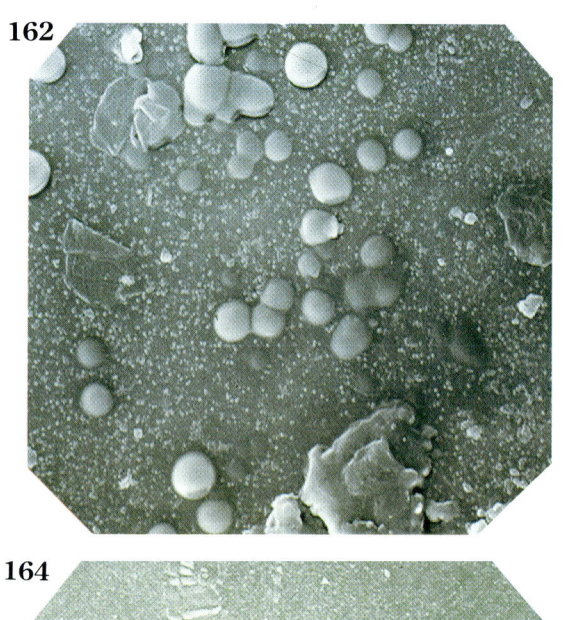

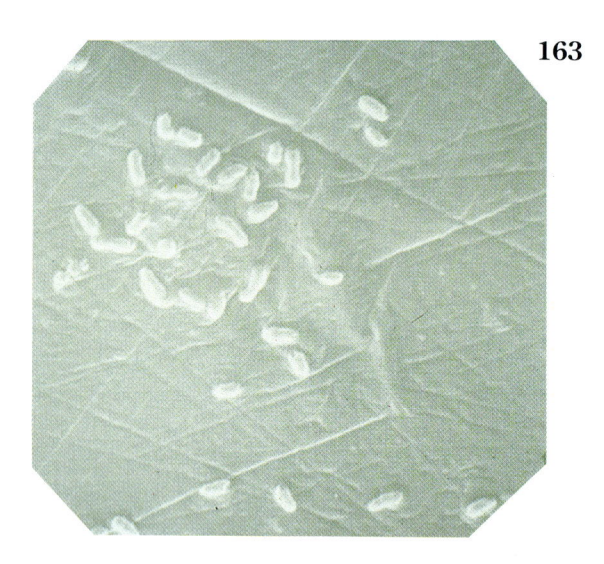

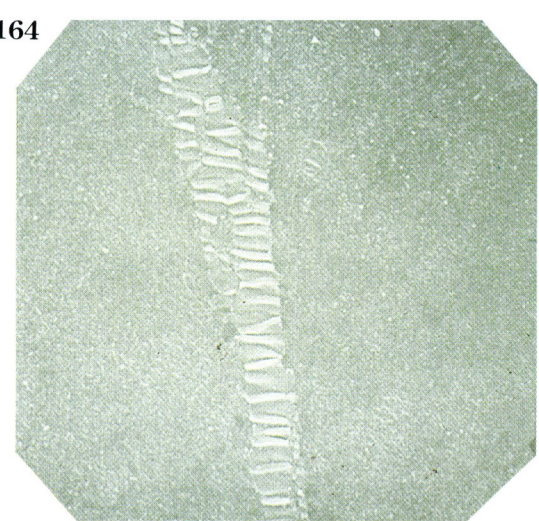

162 The round bodies could be one of several things. Primary bodies of the polymer material are one possibility. Powder particles contaminating the surface or *Candida albicans* (yeast) infection are others. Powder particles often have a 'spiky' surface appearance. (M. Piccolo and R. Boltz)

163 Bacterial contamination. The surface shows bacterial contamination. (M. Piccolo and R. Boltz)

164 Linear deposit, most likely a coating that has become rucked, forming steps. (M. Piccolo and R. Boltz)

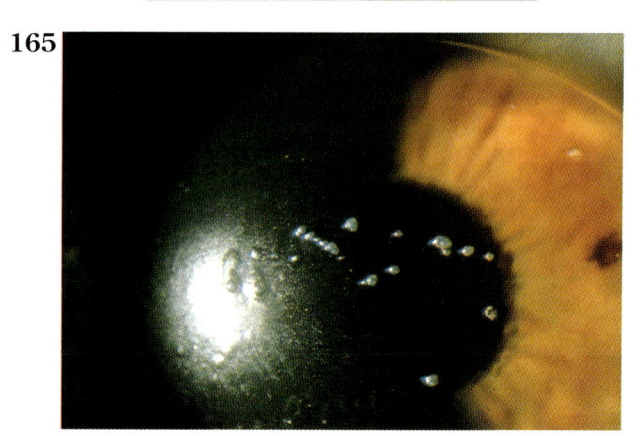

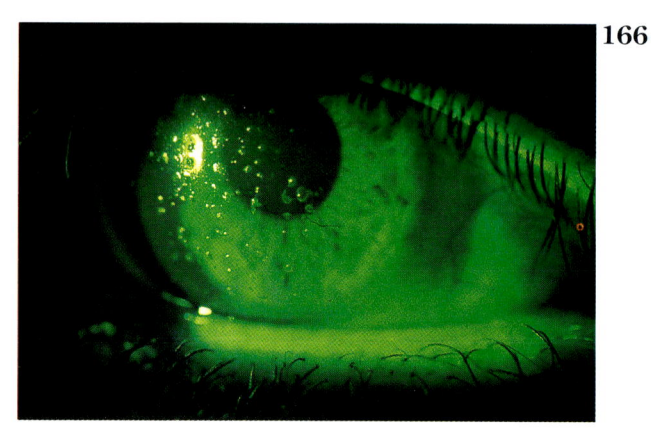

165 & 166 Mulberries. Small mucolipid conglomulates (mulberries) on the lens surface.

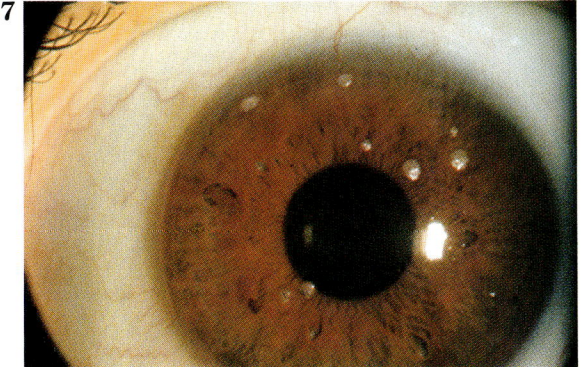

167 Larger mulberries. Larger conglomerulates on the lens surface.

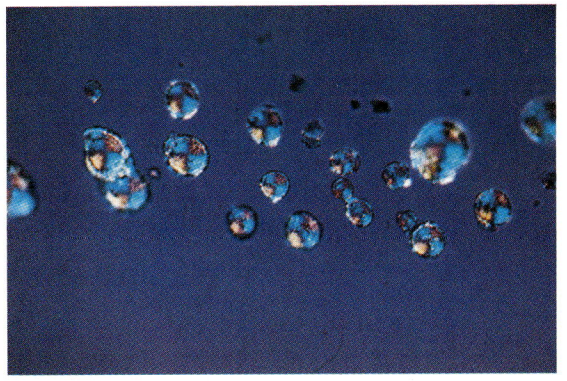

168 & 169 Broken up mulberry, showing bifringen effect due to the highly refractile lipid layers.

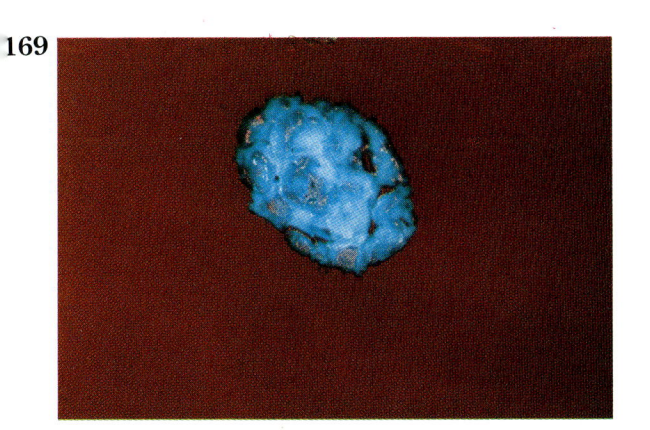

170 Surface appearance of a mulberry.

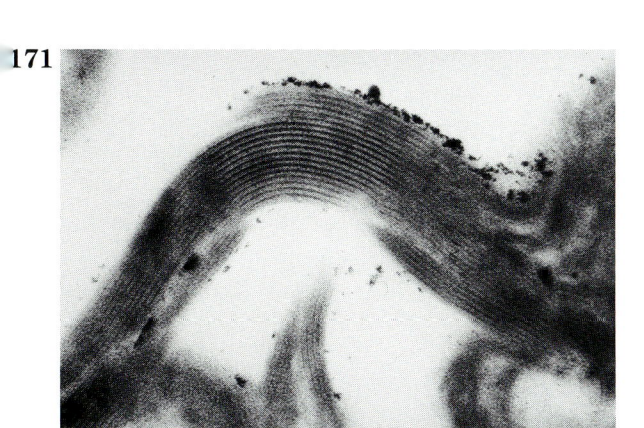

171 High-power section of a mulberry. The lamellae are phospholipid bands. The black granules are calcium salts. Inferior to the lamellae is polymucosaccharide. (R. Tripathi)

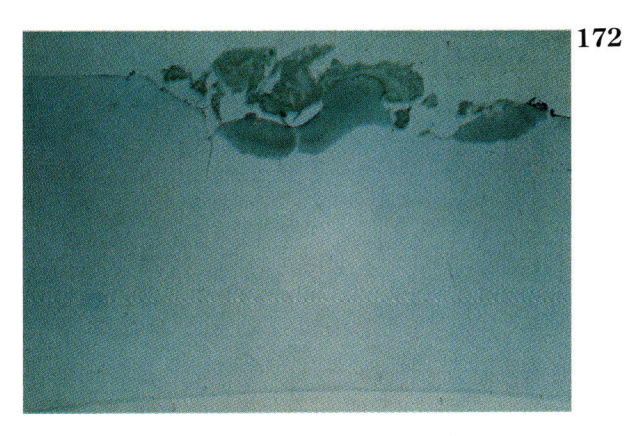

172 Section of a deposit to show how the broken polymer surface may be the nidus of subsequent lamellae. Removal of such deposits leaves a spoilt surface. The cause of surface deposits is drying of the lens surface during wear, permitting a continuous accumulation of protein and lipid on the microcrater-like surface of the lens.

Future methods of lens surface investigation:
- ESCA Electron spectroscopy for chemical analysis.
- XPS X-ray photoelectroscopy for surface molecular analysis.
- SIMS Secondary 10n mass spectrometer for surface film analysis without destruction.

Fungal and bacterial contamination

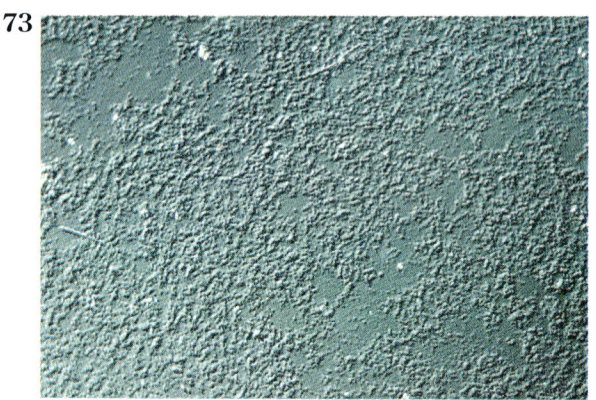

Over 30 per cent of cases and *used* solutions have been reported as contaminated. Therefore, the possibility of eye infection is forever present.

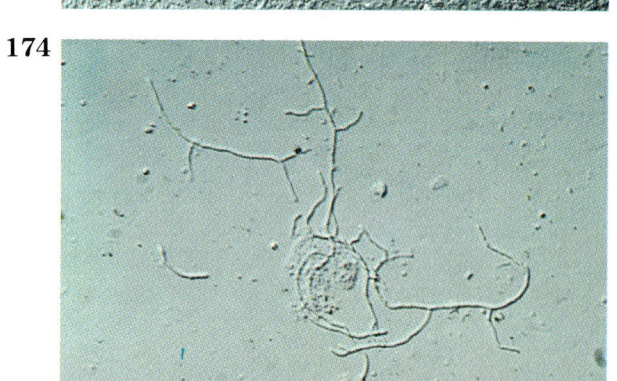

173   Lens surface bacterial contamination
—*Pseudomonas aeruginosa* was grown from the case.

174   Fungus mycelium on the lens surface.

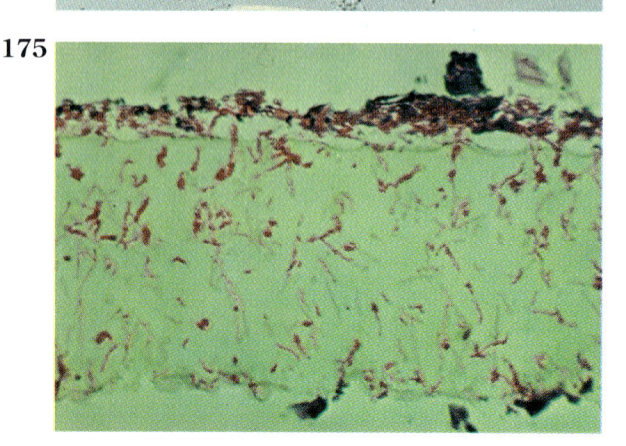

175   Lens showing mycelium in its substance.

176a & 176b Drying of the soft lens surface during wear. This is commonly seen on coated and contaminated lenses.

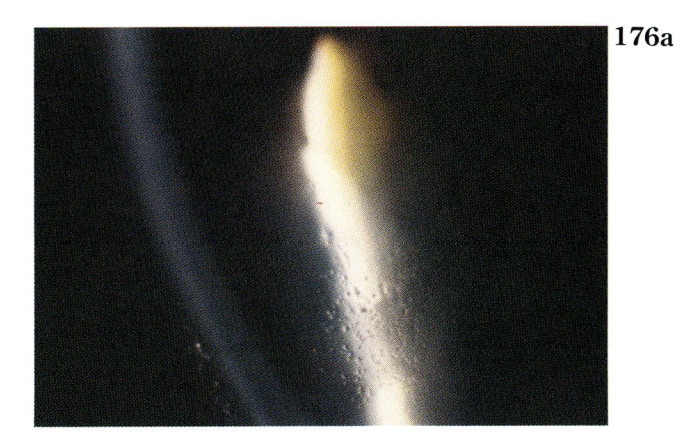

176a

176b

177 An unworn, fungus-infected lens from an infected lens case.

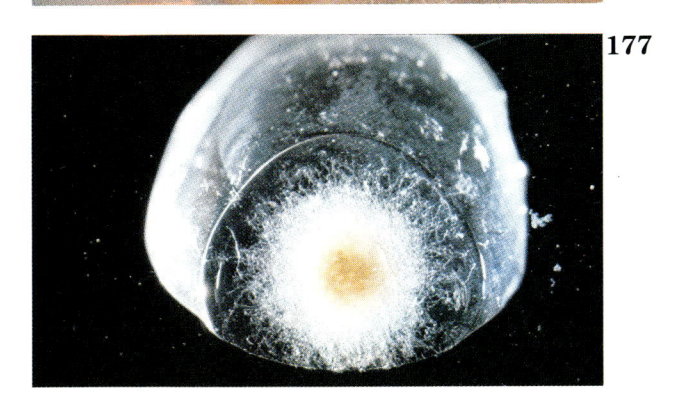

177

178 Cysts and trophozoites of *Acanthamoeba* adhering to the surface of a new, unworn soft contact lens. (× 525) See page 179 for clinical details of *Acanthamoeba* keratitis. (R.C. & B.J. Tripathi and R.H.G. Monninger, Vortrag gehalten auf den 86, Tagunrg der Deutscher Opth., Gesellschaft (Berlin).

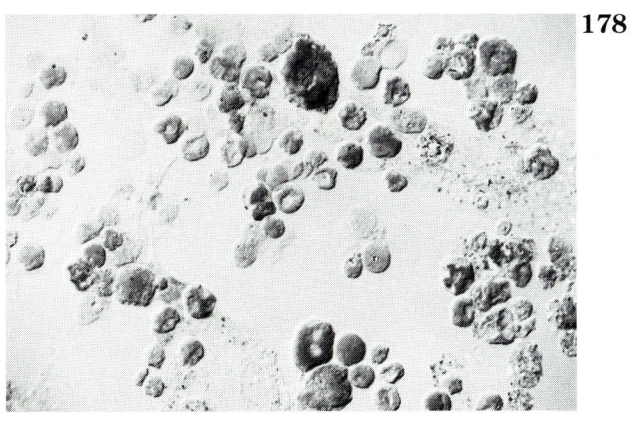

178

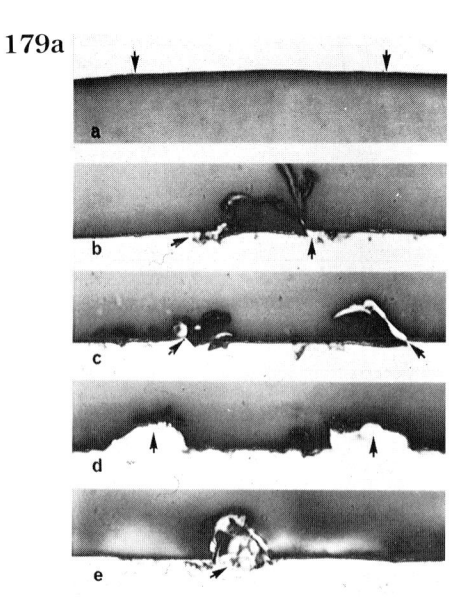

179a **Light microscopy** of a high water content contact lens. The patient suffered from suppurative keratitis. (a) The posterior surface is intact. (b, c, d, e) The anterior surface, showing cracks, craters and surface tears.

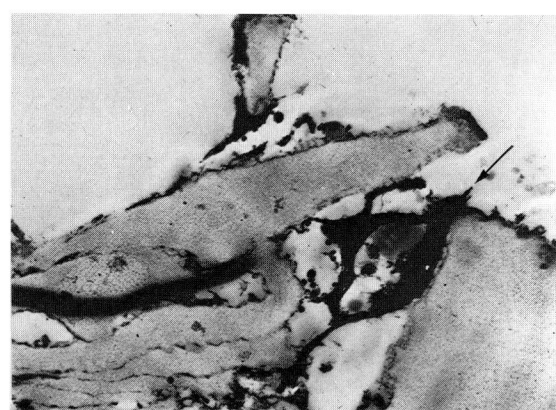

179b **Yeast-like infection.** Same lens as in **179a** showing a yeast-like infection in the cracks of degenerate polymer. (R. Tripathi)

Soft lenses for disposal

This chapter has shown that the best and safest lens is a new, unworn lens. After use, the lens starts to deteriorate and is spoilt and contaminated at variable rates by the following:

- The methods of cleaning, disinfection and storage.
- The degradation of the lens surface and substance from manual trauma and the environment (e.g. drying, material ageing and weathering).
- Contamination by micro-organisms.

Lenses should be changed frequently to remove the hazards of wearing spoilt lenses. It is appreciated that there are instances where individuals can wear the same pair of lenses for several years, but a lens can be spoilt after only a few weeks of wear. The logical conclusion is to dispose of a spoilt lens even if it has only been worn for a short period. Thus a 'disposable lens' is the same as a 'normal' lens, but it is the method of use that has attracted the term 'disposable lens'. A thin, high water content lens does not require cleaning after spoilage, only *disposal*.

Advice to the extended wear patient:

- The number of new lenses issued per annum must be tailored to the individual such as his tear flow quantity and quality, and the environment in which he lives and works. But in general lenses should be changed every one to two weeks.
- Note that the hazards of insertion infection, compromized eye tissue, and opportunistic micro-organism infection will remain even with frequent changes to new lenses.
- Do not clean lenses, but use a new lens and only store lenses in solutions advised by the manufacturer.

Advice to the daily wear patient:

- The same schema is followed, only the lenses should be removed at night, rinsed and stored in the disinfectant solution, and in the morning rinsed with sterile saline, not cleaned, and inserted. A dirty or spoiled lens is replaced with a new lens.
- Lenses should be changed every two to four weeks.

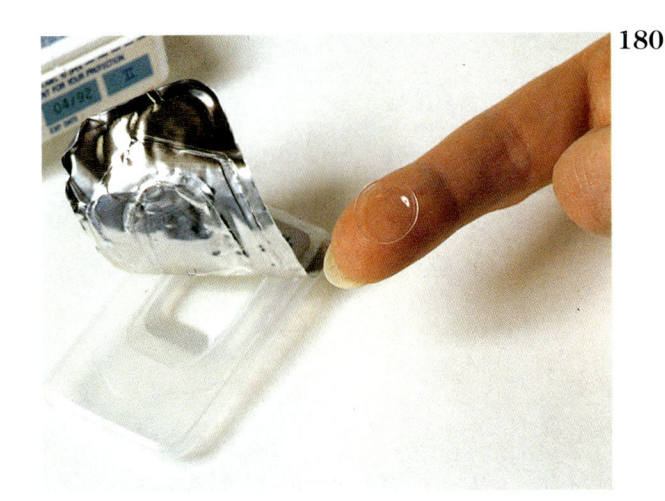

180 A lens removed from its sealed case ready for insertion into the eye. Cases containing several lenses are issued to the patient.

Properties of a disposable lens used for extended wear:

- High Dk/L.
- Of sufficient tensile strength to last two weeks' wear.
- Packed cases are water and air tight and disposable after opening.
- They must be sterile whilst in the case.
- They must be an economical proposition to the patient.

6 Fitting of contact lenses

General principles

General principles applicable to all contact lenses:

- A lens should never seal onto the eye.
- The peripheral fit should permit some tear flow under the lens when the lens moves on the eye.
- Whenever the upper lid covers the lens then the forces applied to the lens should balance opposing forces acting on the lens so that it is not dislodged.
- Lens stability—maintainance of the fit.
- Lens centration—the optic of the lens should be centred on the eye's vision axis.
- The optic portion of the lens should be placed to give optimal single and binocular vision.

There are descriptively two extremes of fit:

- Static fit—the lens fit is fixed relative to the eye.
- Dynamic fit—eye and lid movement produce lens movement nonrelative to the eye.

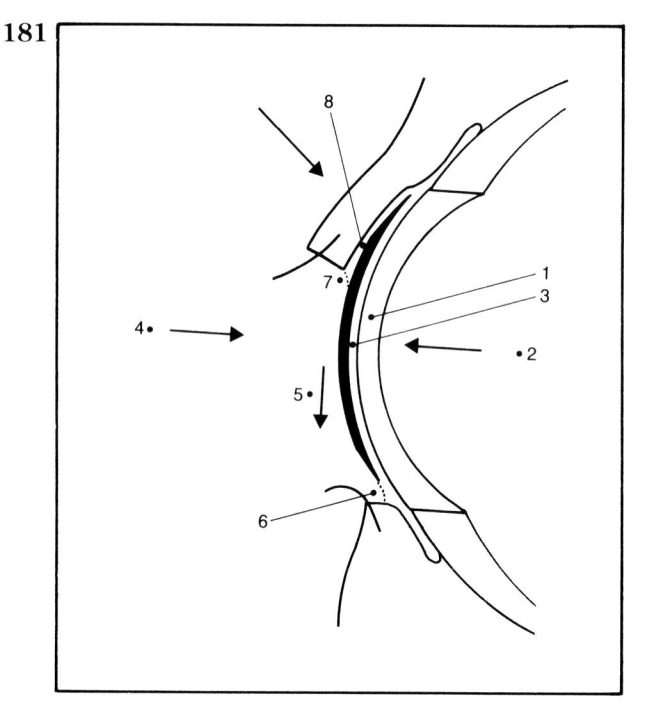

181 Directional forces affecting fit. 1. Corneal rigidity. 2. Intraocular pressure. 3. Adhesion of lens to the eye. 4. Atmospheric pressure. 5. Mass of lens and gravity. 6. Meniscus tension below the lens. 7. Meniscus tension above the lens. 8. Upper lid conjunctival adhesion and muscle pressure.

Lens stability

182 Lens stability factors relative to hard and soft lenses. Soft lenses obtain stability from their area of contact, which is large compared to corneal lenses. Lid movement and lid adhesion only slightly affect this. Hard corneal lenses obtain stability by conforming to the corneal shape over changing zones of contact. At least three separate zones of contact are required to ensure stability (including upper lid adhesion).

Note that an aspheric back surface is more likely to seal on the cornea (fixed stability) than a multi-spherical back surface given equal total sagitta.

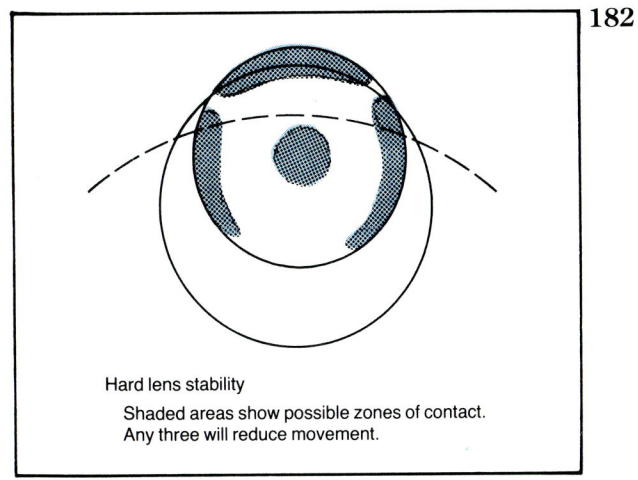

Hard lens stability
Shaded areas show possible zones of contact.
Any three will reduce movement.

Finding the fitting curve from eye models

183 Shadowgraph of model. Shadowgraph of the anterior segment of the eye using a plaster model made from an alginate impression of the eye.

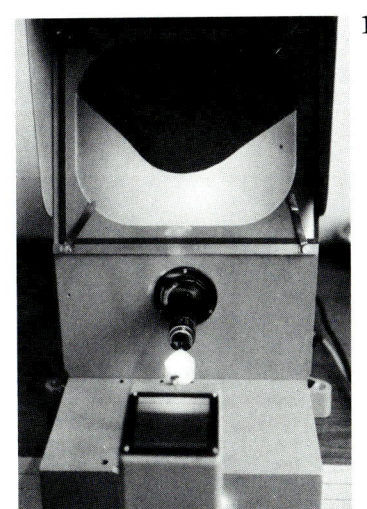

184 A traced drawing of the eye shadowgraph with the sagitta measured over a series of chords. By the technique using several meridians, an average geometric back surface of any diameter lens can be designed for the human eye.

185 Further analysis for finding a fitting curve for the eye shape shows that central corneal chord CC (2-4 mm) is spherical (centre at 1) within the tolerances of contact lens manufacture ($\pm$ 0.02 mm radius). Areas outside the central zone COC can be, on the left side, approximated to a spherical curve of flatter curvature (centre at 2) and scleral AB (centre at 5), but not on the right side, which requires an offset spherical or conical shape to fit CD (corneal) and DF (scleral). Since the cornea and anterior segment shape is a tilted ellipsoid, a regular geometrial fit is *not* possible (but is not required). All contact lenses are fitted with a dgree of misfit to produce a functional result.

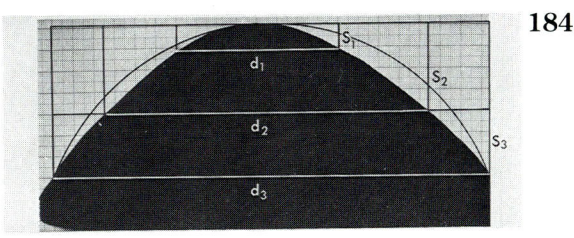

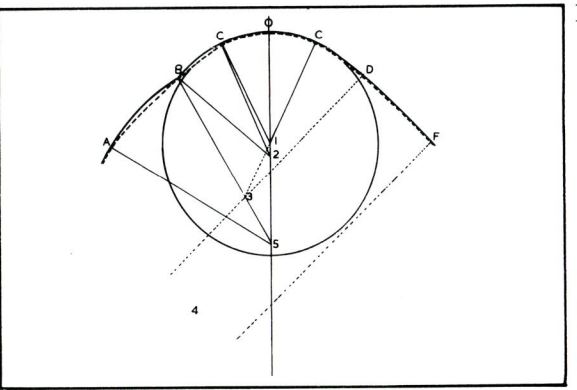

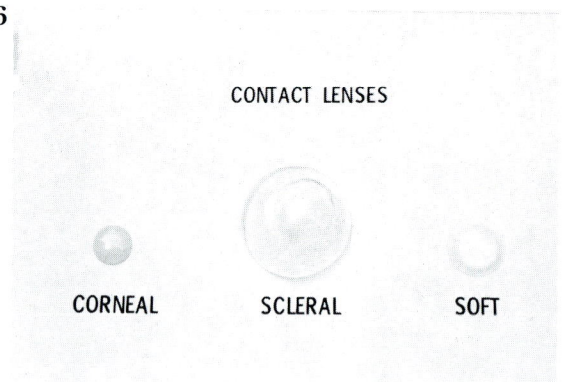

186 In practice there are three main types of lenses:
- Corneal rigid lenses
- Scleral rigid lenses
- Corneo-scleral soft lenses.

Fitting corneal hard lenses

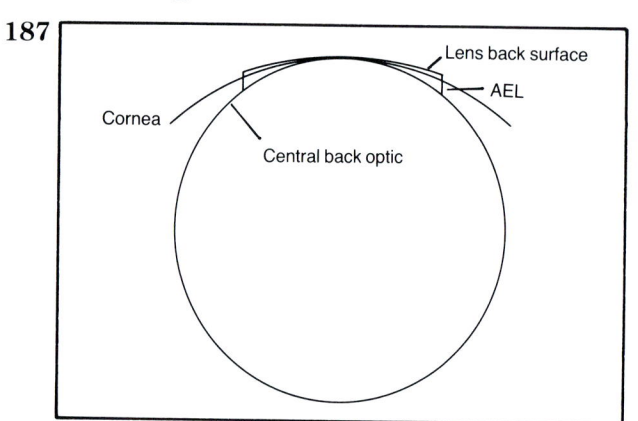

187 Corneal hard lens fit (diameters 7.5-11 mm). Relationship of the lens back surface and central back optic curve (base optic) to the cornea.

In general all fits are on average flatter than the central corneal average keratometry. Thus, although a central fit may be steeper than the central cornea, the peripheral is flatter.

The edge of the contact lens has a clearance from the cornea which can be controlled by the amount of axial edge lift (AEL) given to the back surface. Corneal contact lens back curve design can be given a fixed amount of edge lift to make trial fitting easier.

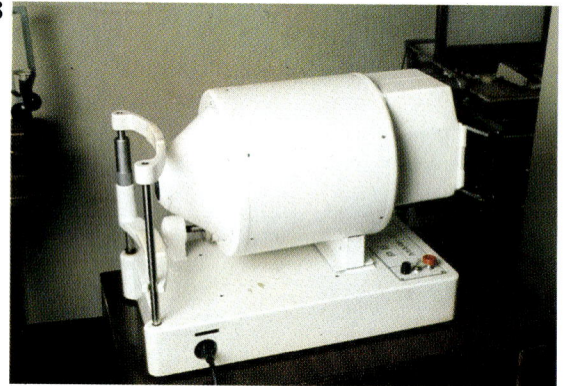

Fitting procedures

Keratometry:

- Central and where necessary 5^0 paracentral.
- Automated keratometry: Hughes system—giving a central reading and the shape factor. Photokeratometry—giving equivalent central readings and shape factors (e.g. Wessley-Jesson system).

188 Photokeratometry. Instrument which takes a polaroid photograph of the corneal image. (Wessley-Jesson)

189-190 The image is analyzed to give readings over the principal axes. The shape factor is then analyzed and departures from the normal noted on the readout. The area of the cornea used is the central 10 mm. From this shape the best fit can be computed from data.

Hard and soft fittings can be ordered from the readings. For hard lenses an allowance of 0.015 mm is made for the tear film thickness.

Automated techniques can work well for the average case but human error in the use of the equipment is sometimes greater than the precision and accuracy of the mechanical device.

The photokeratometer is a very good method for recording corneal shape changes such as in keratoconus and the various refractive corneal surgical procedures.

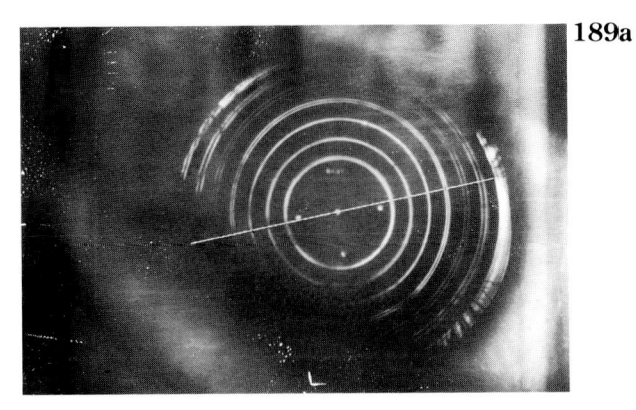

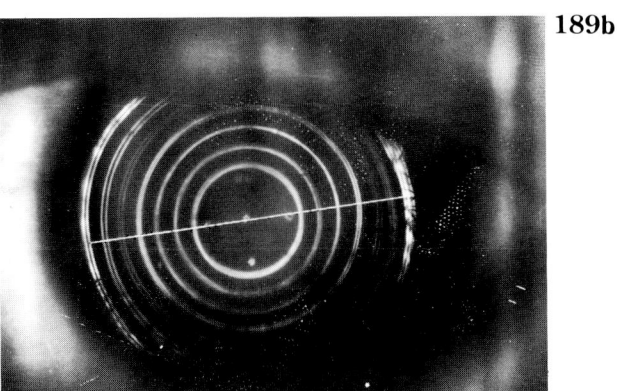

189a

189b

190

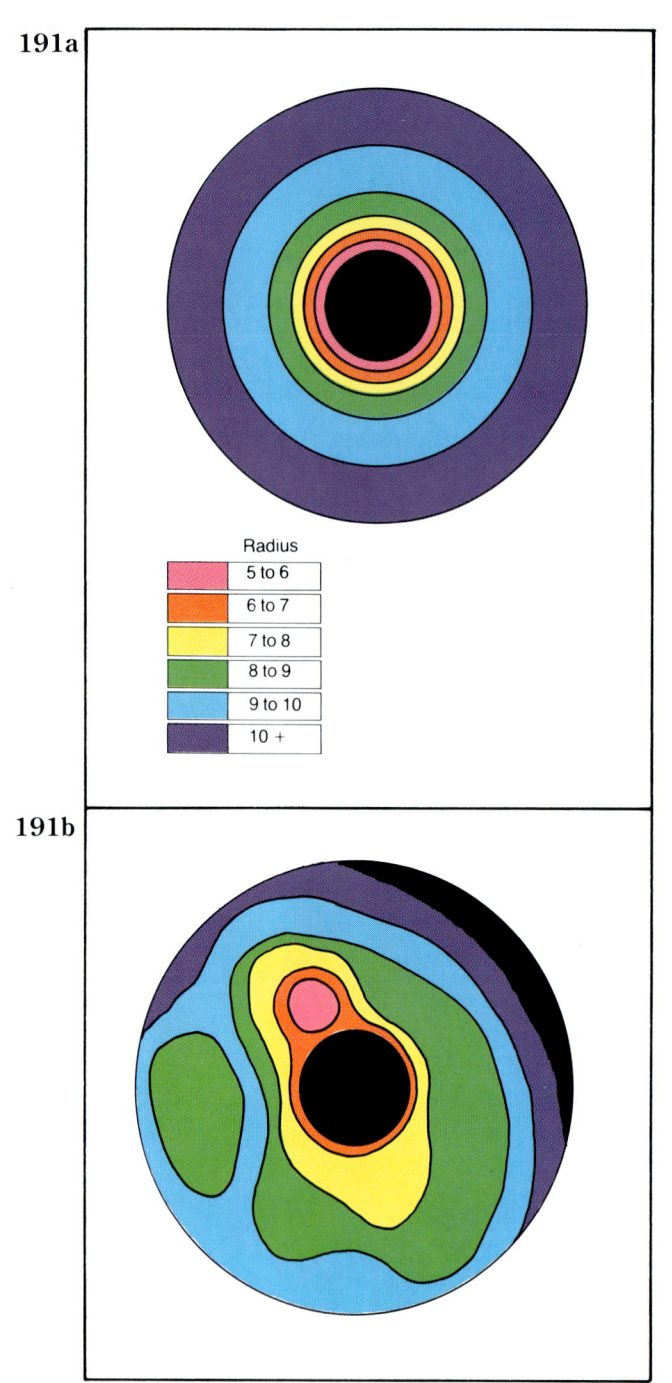

191 a & b Colour coded photokeratograms.
Computers can be used to distribute the results of photokeratometry into zones. S. Klyce has used the computerized zones to produce isometric colour prints. Their greatest value is to describe visually the contours of the abnormal cornea, such as in keratoconus after keratoplasty and refractive surgery. The fitting of a contact lens can be assisted by knowing where steep and flat zones are evident and their extent. Furthermore, the change in the colour contour print can help evaluate clinical progress.

Figure **191 a** shows a colour coding simulation for an aspheric surface and figure **191 b** shows a colour-coding simulation of a graft after keratoconus keratoplasty. (The figures use a limited number of colours by way of example as compared with the actual system which, with different zonal bands and more colours, can be more detailed. (Stephen A. Dingeldein and Stephen D. Klyce, 'Keratoscope by Computed Anatomy', *Cornea* 7 (3): 170-180, 1988.)

Lens power

Power of the contact lens. This is calculated from the spectacle lens refraction (F_s) and the back vertex distance (BVD). Except in those instances where toric powers are used, the average spectacle refraction is used. The contact lens power is therefore the effective power of the F_s in the plane of the cornea (ocular refraction). This is expressed as:

$$P = F_s/1-dF_s$$

192 & 193 Over-refraction. This is the effective power at the cornea of a spectacle correction lens used in addition to the contact lens. This procedure is used to find the correct power when fitting is done using a trial set of contact lenses, or when following up a patient wearing contact lenses. Effective power calculations are only necessary for $F_s > \pm 4d$.

Note that the need to use cylinders in the over-refraction will indicate the existence of either residual or induced astigmatism (see *Toric surfaced contact lenses*—page 79).

N.B. In the instance of a scleral lens with a thick tear lens (b), the power of the lens (a) at P_1 and the tear lens have to be taken into account (see also **189** and **190**).

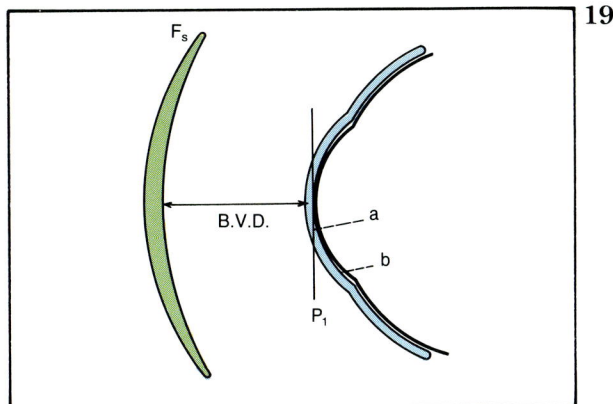

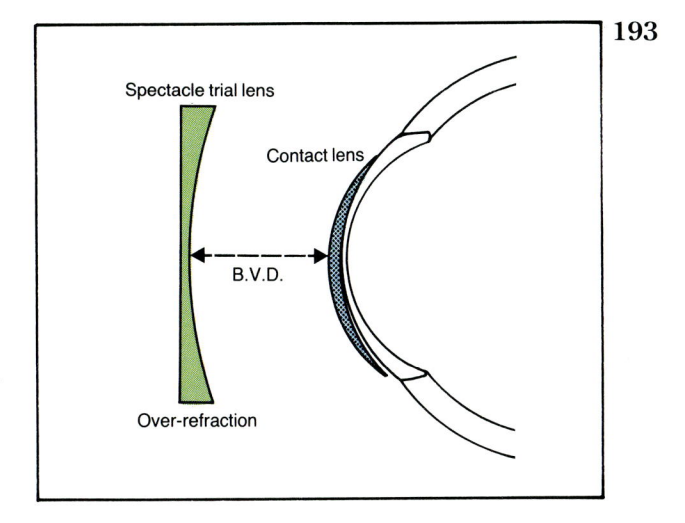

192

193

Trial lens fitting

The same manufacturer should produce both the trial and issue lenses, and all modifications, except edge polishing is to be done by the manufacturer.

- Trial lenses are standard sets of lenses.
- A stock of several lenses over a complete range of fit, size and power is used by the practitioner to:
    1. Assess fit, acuity, and initial tolerance for trial periods of wear.
    2. Supply lenses for wear.
    3. Replace lenses.

If there is to be a difference between rigidity of the corneal hard lens used for fitting and the issue lens, it should be remembered that: higher Dk materials can warp and flex when thin, whereas PMMA lenses, even with centre thicknesses of 0.08 mm, remain rigid upon the eye. To avoid lens flexure upon the eye, HGP lenses are often of a thick design which to a certain extent negates their usefulness. HGP lenses of low minus power are often 0.13 mm thick at the centre. To avoid the problem of warpage, HGP thin and small diameter lenses are fitted steeper than PMMA lenses, especially if corneal astigmatism is present. Some practitioners prefer to take the alternative approach and deliberately fit large and flat HGP lenses and thus obtain rigidity in design by the sheer mass of the lens. Such lenses are unlikely to seal on the cornea.

Table 5. A guide to trial fitting sets for lenses of gas permeable and non-gas permeable material (PMMA)

Purpose	BCOR	BCOD	TD	AEL	T_c	T_e
A. Low minus or plus small corneal	7.0-8.50	7.0-8.50	7.0-8.50	0.14 (PMMA) 0.07 (GP)	0.10 Minus (PMMA) 0.12 Minus (GP) 0.25 Plus (PMMA) 0.35 Plus (GP)	0.16 (PMMA) 0.16 (GP)
B. Conventional size corneal -20.0 and $+20.0$	7.0-8.7	7.0-8.0	9.0-10.3	0.15 (PMMA) 0.07 (GP)	0.08 Minus (PMMA) 0.17 Minus (GP) 0.30 Plus (PMMA) 0.35 Plus (GP)	0.18 (PMMA) 0.18 (GP)
C. Keratoconus two powers $-4.0\%-15.0$ (also grafts)	5.5-7.5	6.0-7.0	9.0-10.0	0.05-0.10	0.10 (PMMA) 0.17 (GP)	0.16 0.16
D. Corneo-scleral plano & -14.0	7.8-9.3	8.0-8.6	11.5-13.0	0.25-0.35	0.12	0.20
Toric truncated Bitoric GP Power compensated		Suggested difference in back optic radii: least 1 mm with 1.5 prism d. base down. Size 9.70 and axes marked. Bitoric set requires no truncation.				

NOTES

BCOR, back central optic radius; BCOD, back central optic diameter; TD, total diameter; AEL, axial edge lift; T_c and T_e, centre and edge thickness.

A. Negative peripheral front surface and front reduced optic for high plus lenses. Smaller sizes can have single cut back surface and edging.

B. There will be thickness variation dependent upon the material and method of manufacture.

C. Reduced front optics for the higher powers.

D. Three to four fenestrations 2 mm inset from edge. Advise GP material only except for prosthetics. These lenses only for keratoconus, keratoplasty and aphakia.

Assessment of fit

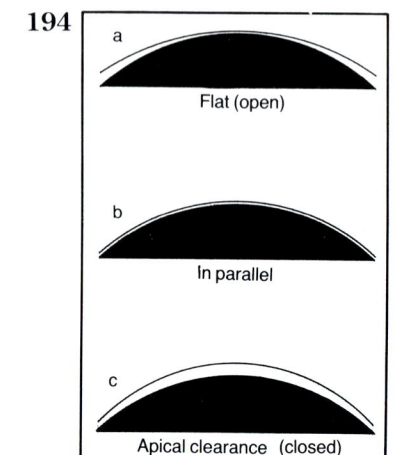

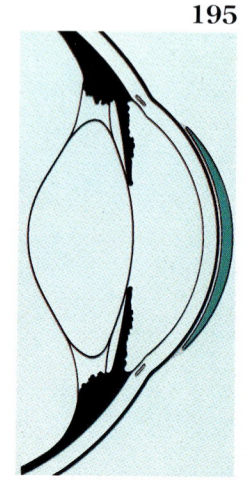

- The assessment of lens stability and centration is by naked eye observation of the lens in white light and using a low magnification.
- To assess the retro-lens tear fluid distribution, stain the tear film with a fluorescein drop or paper and then use blue light illumination and an orange filter for the observer.

194 & 195 Basic fits of the hard corneal lens central area.
a) Flatter than the average keratometry reading—open at the periphery.
b) Parallel to the average keratometry reading—open and closed at the periphery.
c) Steeper than the average keratometry reading (apical clearance)—closed at periphery.
Such a lens, if of HGP material, could seal on the cornea and be of a static fit.

196 Fit diagram. *Right* shows the fluorescein tear film with a parallel fit. Note that if there is *no* fluorescence, then fluorescein concentration is likely to be less than 10^{-6}

Left shows a closed central fit and clearance from the cornea. Contact with the cornea is in the intermediate zone. The periphery is open. Excess intermediate contact can result in arcuate corneal epithelial staining.

197 Parallel fit. Slit lamp appearance of a plus power lens to show parallel fit (Menicon 9.30 mm gas permeable lens).

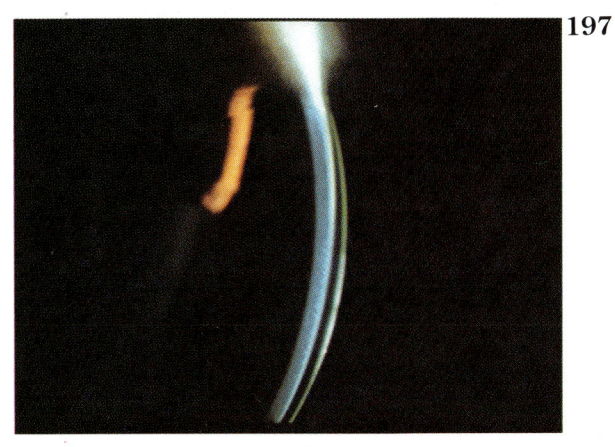

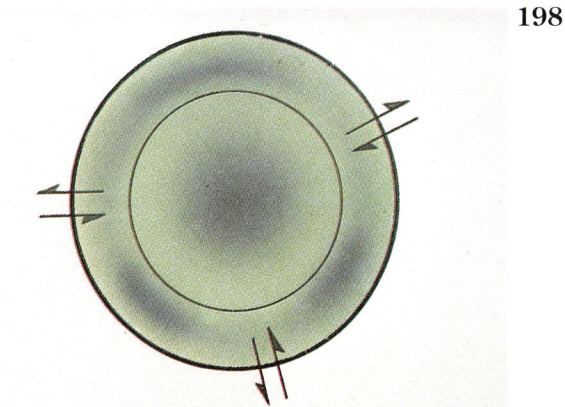

198 Tear fluid flow under a contact lens:
- Central area—minimal apical clearance
- Intermediate area—three zones of contact
- Periphery—tear fluid movement

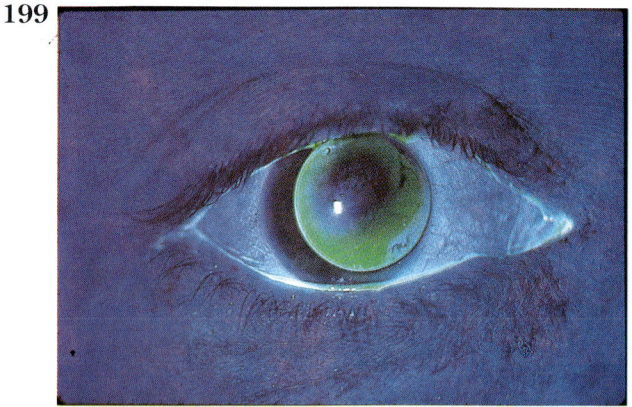

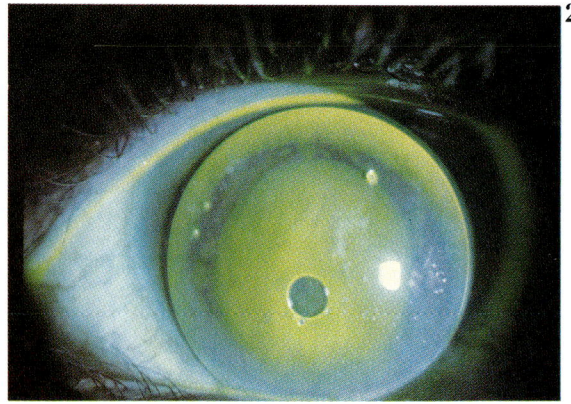

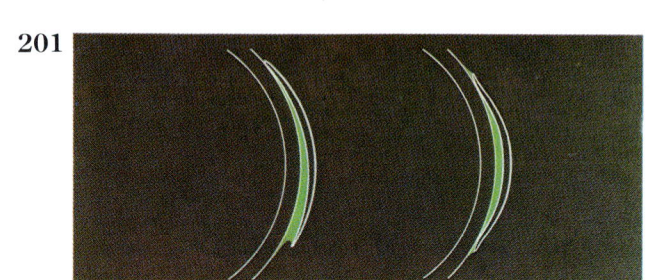

199 Adhesion from the upper lid conjunctivae to the contact lens and a loose, open fit. This fit will be dynamic because the lens will move with the upper lid blink.

200 Excessive central clearance with a trapped air bubble. This is a sealed fit an the cornea is at risk since even with a high Dk material negative pressure is likely to develop and there is a risk of hypoxia.

201 Diagrams. *Left* is diagrammatic of **199**. *Right* is diagrammatic of **200**.

Interpalpebral lens fit

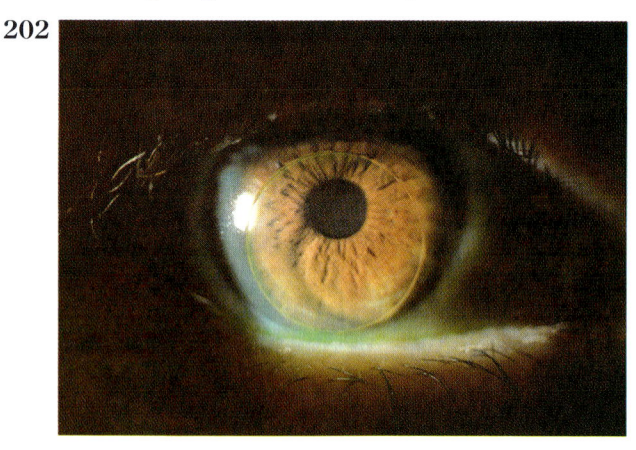

An interpalpebral lens fit is a static fit lens that obtains no lid support and is usually therefore a small diameter lens (less than 8.50 mm). It is used to reduce hypoxia problems and corneal tolerance sensitivity, but a poor edge design results in lid intolerance and a complete loss of blink and tear wetting.

202 Small corneal lens of 7.8 mm diameter.
Example:
   Corneal average keratometry = 7.7
   Contact lens back curve = 7.7:7.70/10.50:7.90
   Single cut lens with edge bevel
     $T_c = 0.10$ mm $T_e = 0.16$ mm $P = -4.0d$

Hard lens centration

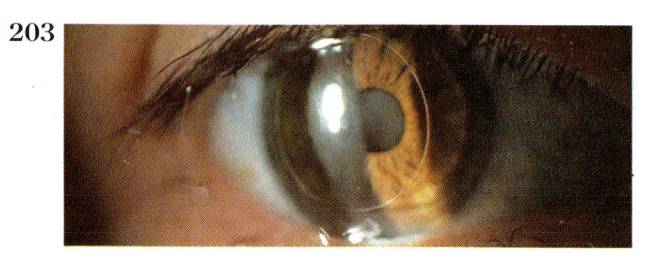

203 This fit shows good centration on the eye even through the versions for distance fixation.

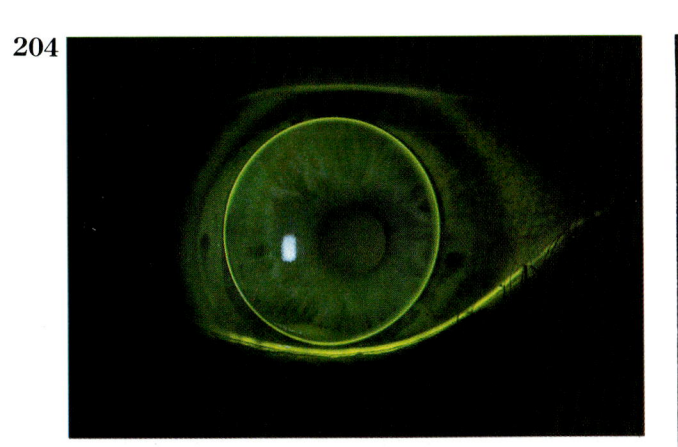

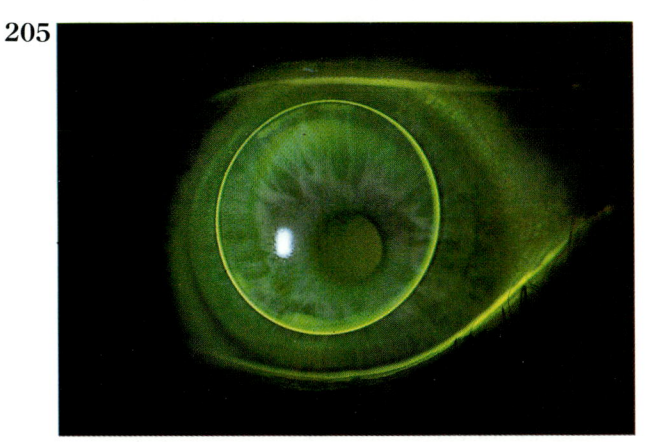

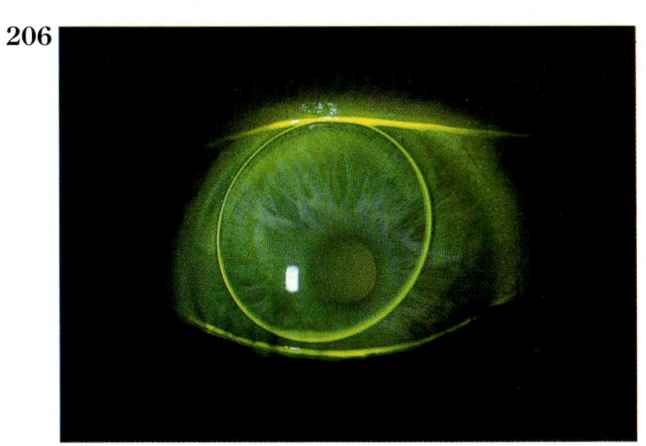

204–207 Change of version to the reading position and lens decentration. This is a good 'on keratometry' fitting of a low minus power small diameter lens (8.75 mm). In the three positions, note that the centre of the lens is not in line with the pupil centre but the vision was not affected—the problem of poor vision with decentration arises when the lens is of high power and the optic too small.

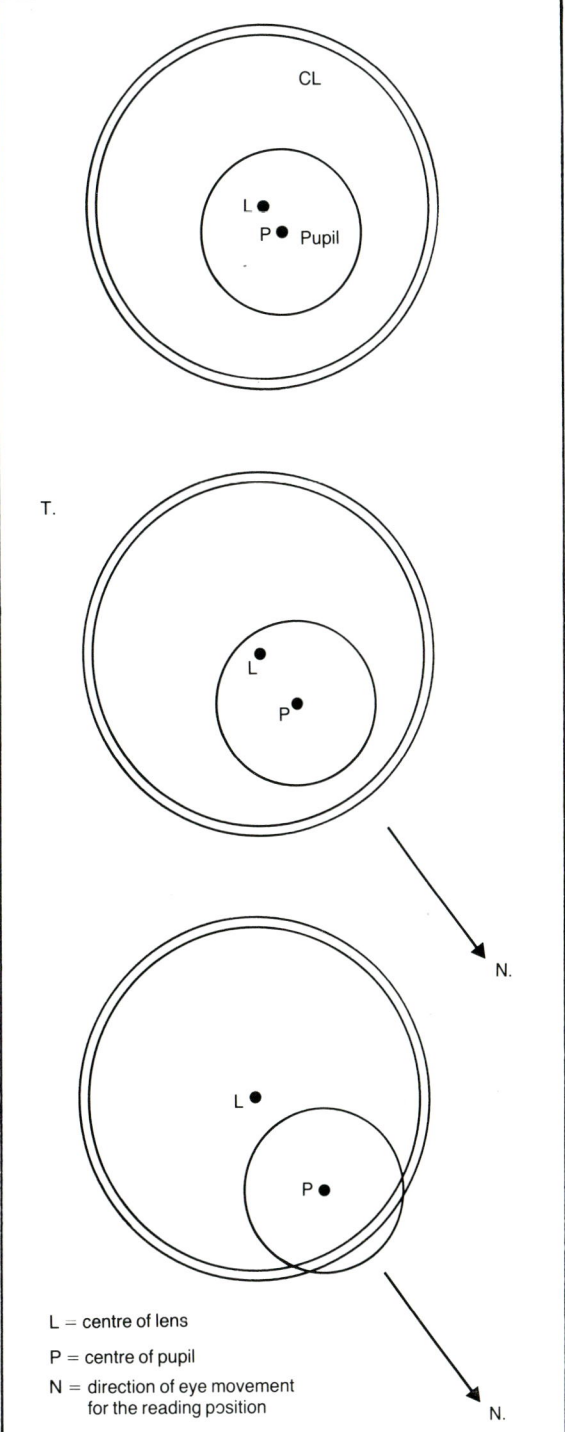

L = centre of lens
P = centre of pupil
N = direction of eye movement for the reading position

75

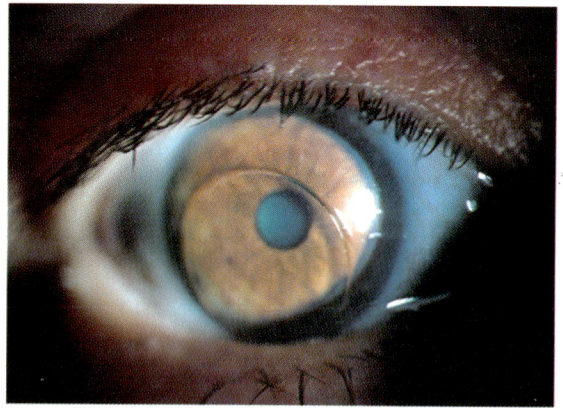

208 This small contact lens was fitted too flat and therefore it sagged down. However, the patient tolerated the fitting very well. Unless there is a sufficiency of tears, this fitting can be associated with corneal dessication.

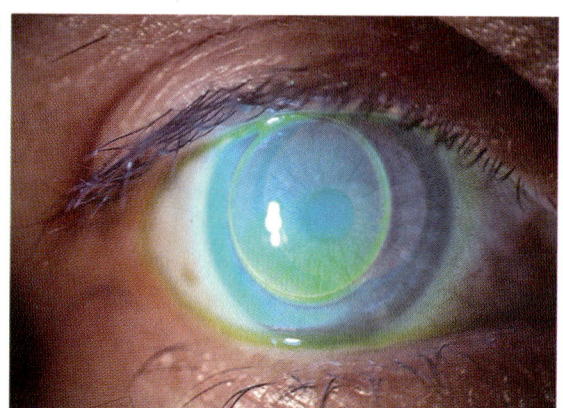

209 Simplified small lens fit design Rx:
Back central radius = Av. K + 0.2 mm
Diameter = Av. K + 0.2 mm
An edge bevel is added. Such lenses must be thin (0.10 mm or less). GP materials may not be of use for such lenses and PMMA is preferred.

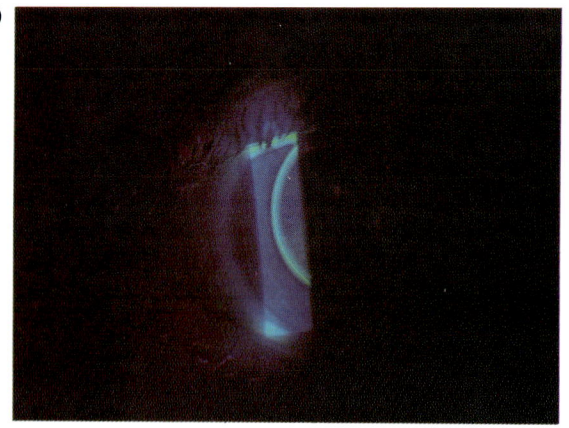

210 Small lens fit and parallel fit with good edge lift.

Corneal intermediate sized lens (9-10.5 mm in diameter)

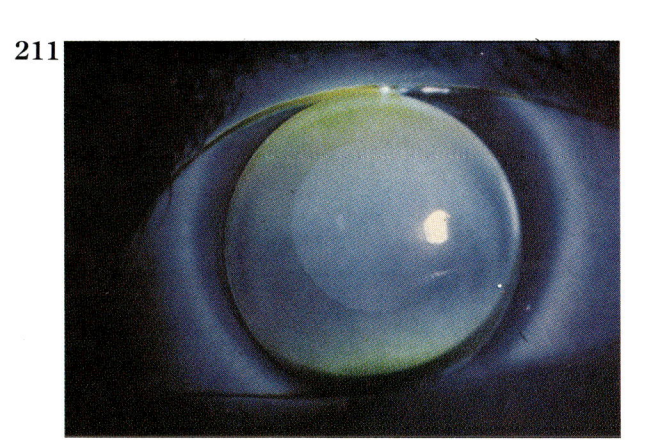

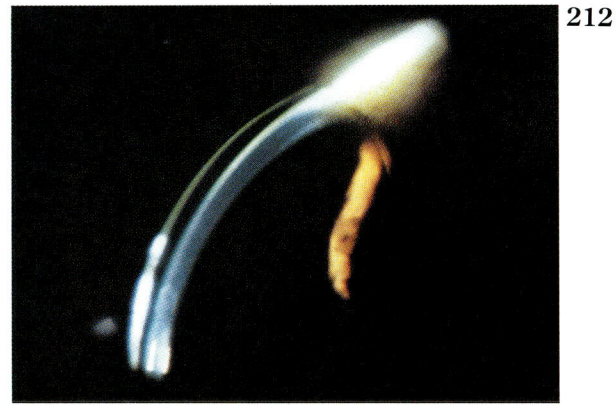

211 & 212 **Flat fit lens with an open periphery** and a low plus power (GP Menicon).

213 **Good edge fitting** in a plus power lens.

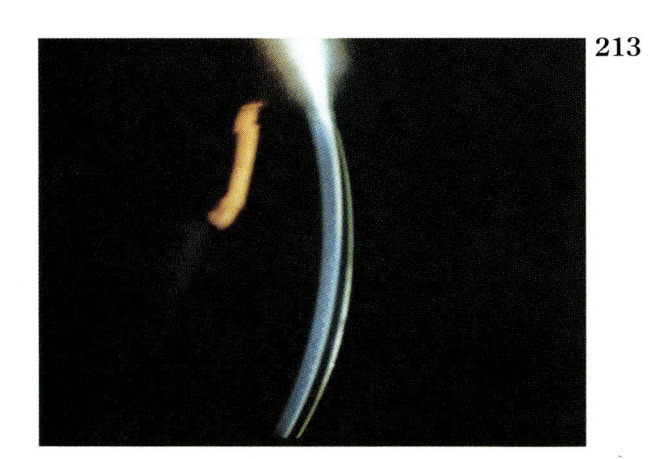

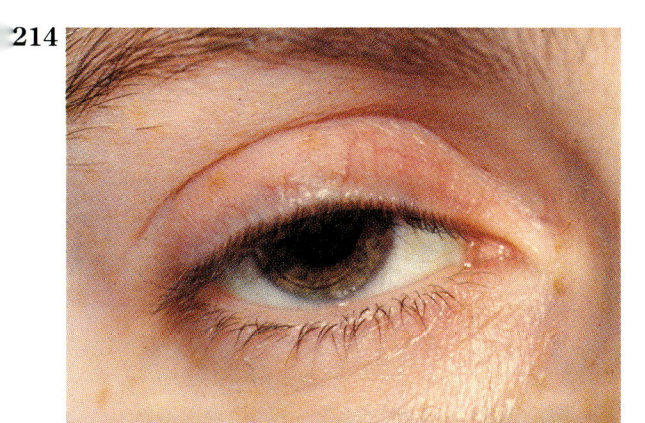

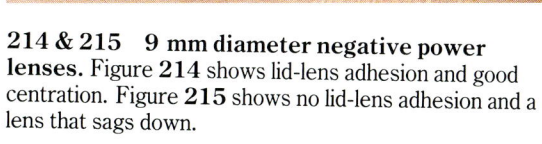

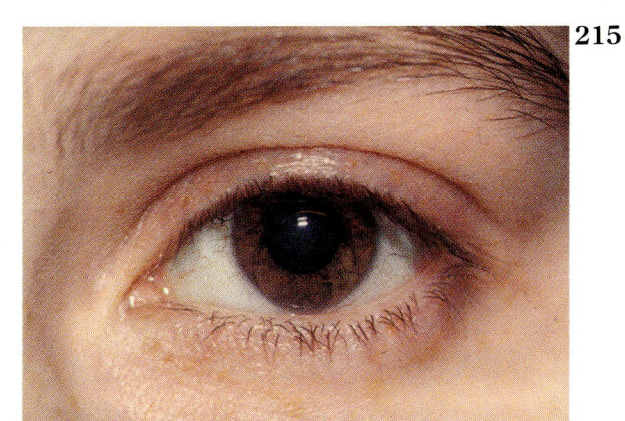

214 & 215 **9 mm diameter negative power lenses.** Figure **214** shows lid-lens adhesion and good centration. Figure **215** shows no lid-lens adhesion and a lens that sags down.

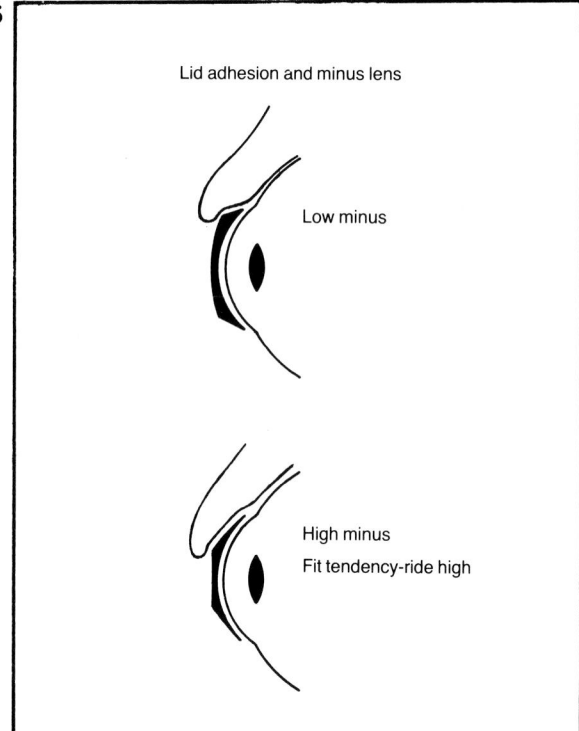

Lid-lens adhesion

216 Upper lid-lens adhesion. The upper lid is normally in close apposition to the surface of the eye and the pressure of the normal blink does little to disturb the tear film. When the upper lid rides over the contact lens, unless the other forces holding the lens on the eye are greater than the forces of the blink, there is a tendency for the lens to move with the lid.

To enhance this effect of upper lid-lens adhesion, the form of the peripheral portion is made with a negative front surface. (This type of design is best exemplified by the reduced optic in a plus powered lens.)

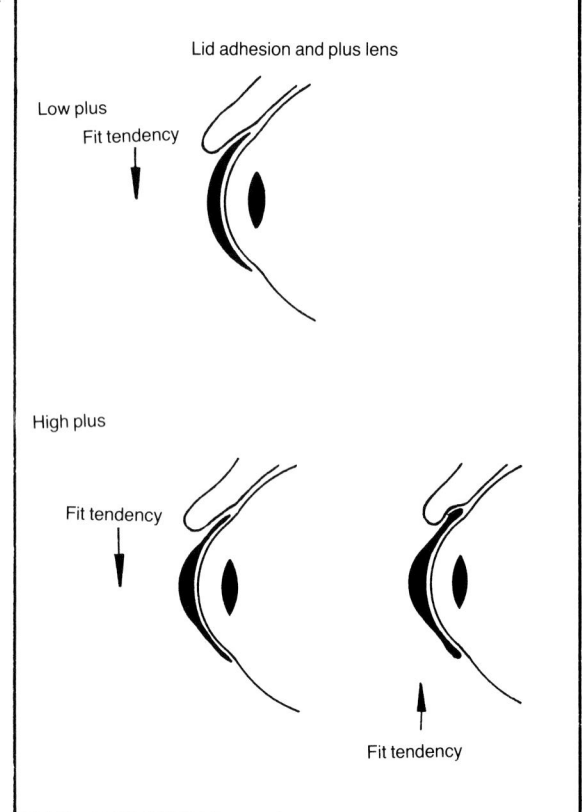

217 Lid-retaining effect with plus lenses that have a negative type carrier. Use of an aspheric front plus surface, while reducing the thickness of the lens, can lose the advantage of the negative carrier effect.

Toric surfaced contact lenses

Principles in the use of toric surfaces:

- To centre a lens on an astigmatic surface.
- To improve retro-lens tear flow (back surface toric).
- To produce greater rigidity of form (bitoric).
- To correct residual and induced astigmatism.

The toric surface can be confined to the peripheral portion only. A toric back surface in the instance of a hard lens will *induce* astigmatism. This can be corrected by using a compensatory front toric surface. A hard lens may correct almost all the anterior corneal surface astigmatism but leave the posterior corneal and lenticular astigmatism uncorrected. This can then be corrected by using the front toric surface or additional toric power on the back surface.

The astigmatism left uncorrected by a spherical contact lens is called the 'residual astigmatism'.

The use of a back toric surface on an astigmatic cornea may not be sufficient to stabilize the lens, so stabilization of the lens has to be considered. Stabilization means keeping a fixed position relative to the corneal meridian, whereas centration refers to the optical or vision axis of the eye. Lenses with back and front toric surfaces are called bitoric contact lenses.

A soft lens placed on an astigmatic cornea will mould to its surface and the corneal astigmatism, in the case of a thin lens, will not be corrected. A thick, soft lens introduces a rigidity factor and the astigmatism will then be partially corrected.

The soft lens to correct astigmatism must have a stabilizing factor introduced in addition to a toric surface to correct the residual astigmatism. This, in the case of thick, soft lenses (greater than 0.12 mm = T_c), should be at the posterior surfaces and, in the case of thin, soft lenses, which have little rigidity factor, it is immaterial whether the stabilizing factor is at the front or back surface.

218 Spherical back surface lens on an astigmatic cornea. The 10^0 meridian is the flatter meridian. The residual astigmatism can come from the posterior cornea and/or lens. Note that the back rigid spherical surface corrects the astigmatism because it negates the refraction of the cornea (in theory only 4/5ths of the refraction).
RIs are as follows:
Hard lens 1.50
Tears 1.33
Cornea 1.37

219 Fluorescein pattern of **218**—the lens back surface is fitted to the flatter meridian (a parallel fit at 10^0).

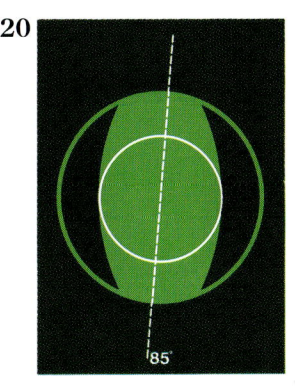

220 Steeper meridian. Diagram of the fluorescein pattern when fitting a lens to the steeper meridian.

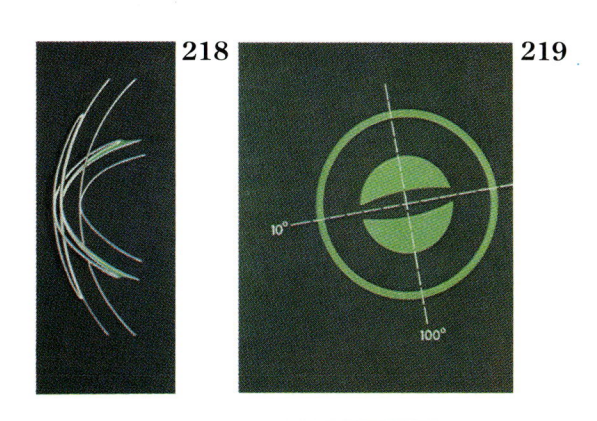

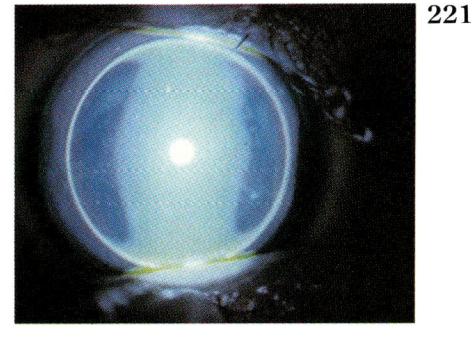

221 Steeper meridian. Photograph of the same type of fitting as shown in **220**.
N.B. Fitting to the steeper meridian is advised for the thin, gas permeable materials using small lenses which are under 9 mm in diameter).

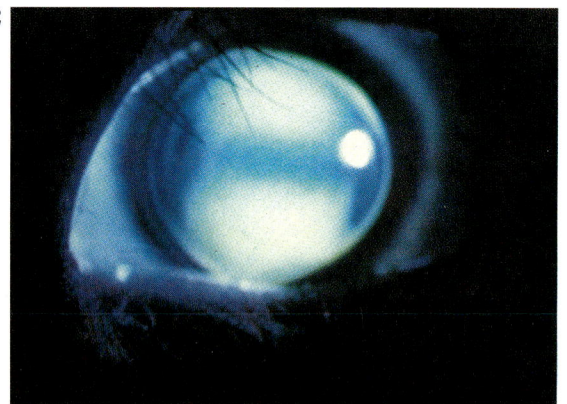

222 Fit with peripheral back toric and central spherical back optic zones.

N.B. Differences in the meridians of less than 1 mm produce unequivocable results.

Example of Rx writing of such a lens:
Back surface = 7.80 : 8.00 / $\underline{9.60}$: 9.30 / 12.00 : 9.50
10.60

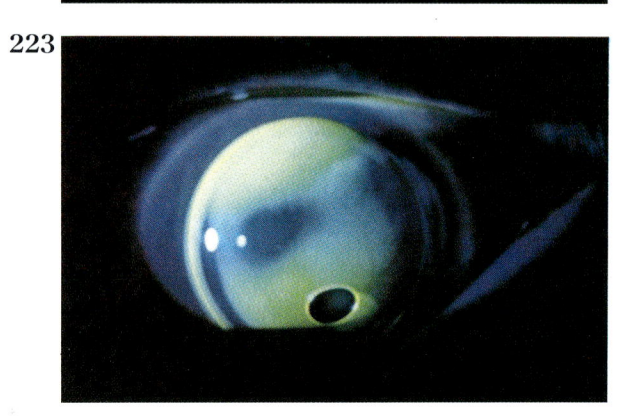

223 Example of a poor lens fit.

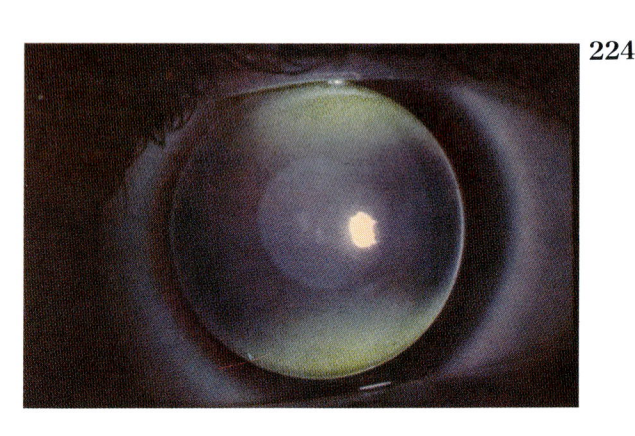

224 Good back fit with a back toric lens surface (bitoric contact lens).

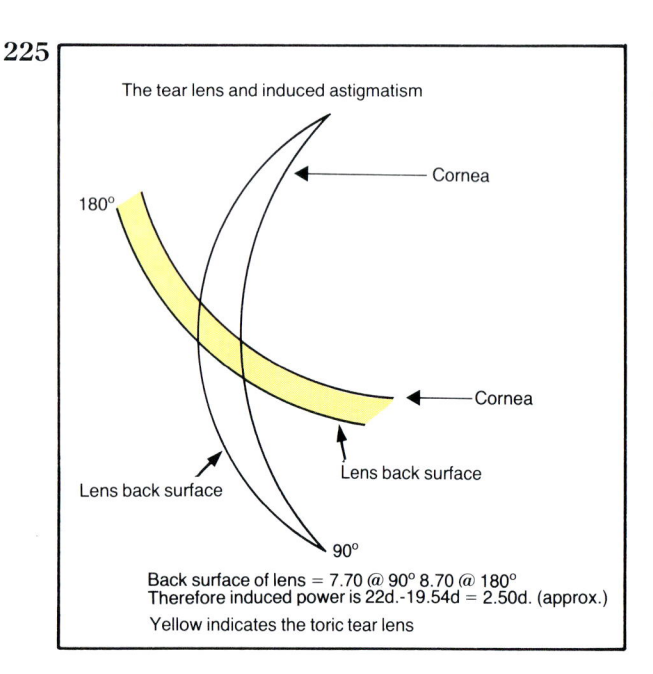

Induced astigamtism of a toric back surface (225)—example of calculation:

Back surface central toric curvatures:
7.7 at 90°/8.7 at 180°
RI of lens = 1.50 RI of tears = 1.33

Power in the 90° meridian of the lens on the eye =

$$\begin{array}{cc} (1) & (2) \\ \dfrac{0.17 \times 10^3}{7.7} \quad \text{at } 180° & \dfrac{0.17 \times 10^3}{8.7} \end{array}$$

Astigmatism = (1)−(2) = 2.55 d
Depending upon the refraction it could be −2.55 cyl. at 180°.

(Residual astigmatism always tends to be negative cyl. against the rule (at 90°) or plus cyl. with the rule.)

To complete the theoretical fitting, the induced astigmatism is found and corrected by the front toric

Diagram 225: The tear lens and induced astigmatism
Back surface of lens = 7.70 @ 90° 8.70 @ 180°
Therefore induced power is 22d.-19.54d = 2.50d. (approx.)
Yellow indicates the toric tear lens

surface in addition to the power required for the ametropia. The bitoric lens should have the axis marked to check stabilization on the eye.

In practice, all the details that are required from the practitioner by the manufacturer are:

- Refraction and BVD.
- Keratometry.
- Toric back surface required and diameters.
- Type of stability required, e.g. prism base down and/or truncation.
- Optimal thickness.

The manufacturer will make the necessary computations for the bitoric lens.

For the best results a set of bitoric hard lenses should be used and the over-refraction calculated after obtaining the best fit. If the bitorics are of the compensated power type then it will be mainly the remaining spherical and residual astigmatism to correct.

Lens stabilization

Reasons for stabilizing a contact lens:

- To achieve centration of a toric surface or any surface that displaces on rotation of the eye.
- To maintain position for multi-vision lenses of segmental type.
- To produce prismatic effects.

Methods of stabilization

Table 6 Prism ballast.

	Powers	
	0 - -8.0	-8.0 and over
For negative lenses	$1^\triangle$	$1.5^\triangle$
For plus lenses use negative peripheral optics carriers	$2^\triangle$	$2^\triangle$

The prism ballast is often combined with a truncation. Plus lens stabilization is a difficult fitting to achieve.

- **Prism Ballast (226)** of $1^\triangle$ to $2^\triangle$ with the base down.

- **Toric back surface:** the fit is parallel to the corneal astigmatic surface. *N.B.* An aspheric back surface simulates a toric form at its periphery.

- **Oval shaped lens (227).**

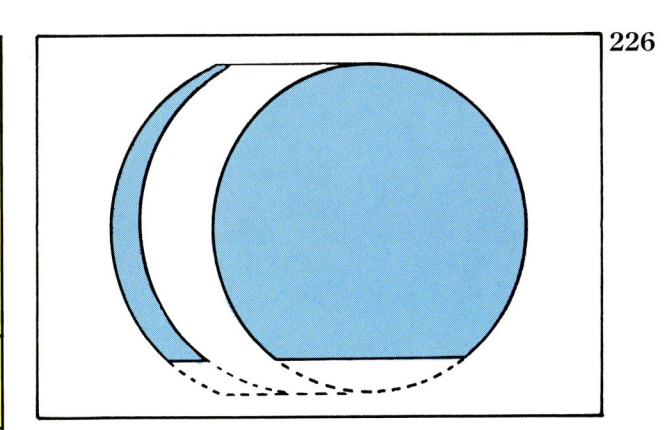

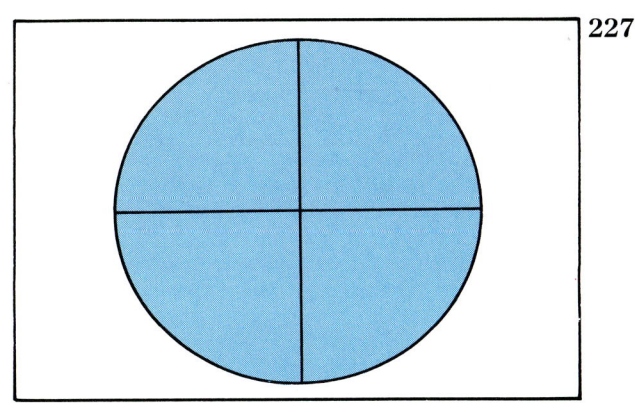

226

227

228

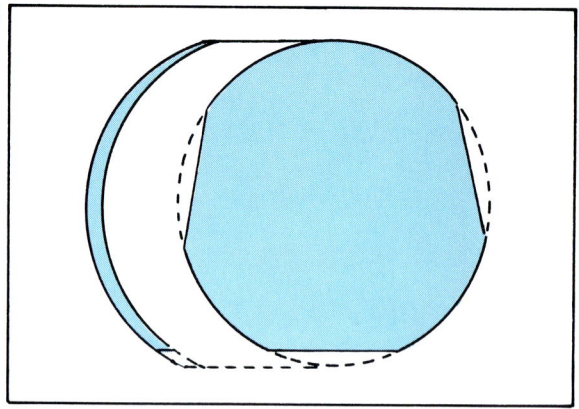

- **Truncations (228)** can be below and/or at sides of the lens. *N.B.* Combinations of the above are often used. Truncations with prism ballast can result in thick inferior portions that are poorly tolerated in both hard and soft lenses.

Table 6a Truncation insets. For corneal lenses covering two-thirds of corneal surface, the following is advised:

Lower lid position		Truncation
1 above limbus	—	1 mm inset
2 at limbus	0	0.5 mm inset
3 below limbus	+	no truncation

229

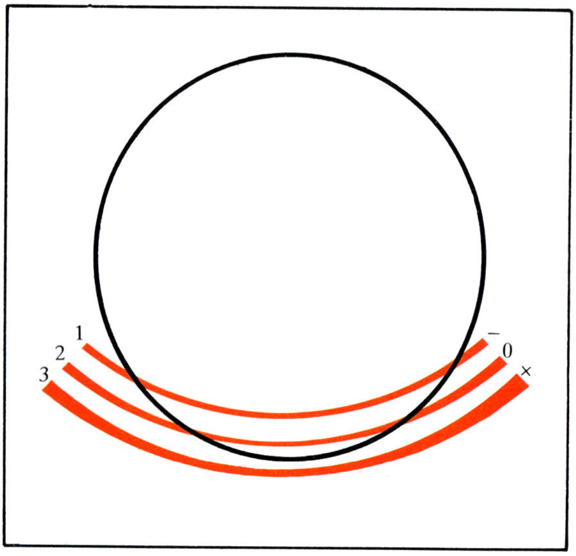

229 Three positions of the lower lid with the eye in the primary position. For position **1** a truncated hard corneal lens would gain lid support but not for positions **2** and **3**. (For a truncated soft lens of 14 mm diameter a 1 mm set in truncation is likely to be of no value for lid position **3**.)

Another method of stabilization includes normal centration through at least three zones of contact, e.g. central and two peripheral zones of contact; three peripheral zones of contact; or two back peripheral and upper lid front contact (see **198**). Upper lid lens adhesion is yet another method of lens stabilization (see *Multi-vision contact lenses*).

Multi-vision contact lenses (bifocals and multifocals)

Multi-vision lenses are used with limited success. However, to achieve presbyopic near correction the following methods can be used:

- Mono-vision, i.e. one eye corrected for distance the other for near or intermediate distances. (Add + 0.50d. to distance if acceptable.)
- Near vision spectacles—the simplest method.
- Concentric bifocal and multifocal powered lenses—the centre zone can be for distance vision and the periphery for near vision, but some lenses use a small central zone for near vision and the remainder of the lens for distance vision.
- Simultaneous vision contact lenses—concentric distance and near diffractive (microfresnel) zone lenses.
- Alternative vision lenses—solid segment designs and fused segment designs.

(The latter groups are often ballasted to give centration and assist transference from the distance to the reading positions of the eye. Note also the lid adhesion function in holding the lens as the eye achieves the downward reading position.)

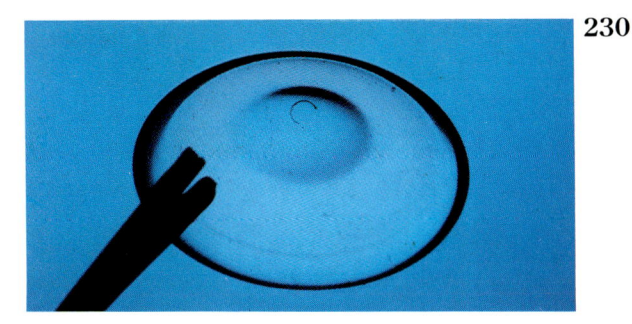

230 Concentric vision bifocal lens.

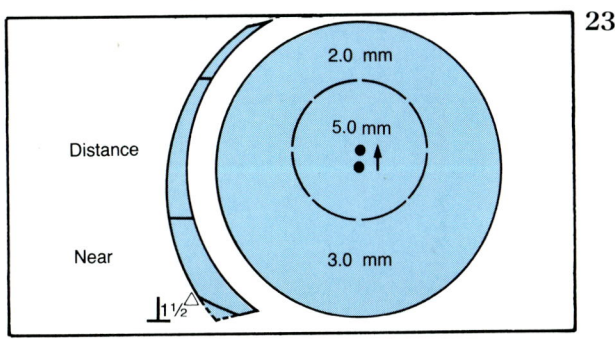

231 **Only a 5.0 mm diameter** is used with this design for the distance (decentred) vision with a prism ballast placed inferiorly to assist optical centration. Truncation is avoided by thinning the antero-inferior portion of the lens. This design is also applicable to the larger soft lens. The peripheral fit must be loose to allow transference of the lens from distance vision to the reading position.

Simultaneous vision lenses

The application of Fresnel and other basic prinicples of diffraction gratings to contact lenses is an interesting development.

Gratings (echelons) of high resolution with exact phasings are required. When angled, such gratings produce interferometry patterns with good resolution image formation which can be combined with the refraction image formation produced by the contact lens surfaces. Diffraction image formation has been the basis of holographs using incoherent light but here the light source is coherent light. The present developments are based upon the Cohen and Pilkington patents. (Allen Cohen, US Patent 4,340,283, Phase shift multifocal zone plate, filed December 1979, issued July 1982; Charms P.W., Freeman M.H., Melling J., Stone J., Walker P.J.C., *The development and clinical performance of a new deffractive bifocal*, Contact Lens Optometry Today, 87, 27 (22), 721-724.

In one type of lens the echelons cover most of the back surface of the soft hydrogel material; and in another type of lens, the diffraction zone is limited to the central 5 mm diameter zone of the hard gas permeable material which is 9.5 mm in diameter.

232

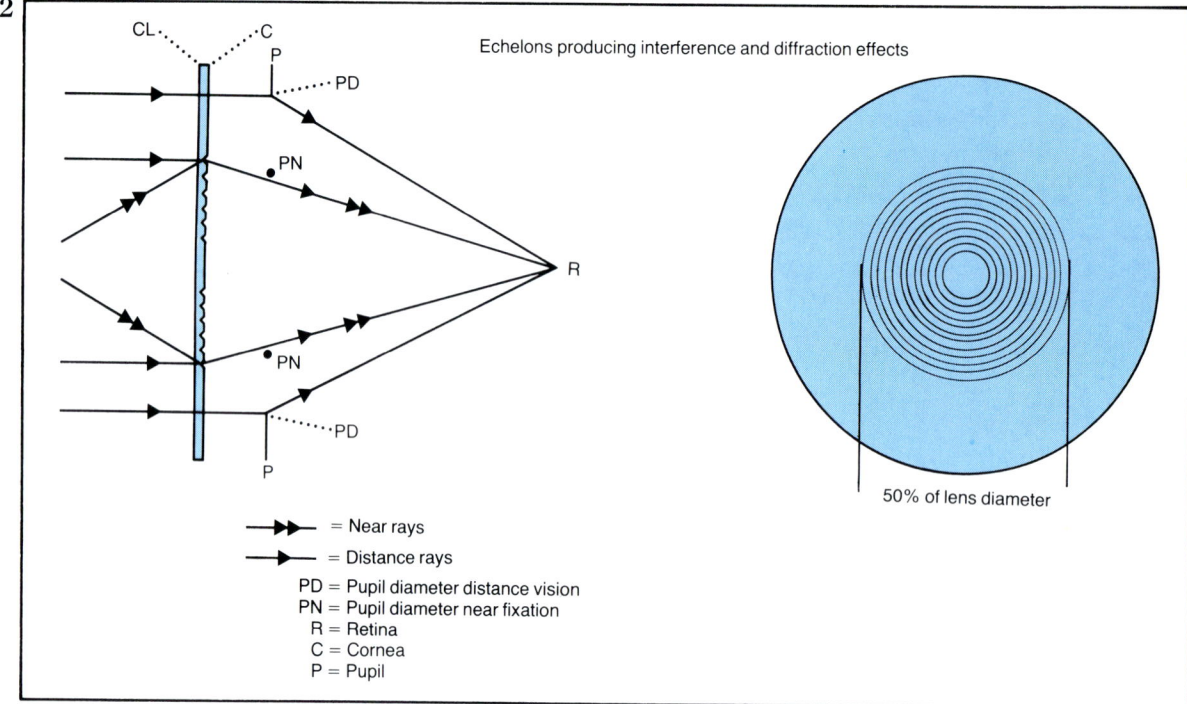

Echelons producing interference and diffraction effects

⇒⇒ = Near rays
⇒ = Distance rays
PD = Pupil diameter distance vision
PN = Pupil diameter near fixation
R = Retina
C = Cornea
P = Pupil

50% of lens diameter

232 The diffraction zone will produce a retinal image for near fixation, as shown by the ray diagram on the left, but if the pupil is not centred on the system, or if the pupil is larger than the diffraction zone, abberations and double image (ghosting) can occur.

This type of lens has to be fitted so as to produce minimal translation of the lens on vergence to the reading position (± 0.25 mm). Therefore a slightly steeper fit than the one conventionally used is advised.

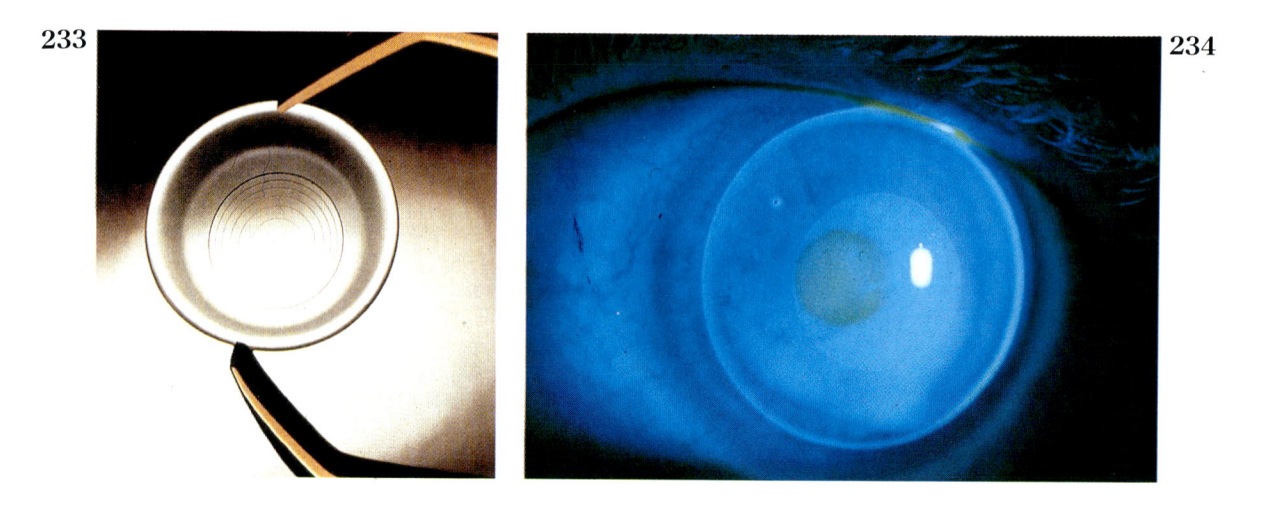

233 & 234 **The Pilkington lens** and the way it fits on the eye.

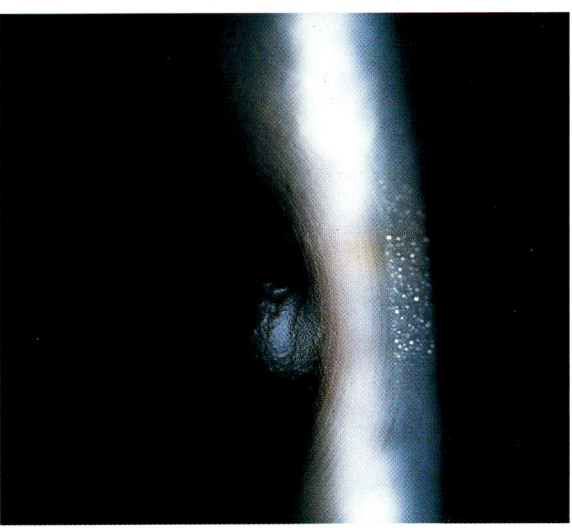

235 & 236 Diffraction zone interferometry pattern of a soft lens (Hydron). (Photographs, Graeme Young)

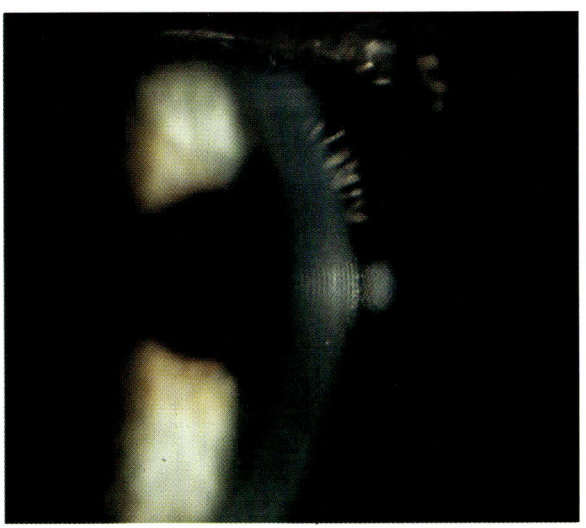

The other problems with this type of simultaneous vision bifocal lens can be lack of contrast in mesoptic states of illumination, haloes and spectroscopic image edging and acuity deficiency. Good binocular vision is required to fuse this type of image otherwise confusion can occur and sometimes monocular spurious steroscopy can result.

Segment design bifocals

A segment bifocal of fused or solid design can be used with some hard materials. For soft lenses, solid designs (concentric and segment designs with prism ballast) are possible.

Hard corneal fitting programme:

1. Fit a spherical powered lens with prism ballast.
2. Modify the peripheral fit until translation is satisfactory.
3. Mark with a red Pentex pencil the area for the near segment. In distance fixation *no* red should be seen.
4. Return the lens to the manufacturer for remaking with a near segment.

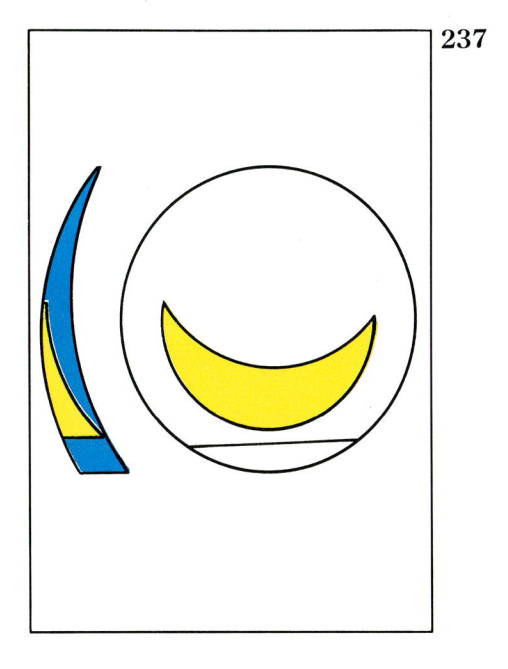

237 Truncation need not always be used. Prism ballast lenses can be made round and the inferior portion thinned away from the front peripheral surface (see **231**).

238 & 239   Correct translation of the lens.
N.B. The function of the upper lid can be more important to hold the lens than the ballast effect.

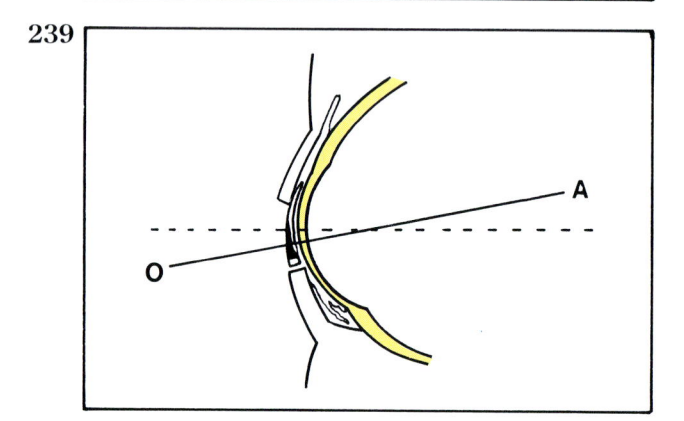

240 & 241   Fused large segment lenses on the eye in the distance and near positions.

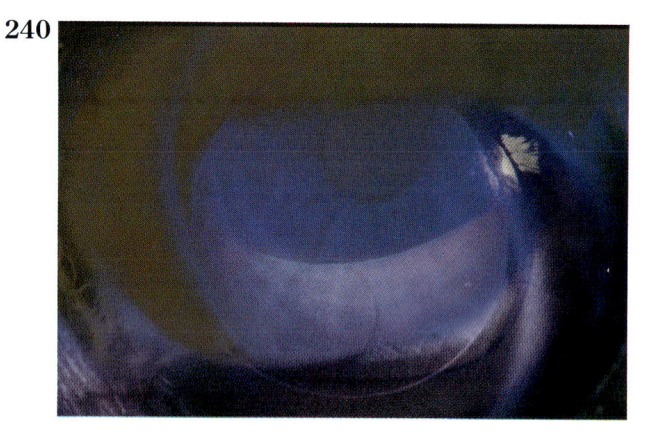

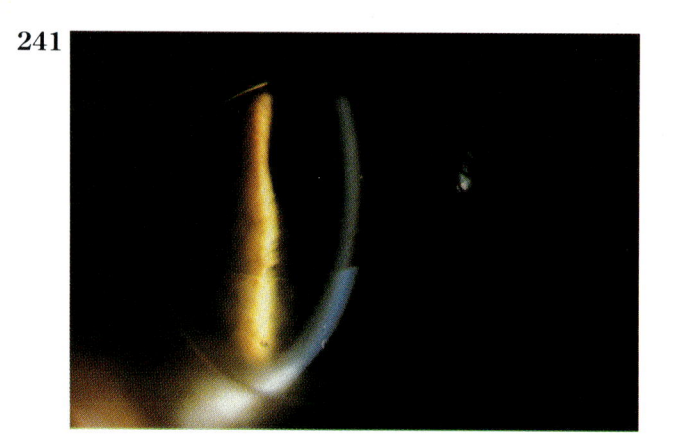

Soft lens fitting—hydrophilic and silicone rubber lenses

Because the soft lens materials have a greater plasticity (flow) than elasticity property, soft lenses have to be made of a larger size than corneal lenses to achieve stability. The introduction of thickness to achieve stability, while permitted in special instances, negates their gas flow qualities and tolerance.

The basic designs used in their manufacture emanate from hard lens design, since in many instances the soft lens passes through a hard, dry state before being equilibrated with water (as in the case of hydrophilic lenses). Moulded lenses and cast lenses emanate from dyes based on lathe cut generation ideology.

The size of a soft lens is related to its fitting tolerances (see Table 7). Thus, if one compares large lenses with small soft lenses of the same thicknesses, then the small lens must have more incremental fittings available than the large. The small lens will move more than the large lens and therefore better edge tolerance is essential for the small one. The larger lens has a greater scleral contact and greater upper lid conjunctival adhesion; both have long-term problems. There are ethnic and sexual differences that make the small soft lens preferable overall to the large soft lens. But given a very thin and highly elastic material, the *one* fit designed lens can be tolerated by the normal range of keratometry readings.

Table 7. Soft lenses: determinants of size and thickness.

Size (mm)	Fitting tolerances	Comfort	Complications
13.50-15.00	Crude	Good	Chronic lid and corneal occlusion problems
11.50-13.50	Fine	Edge design determines comfort	When the lens has a flat fitting, poor edge design causes intolerance and corneal changes

The above supposes all fittings are functional.

Table 8. Thickness. This is related to volume and maximum and minimum zones of the lens. Average thickness should be known.

Power	Thickness	Optics	Complications
Plus	Centre and front optic junctional thickness must be controlled	Reduced optic necessary	Central corneal occlusion
Negative	Peripheral thickness must be controlled	Reduced optic necessary	Limbal occlusion

When fitting, the gas flow through soft lenses is an important consideration. Therefore great care is necessary in controlling the distribution of thickness according to the power of the lens (see Table 8 and Chapter 2).

Fitting principles

For soft lenses there must be:

- Optical centration
- Minimal movement
- Minimal thicknesses
- Loose edges
- Non-adherence of the lens to the eye tissue
- Normal tear film integrity and thickness on the edge and front surface of the lens

242

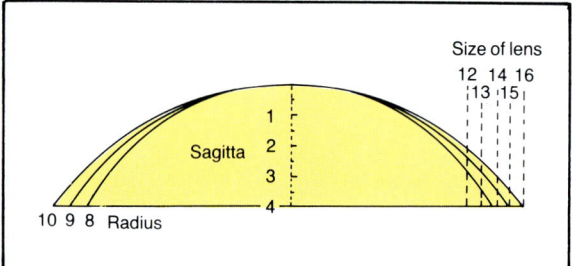

243

244

Sagitta	Total diameter of lens					
	12	13	14	15	16	mm.
2.25	9.10					
2.50	8.52	9.90				
2.75	7.95					
3.00	7.10	8.70	9.85			
3.25	6.40					
3.50		7.85	9.10	9.90		
3.75						Radius
4.00		7.00	8.40	9.45	10.00	±0.20
4.25						
4.50			7.70	9.00	9.65	
4.75						
5.00			7.40	8.55	9.50	
5.25						
5.50					9.25	
5.75						
6.00					9.00	

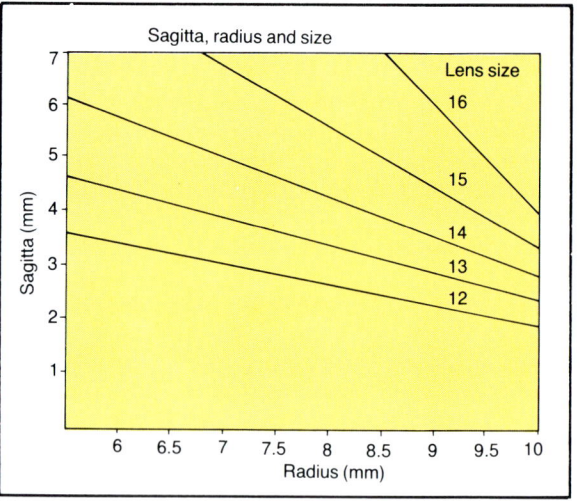

Spherical back surfaces of gel contact lenses in equal sagittal increments

Range of fittings

242 The theoretical relationship of size to back curvature for identical sagitta.

243 & 244 Range of fittings. The examples given are of single curve spherical design, but equivalent bicurve or aspherical lenses are possible. Because of its size, the principle adopted for the soft lens is to use equal increments in sagitta and approximate them to the size and curvature of the lens.

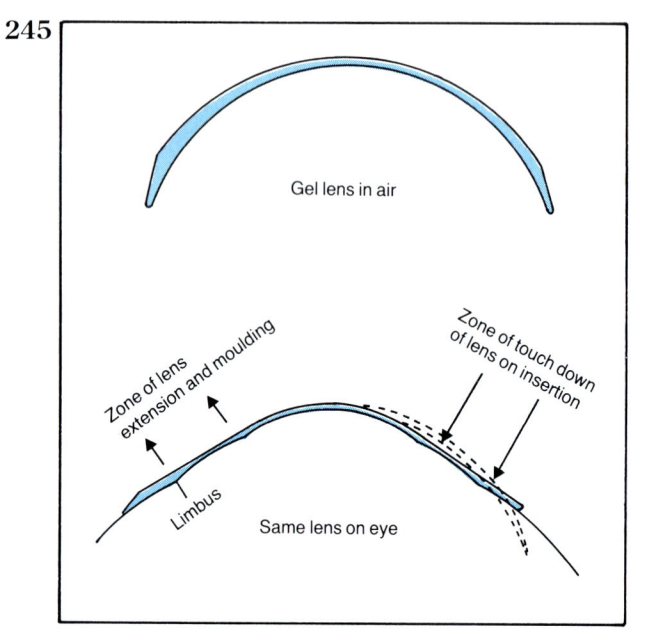

245

245 Flatter scleral position. For any scleral soft lens larger than the limbal diameter, the single back curve lens must have to mould to a much flatter scleral portion (which is small in width but is a relatively important area—**246**). One does this by fitting flatter than the average keratometry by an increasing increment according to the size of the lens.

Note that irrespective of the geometric form a soft lens has *in vitro*, when inserted it conforms to the eye shape to a variable degree. There are many lenses that also have to conform to a scleral fitting, because of their size or movement on to the sclera.

Relationships of areas of contact (see **246**): white central area = corneal contact (12 mm diameter); white and yellow central areas = corneal contact plus ½ mm scleral (13 mm diameter); white and yellow and orange areas = corneal plus scleral contact of 1½ mm scleral (15 mm diameter).

246 Position of the upper lid. If the 12 mm lens is compared with the 15 mm lens then the palpebral-lens conjunctival contact will be four times greater for the larger lens. This can have a bearing on induced conjunctival pathology.

Corresponding fitting back radii of curvatures:

Diameter of lens	Back curve flatter than K by:
12 mm	0.6 mm
13 mm	0.8 mm
14 mm	1.0 mm
15 mm	1.4 mm
16 mm	1.6 mm

This does not make allowance for steep corneas which require fittings steeper than suggested above. The rigidity of the material will also affect the fit and such things as water evaporation.

Soft lenses fitted smaller than the cornea (11.50 mm) will be fitted steeper than the average keratometry.

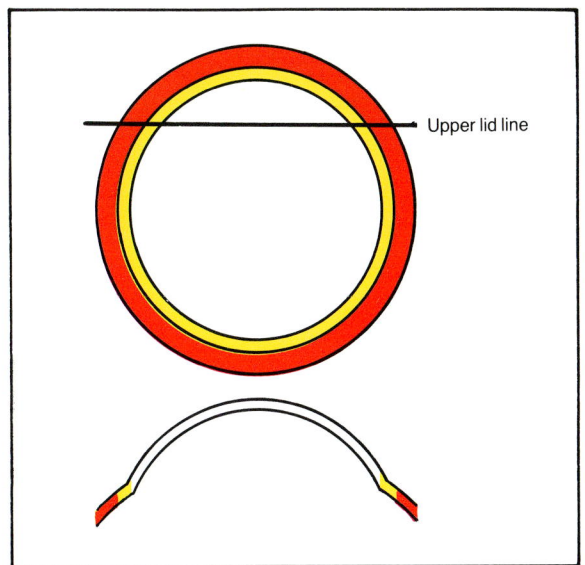

246

Upper lid line

Table 9. Areas of contact with the cornea and sclera.

Lens	Corneal contact	Scleral contact
12 mm	100%	0
13 mm	90%	10%
15 mm	70%	30%

Thus the large scleral lens has a substantial scleral contact.

Examples of fitting

Because of the mouldability of the material and the thinness of most designs in the low powers there are some manufacturers who supply mainly one fit lenses (e.g. disposable system lenses—see page 64).

247 Hydrophilic gel lens (14 mm diameter) on the eye. Movement of the lens 1 mm off the centre by gentle pressure of the lid on the lens should result in the lens springing back into position.

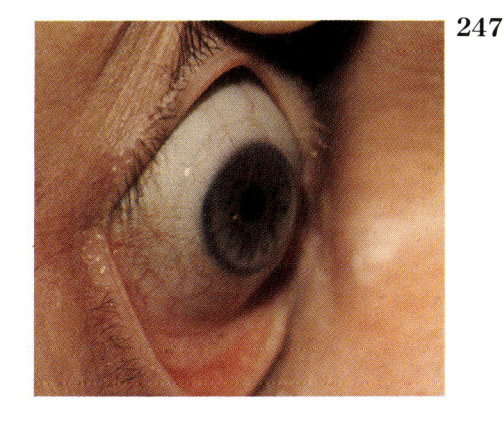

247

248 13.5 mm gel lens with good centration.

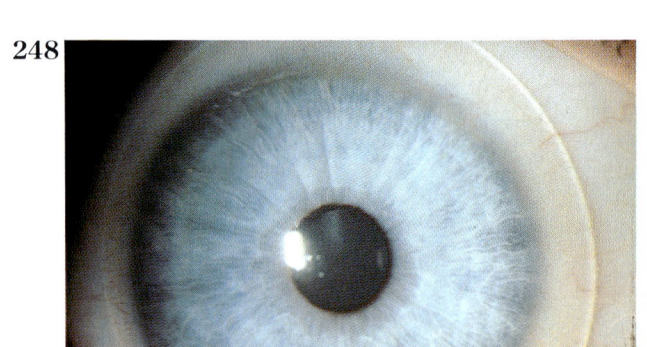

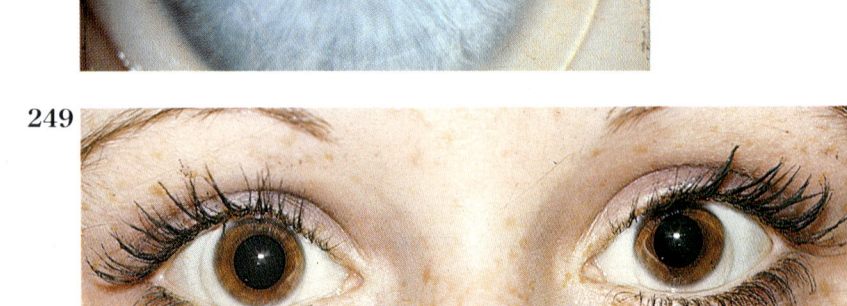

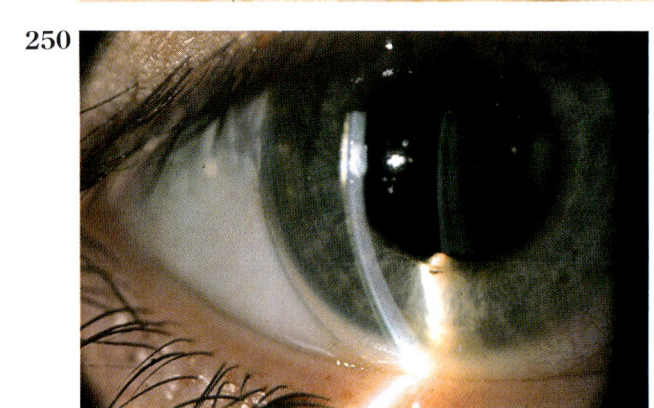

249 & 250 Loose fitting gel lenses. Good tolerance but with high powers and reduced optics can result in poor vision. When this type of fit occurs with aspheric back lenses a steeper fit or larger lens is advised.

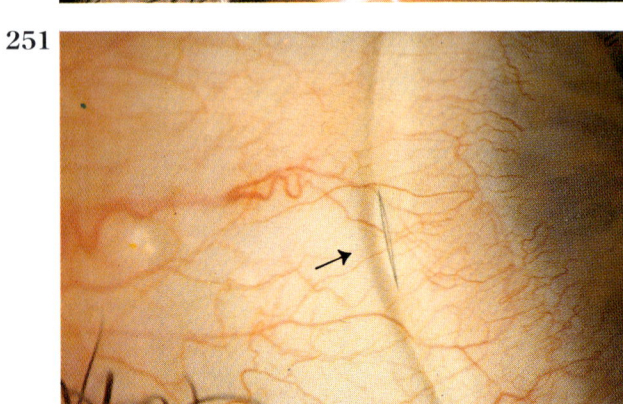

251 & 252 Edge 'lift off' can occur with too flat a fit or excessive eccentricity in back surve design. This can also occur several minutes after insertion due to drying problems and tear deficiency.

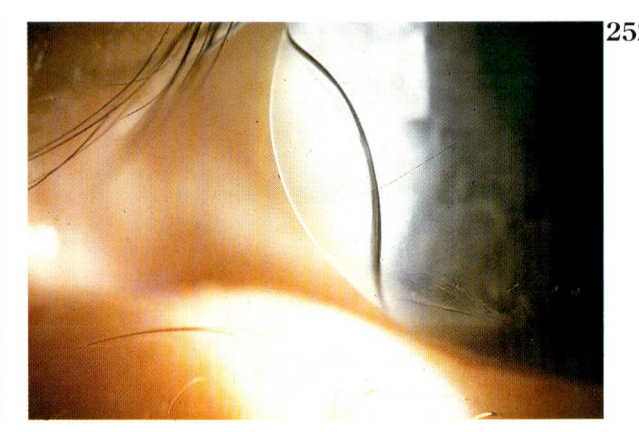

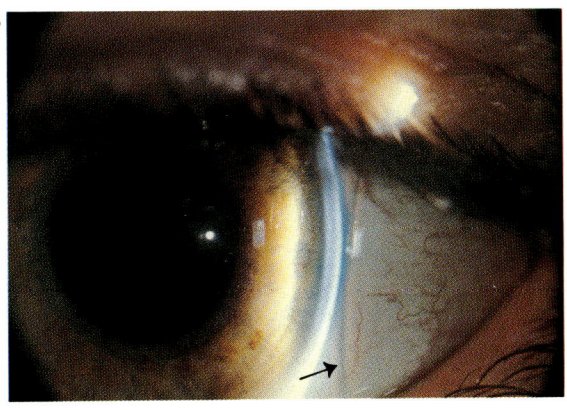

253 & 254 Extended wear lens (water content 80%). The patient dislodges the lens from the cornea at night. In **254** the arrow shows stromal oedema.

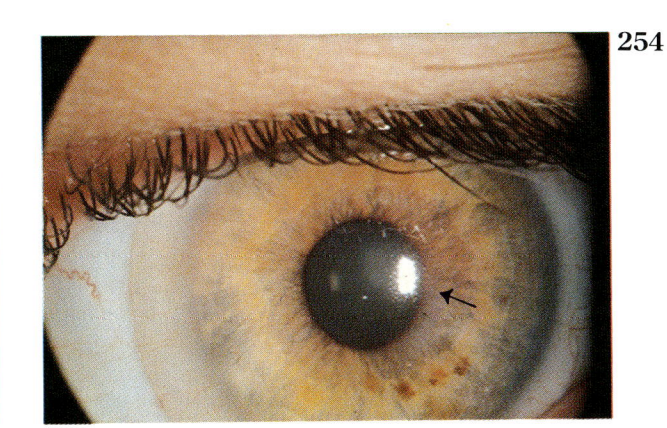

255 A soft lens, smaller than the cornea, made of silicone rubber. The rigidity of the material is greater than that of hydrophilic gel and this permits centration.

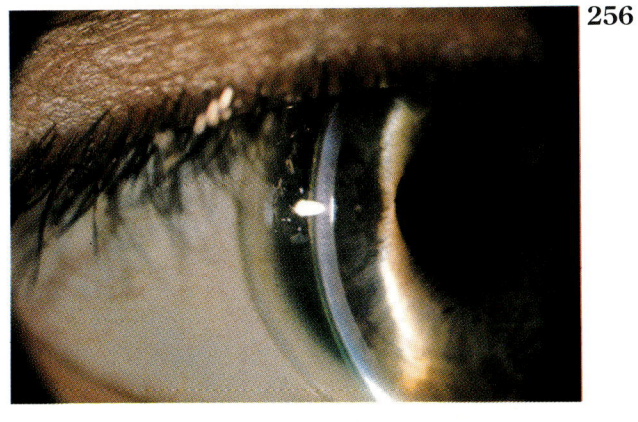

256 Well-centred gel lens. With the slit beam the intermediate area of the lens, as compared with the cornea, is less than a quarter of the corneal thickness (about 0.12 mm).

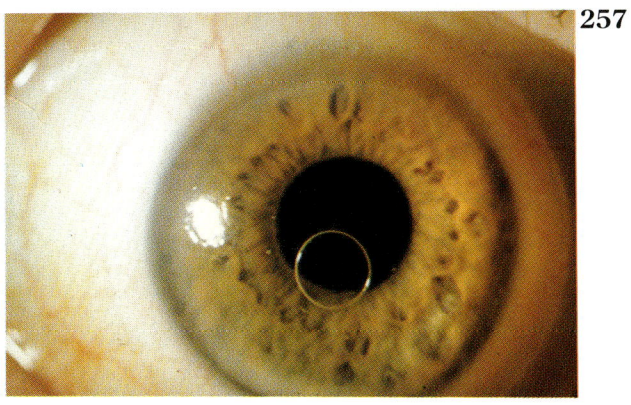

257 Steep fitting gel lens with a trapped bubble of air.

91

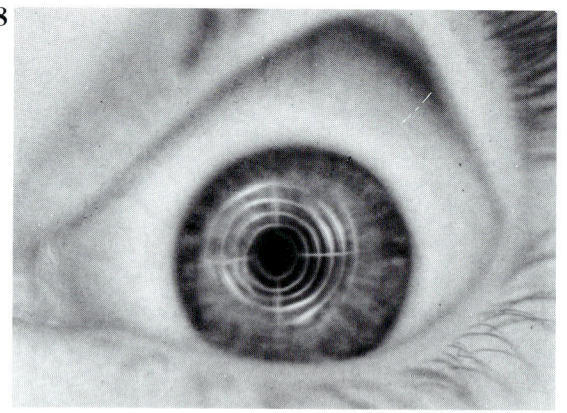

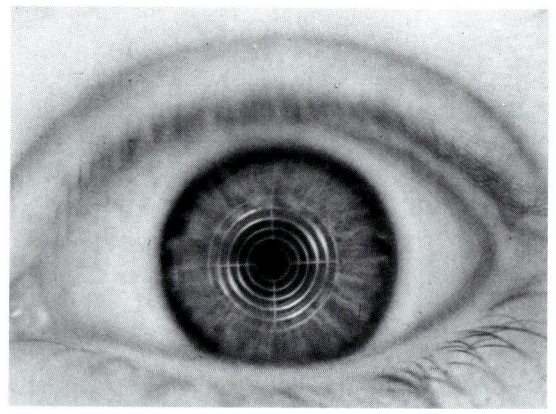

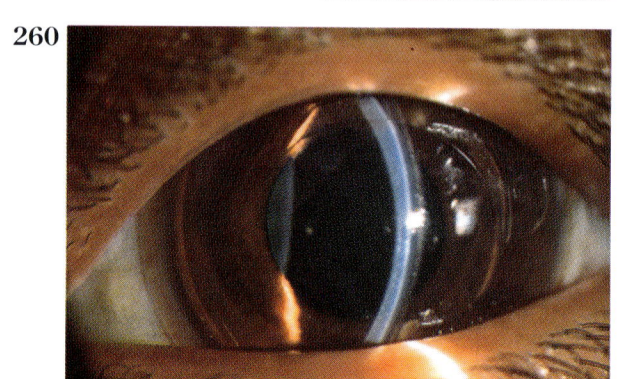

258 Over-lens surface keratometry. Readings can be of value to assess the optical quality of the lens, surface and tear film integrity (the time it takes for the tear film to break up) and also the fit; they are useful to diagnose residual astigmatism. This photokeratogram was of a steep fit.

259 Good PEK photokeratogram over the lens surface.

260 High powered plus lens. The centre of the lens is almost as thick as the cornea.

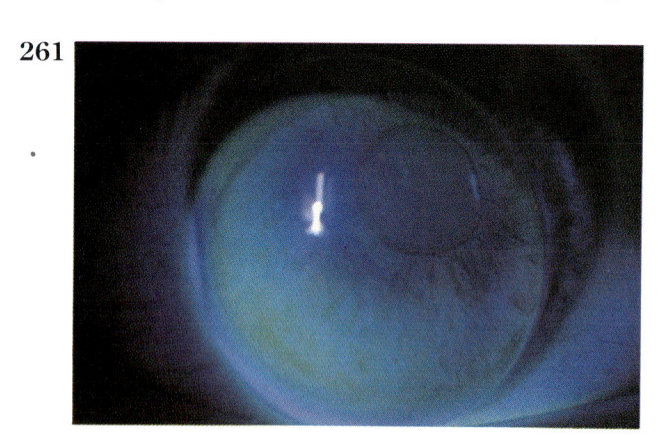

261 & 262 The fit of silicone rubber lenses can be assessed by use of fluorescein since they are soft but nonhydrophilic. The periphery of the lens must be open and excessive movement reduced. Sizes up to 12.5 mm in diameter are available.

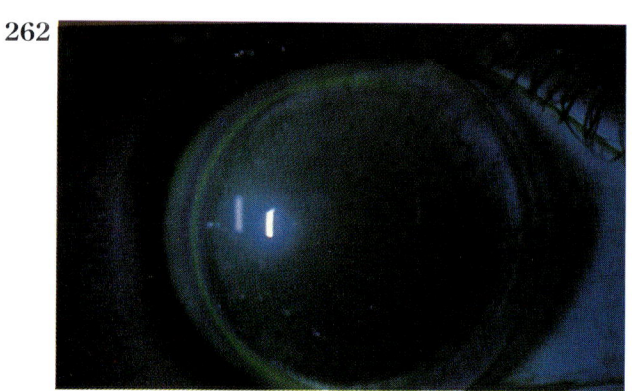

Toric soft lenses

For the toric rigid lens the problems were the induced and the residual astigmatism. However, the spherical back surface had the ability to eliminate most of the corneal astigmatism.

But since the front and back of the soft lens moulds to the corneal astigmatism only toric lens forms are able to correct the astigmatism.

Therefore, to keep in the vision axis all toric soft lenses must be fitted with stabilizing factors, e.g. ovals (elliptical shapes), prism ballast, reduced optics and negative carriers or aspheric back surfaces with front torics (see Table 10).

Table 10. Toric soft lenses.	
Types	Front toric or Back toric — Full aperture or reduced optic powered surface
Stabilizers	Toric back surface Conoid aspheric back surface Truncations Peripheral negative toric forms - reduced optics Prism ballast Ellipsoid (oval) shapes

One or more combinations of the above is required depending upon the position of the lower lid in relation to the limbus. In principle maximal stabilization is required for high lower lid positions. Prism ballast is not always necessary with the truncation of ellipsoid shapes.

263 High and low truncations, depending upon the position of the lower lid.

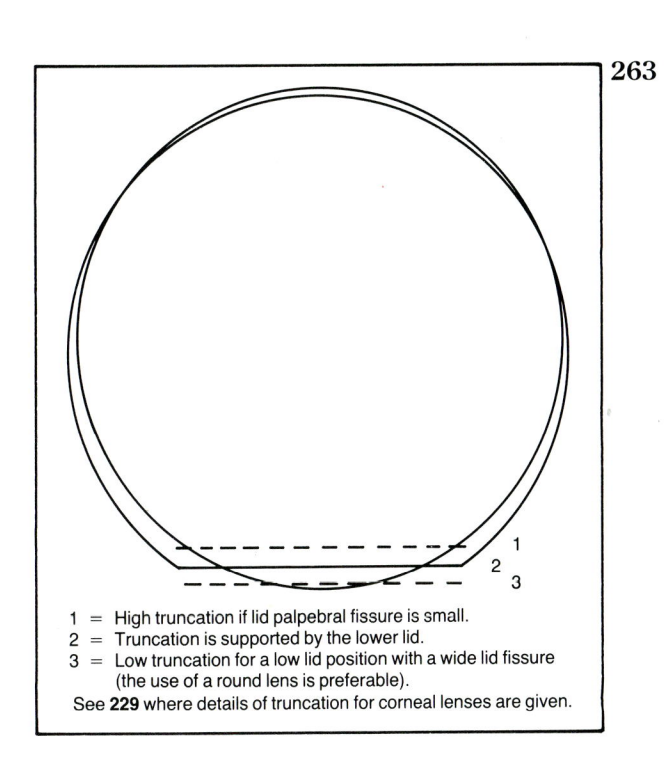

1 = High truncation if lid palpebral fissure is small.
2 = Truncation is supported by the lower lid.
3 = Low truncation for a low lid position with a wide lid fissure (the use of a round lens is preferable).
See **229** where details of truncation for corneal lenses are given.

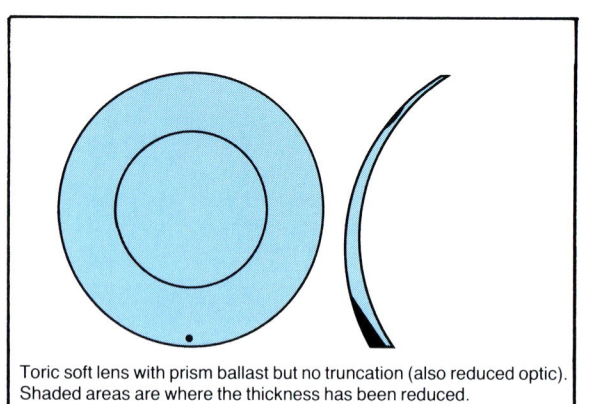

264 **Prism ballast** with *no* truncation but with reduction to the thickness inferiorly. Note also reduction of the intermediate thickness (superiorly). (Compare with **237** for hard corneal lenses.)

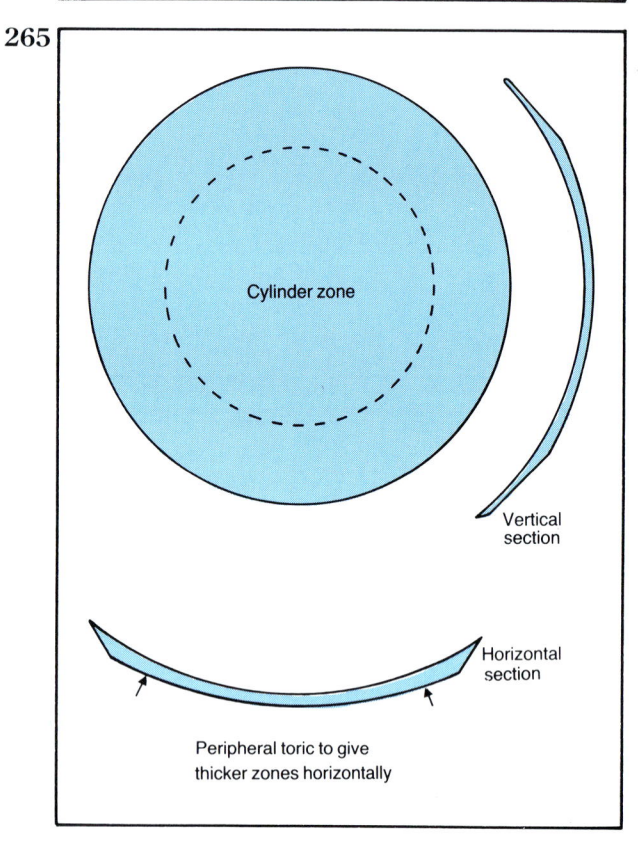

Toric soft lens with prism ballast but no truncation (also reduced optic). Shaded areas are where the thickness has been reduced.

265 **Reduced optic cylinder** in a lens with an increased horizontal thickness (toric negative carrier).

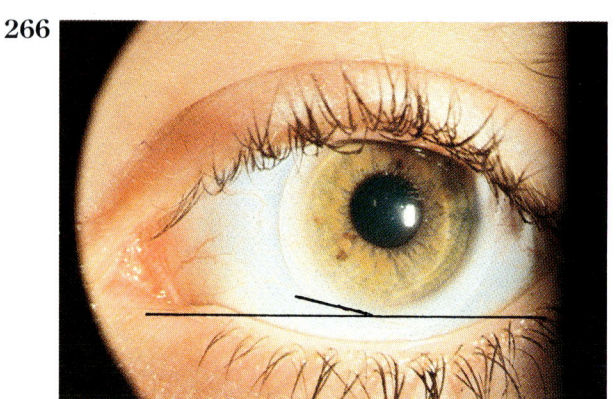

Cylinder zone

Vertical section

Horizontal section

Peripheral toric to give thicker zones horizontally

266 & 267 **Soft toric lenses** showing the angle of mislocation on the eye.

267

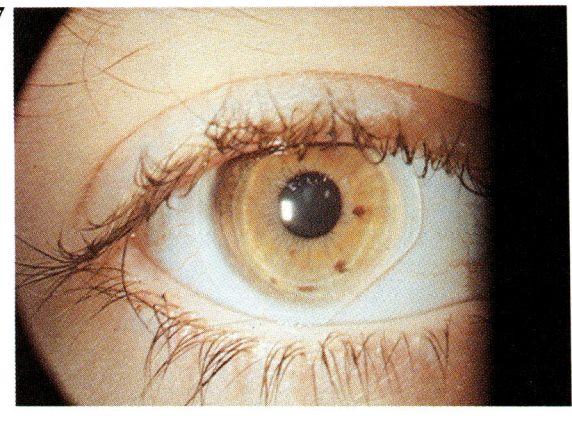

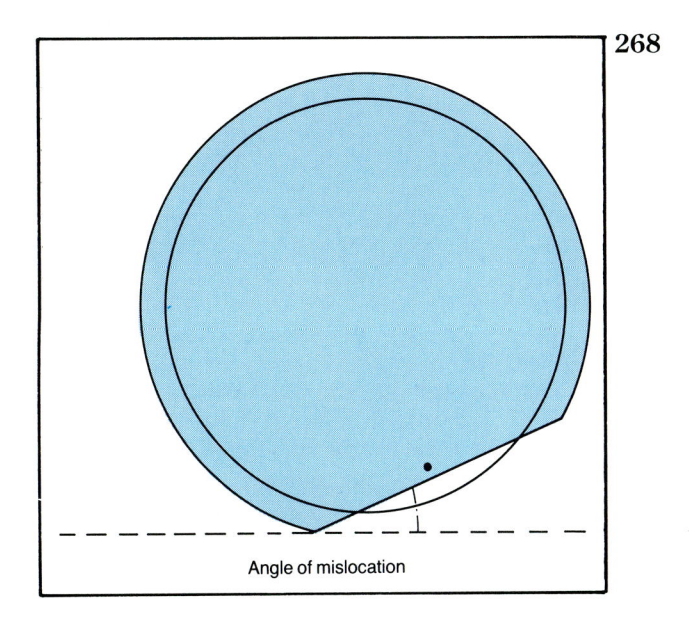

268 Diagram illustrating 267.

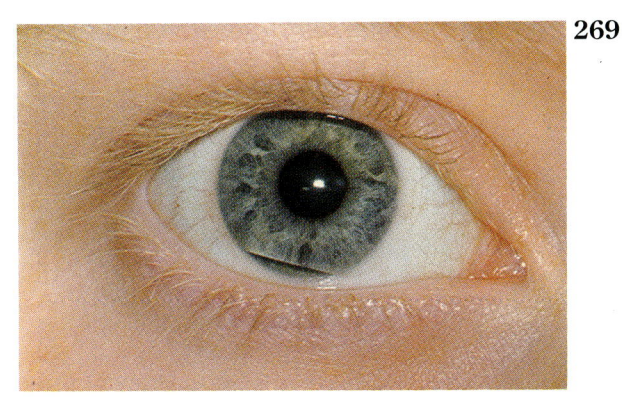

Angle of mislocation

269

269 Truncation is too high and is not advised for the size of lens and position of the lower lid.

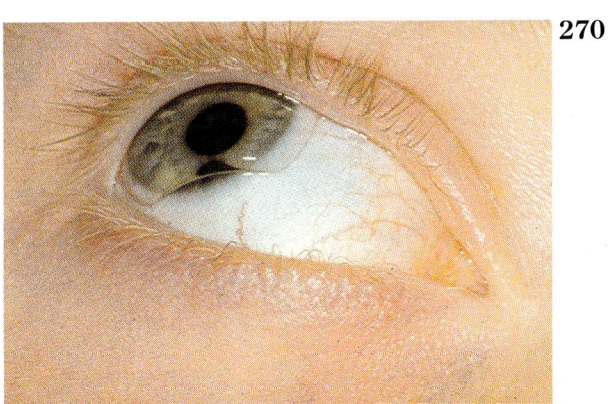

270

270 Good centration even on the versions of the eye and therefore there is good acuity.

Fitting of a soft toric contact lens

a. The manufacturer must give full specifications including the lens thickness and tolerances, so that an accurate substitute can be made and for accurate power control.
b. All lenses are to have their axes marked.
c. Fit a trial equivalent spherical or aspheric lens (supplied by the manufacturer) with the ballast or stability shape to be used for the final lens.
d. When on the eye note the location of the axes of the trial lens.
e. Find the over-refraction of the lens to give best acuity and add a half dioptre to astigmatism (an addition is required for residual astigmatism). Note the back vertex distance.
f. Measure the final lens in a focimeter and relate it to the ordered Rx.
g. Place and allow the lens to settle on the eye.
h. Note degrees of mislocation and non-centring (only 5° or more is significant).
i. Find acuity and over-refraction to give better acuity. (If h. and i. are significant, return the lens to the manufacturer for refit.)
j. Over-lens keratometry readings are of some value if the lens is well centred. Front surface astigmatism of more than 1 dioptre is of significance. N.B. The RI of the lens is *not* that of the cornea, therefore keratometry readings do not correspond to the power of the lens.

Scleral (haptic) lens fitting

These lenses require special technical assistance when fitting and are chiefly used in abnormal eyes. The basic manufacturing method has been described (see Chapter 3).

Making the plaster model of the eye

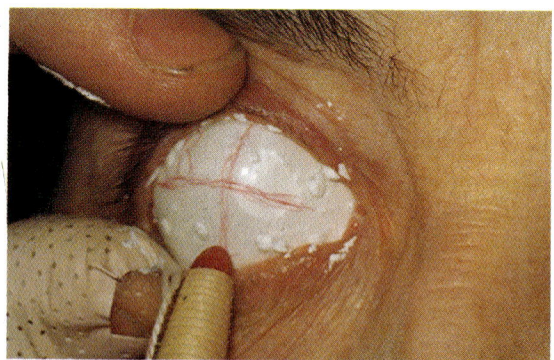

271 & 272 Making the plaster model and plastic shell. The injection tray or shell used for taking the eye impression is inserted onto the eye. The alginate mix is injected or in the case of the shell placed in the shell prior to insertion. (The eye must be anaesthetized with a local anaesthetic drop.) Note that the tray is marked with a wax pencil after the gel has set (**271**) to give correct orientation of the impression. The injection tray is already engraved with vertical and horizontal lines (**272**).

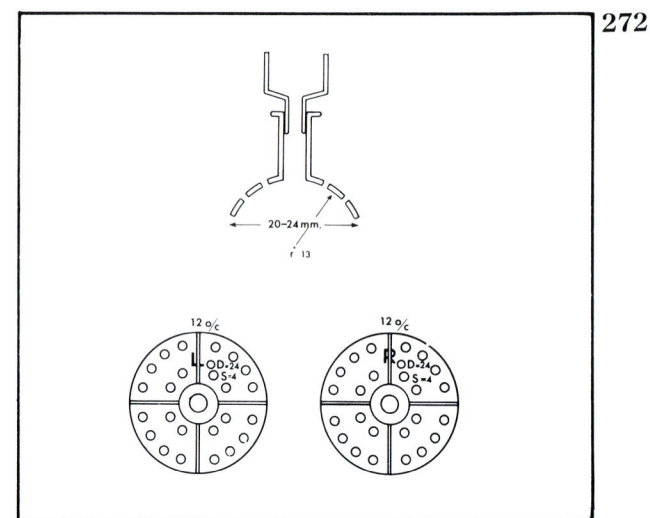

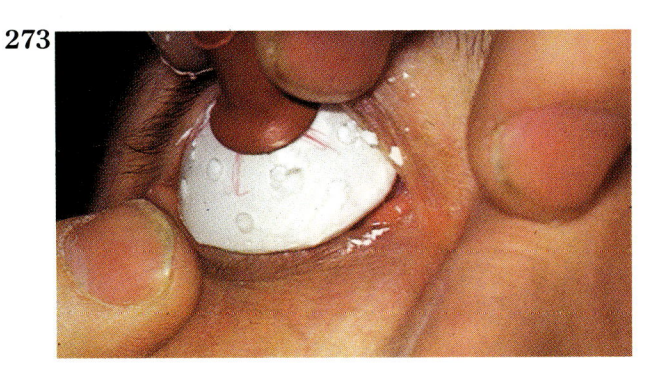

273 The impression and tray are removed. The surface tension is broken by tilting the tray with a large sucker.

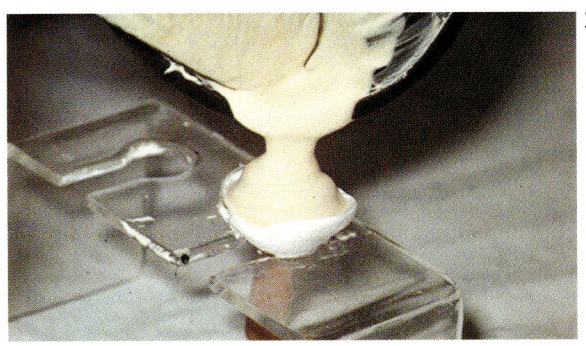

274 & 275 The gypsum (plaster) mix is poured into the alginate impression and allowed to set (**274**). The model of the eye is now separated from the impression (**275**).

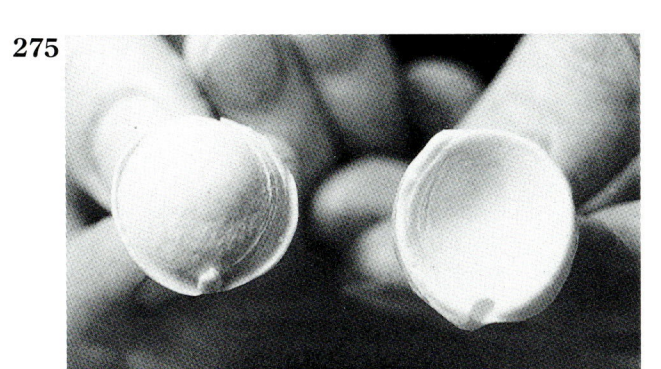

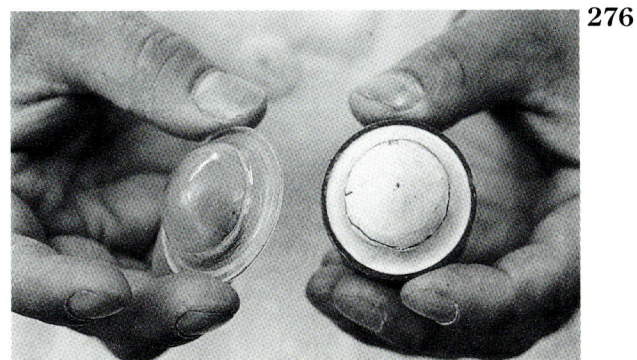

276 The heated plastic (PMMA or other thermolabile plastic) is pressure moulded to the model of the eye and then separated. (Details on the preparation of the shell are to be found in Chapter 3.)

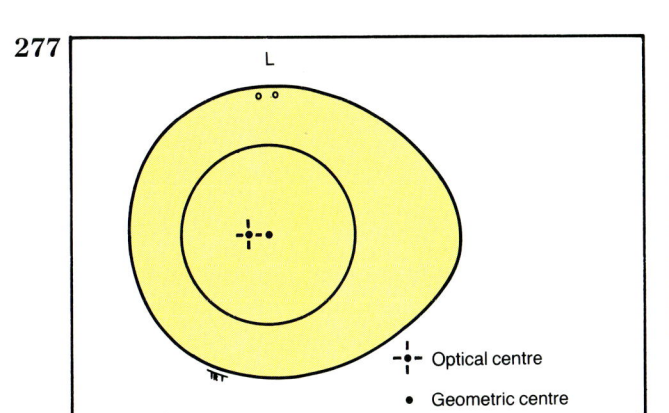

277 Marking the shell. The shell is placed on the eye and the geometric and optical centres are marked. Modifications to the shape are also marked.

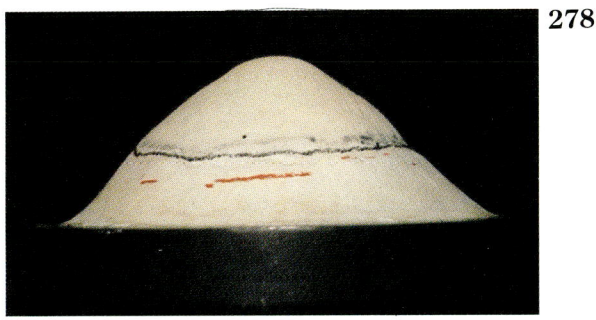

278 If another shell has to be made these markings are noted on the plaster model.

97

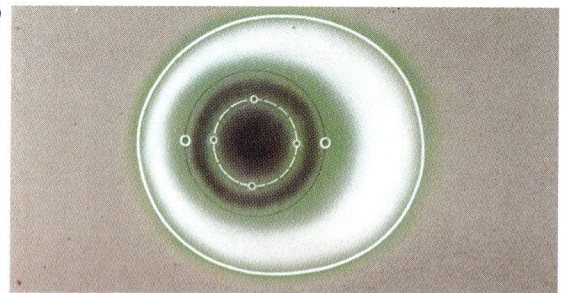

279 Fluorescein clearances. Diagrammatic outline of the desired fluorescein clearances. Note the minimal central clearance. (Intermediate corneal clearance will occur in keratoconus and in graft eyes.) A wide and deep limbal transition area clearance is essential.

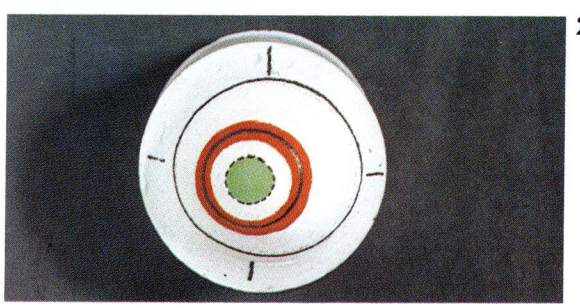

280 Transfer of information. The fluorescein clearance information can be transferred to the model and the manufacturer asked for specific clearances in the preparation of the lens or shell fitting.

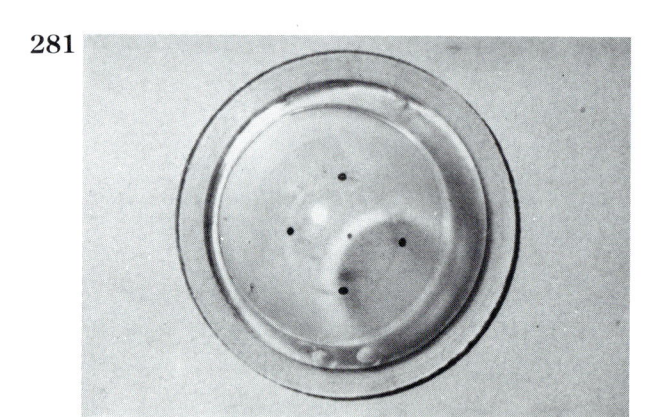

281 Marking of a shell for the optical centre before the lathing of the front and back surface. In this case the lens is a repeat of an existing lens already fitted.

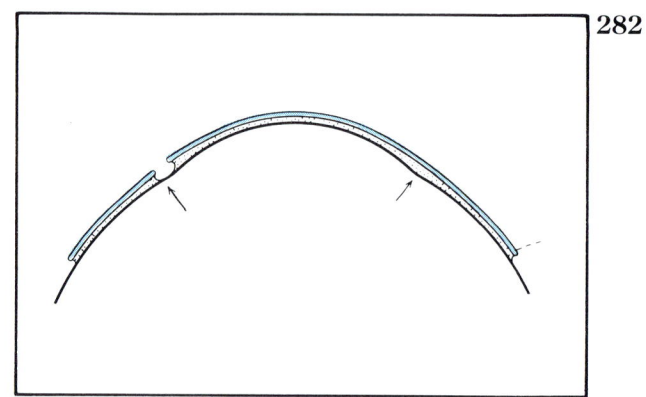

282 Clearance areas in section. How the clearance areas should look in section. Note the limbal clearance and the position of the fenestration. The fitter has to remove material from the haptic portion of the lens to settle it back and to give the required clearances.

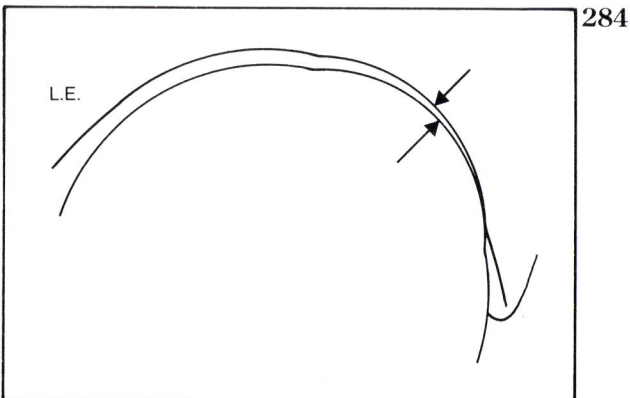

283 & 284 Scleral lens on the eye in the primary position (**283**) and with eye movement the lens will tilt and thus increase the clearance over the contralateral limbal zone (**284**).

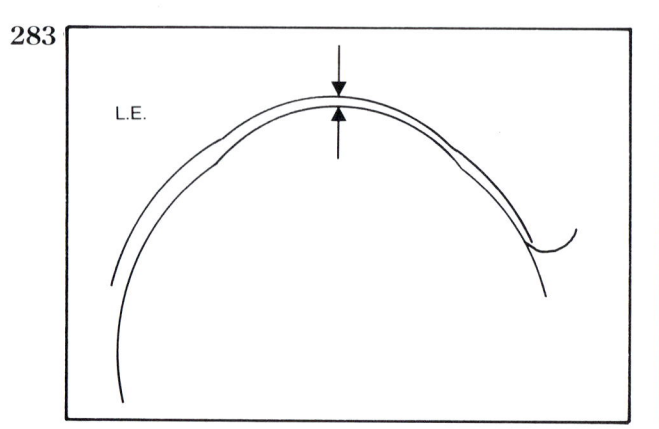

98

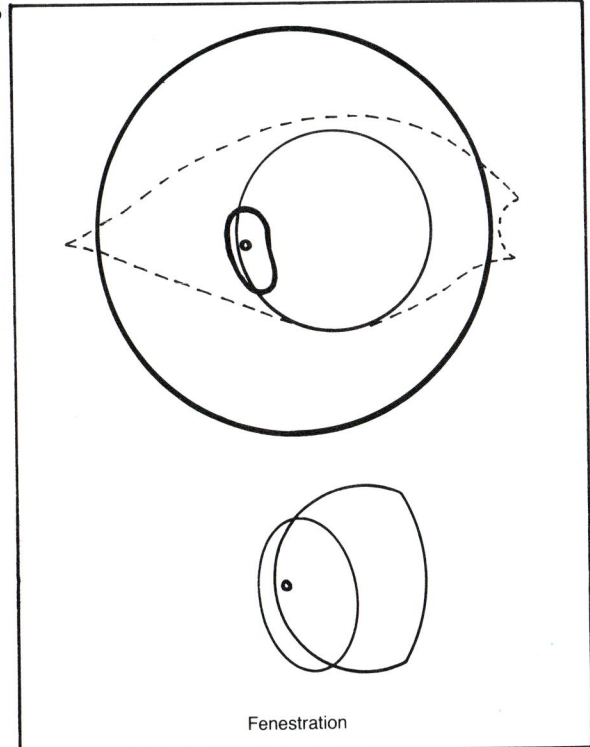

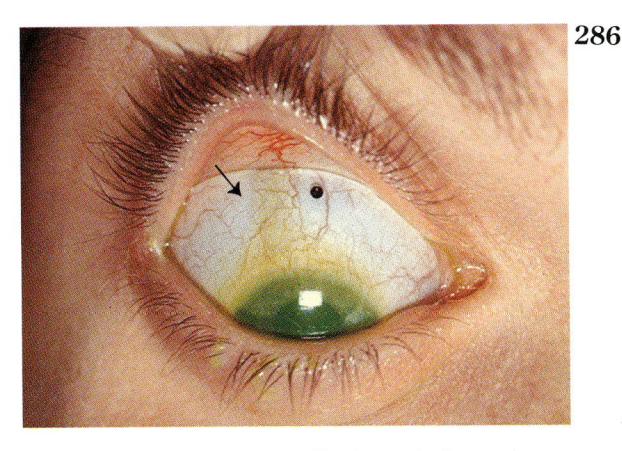

286 **A grooved channel** will alternatively permit tear fluid exchange.

285 **The fenestrated** area will thus draw in a larger bubble of air and provide ventilation.

Preformed geometric scleral lenses

The manufacture of such lenses from hard and soft materials is briefly described in Chapter 3.

287 **A large fenestrated scleral PHEMA** (38% water) lens.

   Horizontal diameter = 25 mm
   Vertical diameter = 23 mm

Electrodiagnostic scleral lens

288 An electrodiagnostic lens with the electrical lead below. Other forms are: Gonioscope lenses and fundus viewing lenses (soft lenses or large hard corneal high minus or high plus lenses are useful for this purpose, specially if the fundus is viewed at the slit-lamp).

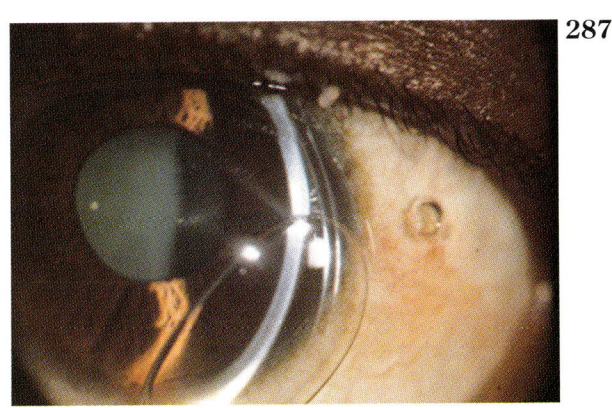

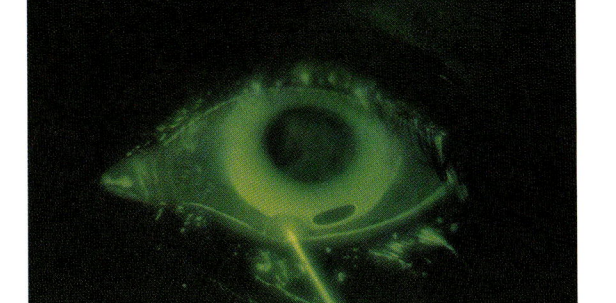

Writing of prescriptions

289

ORDER FORM		Laboratory name		Date:	
Patient's name/No				New Replace	
R Lens type			L Lens type		
Material	Tint		Material	Tint	
Back surface			Back surface		
Front surface			Front surface		
B.V.P.	T_e T_c T_j		B.V.P.	T_e T_c T_j	
Additional comments/instructions					

Notes to figure 289

Specifications of back surface	Back surface fitting curves; one or more curves or continuous (aspheric) curves.
Front surface as determined by optical power	Front surface of one or more curves, the central having a determining optical function.
	Reduced front optic when necessary to produce tolerable thicknesses.
	Central thickness (T_c) and other thickness where specified. For small diameter lenses specify T_c in minus powers
Additional features	Fenestrations. Channels. Slots.
Material	Hard or soft (chemical type) and coated surfaces where applicable.
Solutions used with lens	As specified by manufacturer.
Methods of cleaning and disinfection	As specified by manufacturer.
Tints and colours	Homogeneous tints (transparent). Opaque tints, paintings, or photographic laminates.

289 The contact lens is often ordered over the telephone but a record should be kept separately in the notes. Data can be stored on a program fed into a computer and then immediate information can be obtained on a printout or on the monitor. The upper layout is suitable for a lens order form whilst the lower table details the information likely to be required.

Computer programs

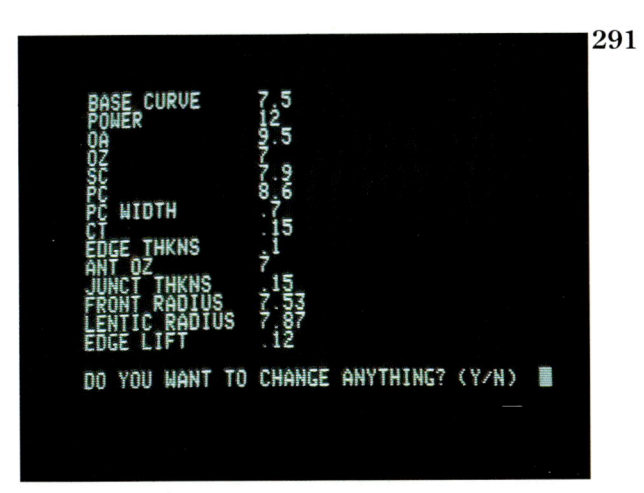

290-294 Computer program can be used for teaching, for manufacture, or to assist in the calculation of contact lens prescriptions. In its simplest form the Rx of any machine-made contact lens must follow geometric formulations and, given essential data, the unknowns can be found using algebra. Furthermore, knowing the optimums for material properties and clinical requirements the data can be controlled so that impossible formulations do not materialize. Finally, the lens form can be shown (**294**). The examples given were worked out from a teaching program by Roger Bolz. They are of course only a small part of the question and answer display that this type of program generates. The screen information shown are not necessarily related and are given as isolated examples. (Computer graphics of lens design are shown in Chapter 2).

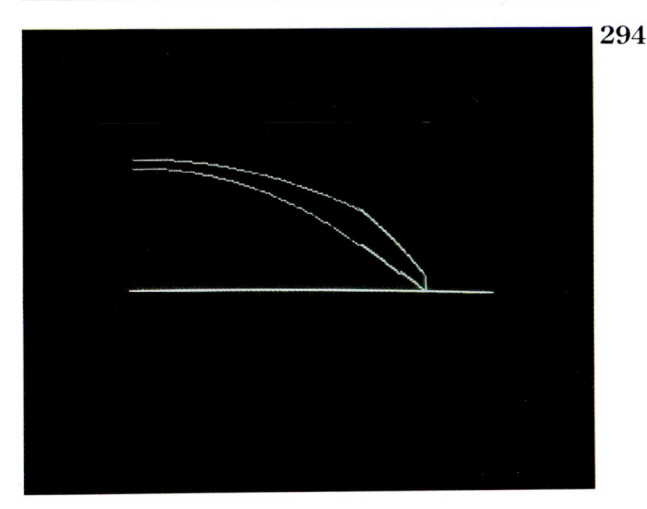

7 Fitting lenses for the abnormal eye

This section includes all those conditions where contact lenses can be considered as part of a treatment and therefore are *not* cosmetic/visual, though in addition, in many conditions contact lenses can be used to gain also a cosmetic or prosthetic effect. This Chapter is concerned primarily with obtaining a therapeutic result and in this respect obtaining better vision or correcting motility problems can be considered therapeutic.

The introduction of practical contact lens fitting commenced in the mid-nineteenth century, when they were used for therapeutic purposes. In the majority of examples that follow it must be realized that the contact lens is part of the treatment, which can be both surgical and medical, systemic and local. Therefore, the contact lens practitioner must work closely with the ophthalmologist and not in isolation.

Indications for fitting

The following group of conditions is not exhaustive—if the lens is considered as just one more tool in a large armamentarium, then other conditions will fall within this context:

- Optical:

    High degrees of ametropia, myopia, hyperopia, astigmatism
    Irregular astigmatism caused by corneal disease
    Binocular vision problems and occlusive therapy
    Subnormal vision
    Photophobia, e.g. albinism, aniridia

- Keratopathies
- Keratodystrophies
- Refractive corneal surgery
- Dry eye, exposure keratitis, symblepharon
- Anterior chamber reformation
- Ocular myopathies

Myopia

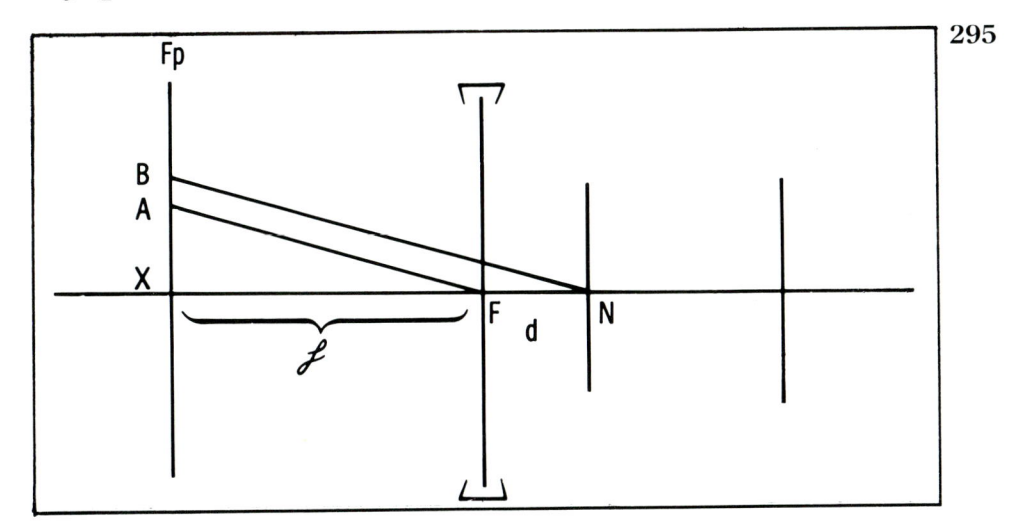

295 High axial myopia. The elongated eye usually has a flatter than normal keratometry and the accommodative power is weak. Therefore, contact lens full correction will require reading spectacles.

The diagram illustrates differences in retinal image size of spectacles (AX) and the contact lens (BX). The magnification is BX/AX = f + d/f = M.

In high axial myopia the magnification by a contact lens as compared to a sepctacle lens can be as high as 20 per cent which is useful if some degree of maculopathy co-exists.

Example: Spectacle lens = −15.0d (f = 66.66 mm)
Spectacle lens distance = 15 mm (D)
Therefore M = 8.17/6.66 = × 1.23 = 23%

296 Accommodation and the myopic correction. The spectacle wearer has the advantage of a base in prism when converging to a near object. A change to contact lenses reveals this need to converge more than with spectacles.

Furthermore, the spectacle lens is several millimetres from the eye and the effective power at the eye for a near object is less than when a contact lens is worn. Therefore, the contact lens wearer has to accommodate more. This state, when occurring in young people, is called pre-presbyopia. A slight under-correction, reading spectacles, convergence exercises or even mono-vision (see Chapter 6) will help. Fitting too flat appears to increase the pre-presbyopic problem and a stable apical clearance lens is preferred.

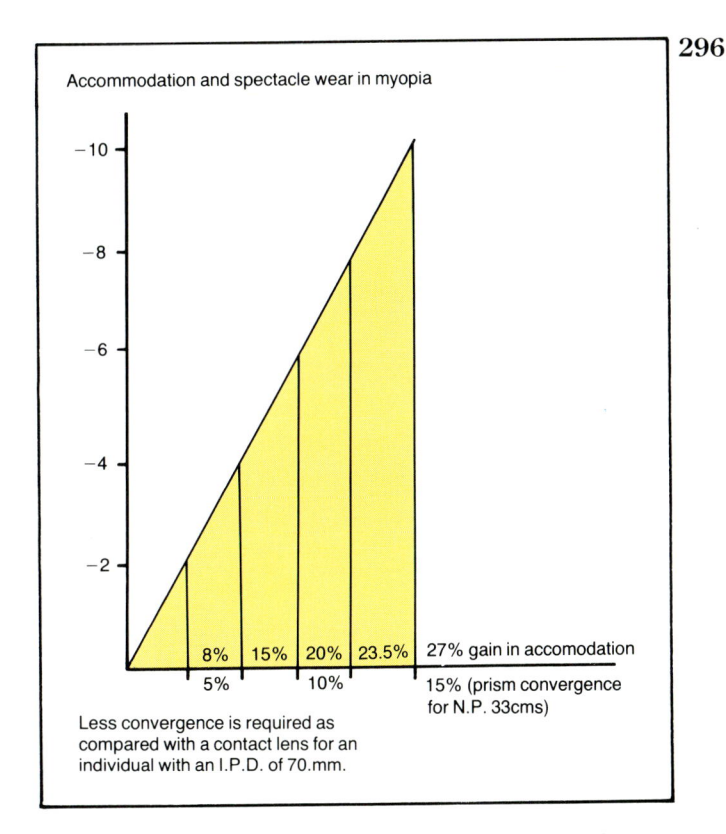

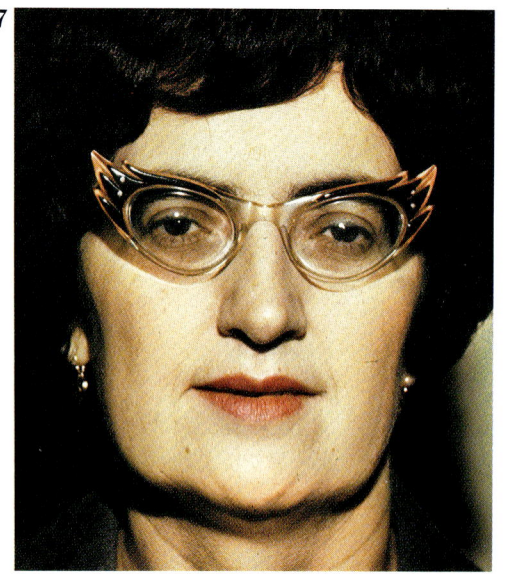

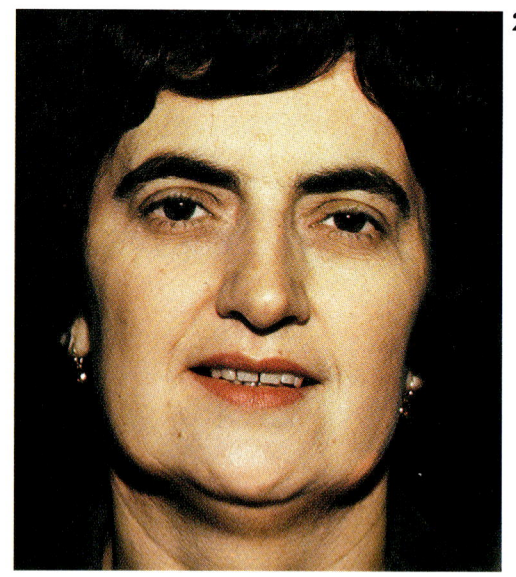

297 & 298   Axial myopia. Woman wearing spectacles and the same woman wearing hard corneal contact lenses.

R&L—19.0d. Spectacle Lens at BVD = 13 mm.
Fitted with corneal CLs—C$_3$ (tricurve back surface).
Back surface = 7.80:7.80/9.0:9.0/12.0:9.30.
T$_c$ = 0.08   T$_e$ = 0.13

Front surface = reduced front optic of 8 mm.
Material Dk = 50. The junctional thickness was 0.32 mm and therefore no lens warping occurred.

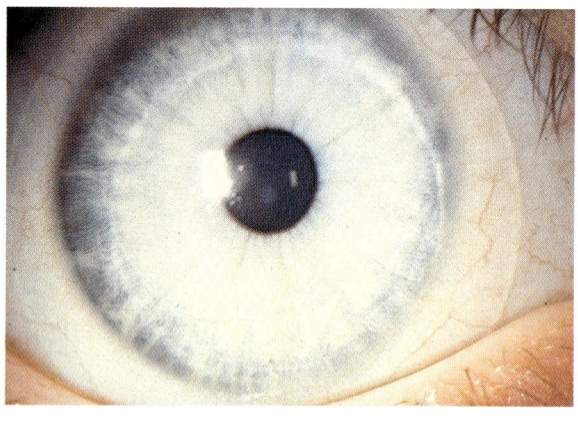

299 & 300   Congenital myopia. (Pierre Robin syndrome in the instance of **299**). In **299** the patient was fitted with high water content gel lenses at the age of four years, for extended wear periods. The patient in **300** was fitted with daily wear 38 per cent water lenses.

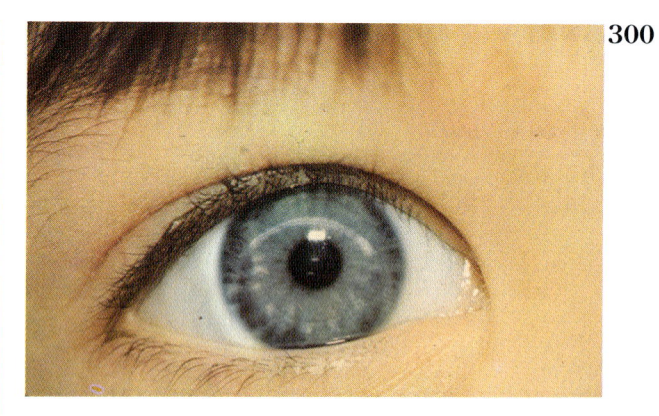

Rx: 8.30/13.0 − 9.0   T$_c$ = 0.10   T$_e$ = 0.12

Both types of congenital myopia can be refitted to gas permeable rigid when the child is old enough to manage the lens care himself.

Binocular vision indications

Some binocular vision indications for contact lens treatment:

- High powers—in instances where spectacle correction produces phorias or tropias.
- Partial and total occlusion therapy.
- Anisometropia and aniseikonia.
- Covergence and divergence excess where over power of refraction correction is required.

301 Anisometropia. The spectacle prism imbalance and the anisiekonia can break down binocular vision. The diagram illustrates one of several solutions to the problem: balanced power spectacles for both eyes with the high refractice error eye wearing the contact lens or with both eyes wearing the contact lens.

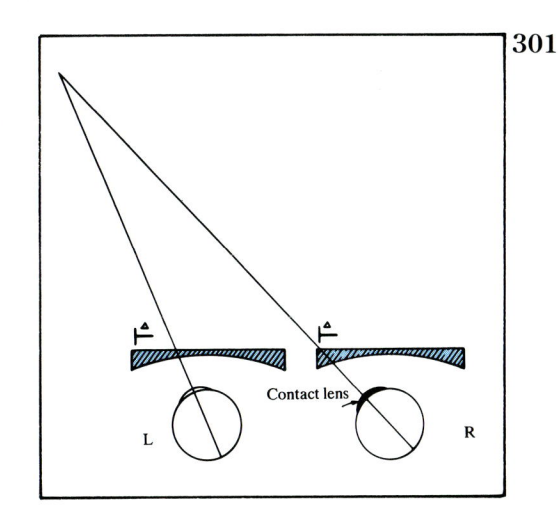

302 Heterophoria and tropias. The example shown is esophoria (with convergence excess), which is correctable by over-correction but, when used with spectacles, results in blurred distance vision. The contact lens over-correction (up to +2.0d) is used in one eye. The contact lens does not result in a prism imbalance whereas the spectacle lens does.

Conversely, in exophoria with myopia a unicular myopic over-correction can be used. A functional result can be studied by looking at the pupil for lack of miotic response on near fixation.

Unless a contact lens is stabilized (see Chapter 6) the use of prisms can only be in the vertical axis. Only up to 3 prism dioptre base up or down is possible.

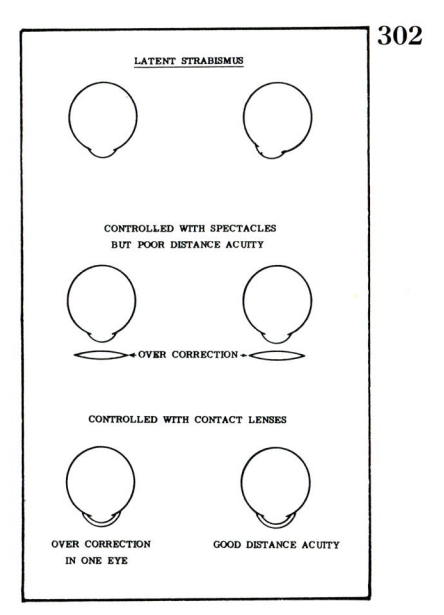

303 Hyperopia and alternating convergent strabismus.
With the spectacle correction − +12° convergence
Unaided = +22°.
With a unilateral lens, over-correct by + 1.5d.
Residual tropia = +7° which also gives a good cosmetic effect.

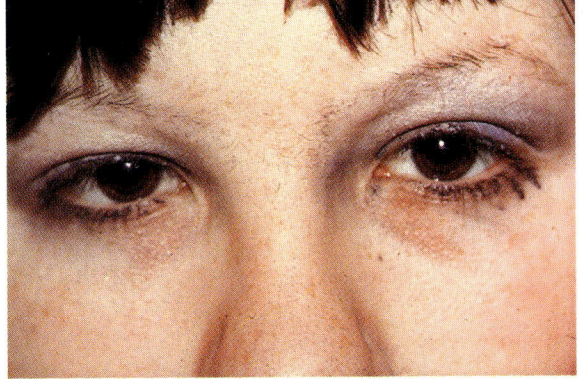

105

304 & 305 Hyperopia and alternating convergent strabismus in an 8 year-old child. Figure **304**—without correction. Figure **305**—with a soft gel lens of +5.0d (full correction).

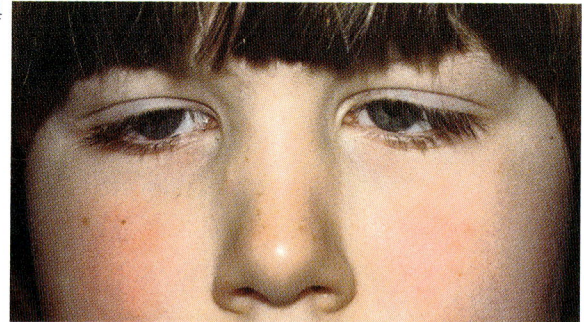

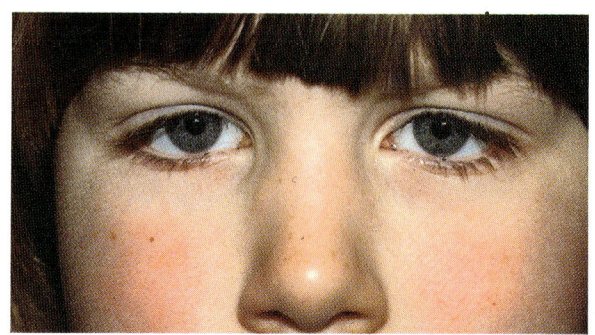

Occlusion therapy

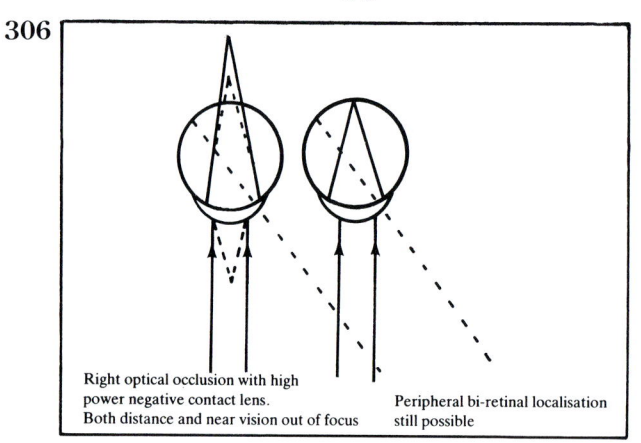

306 **The eye to be partially occluded** is fitted with a very high power plus or minus contact lens (± 15.0d).

Right optical occlusion with high power negative contact lens. Both distance and near vision out of focus

Peripheral bi-retinal localisation still possible

307 Paralytic strabismus and diplopia.

308 **Black pupil to occlude vision.** Same patient as in **307** but wearing an occlusive contact lens (left eye). The fit is poor—not centred—but it is effective.

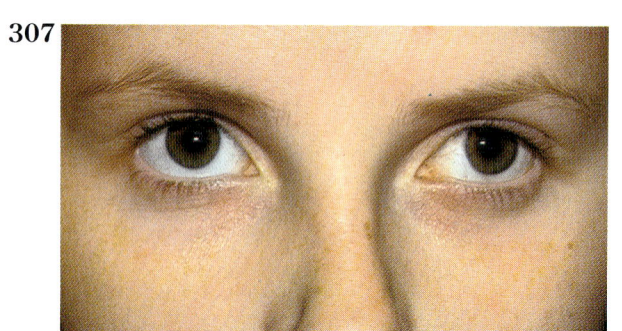

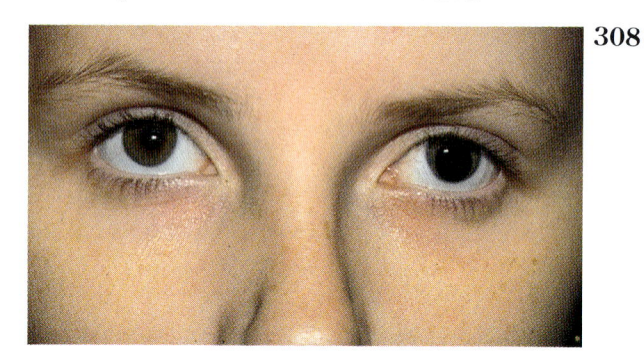

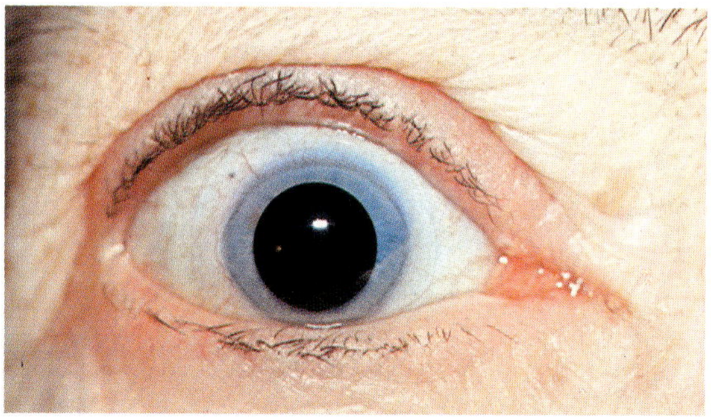

309 **Black pupil in a gel lens** to occlude vision in a patient with insuperable diplopia. The iris is coloured.

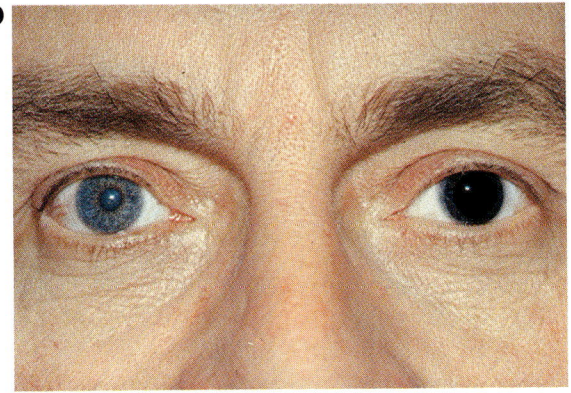

310 & 311 Opaque pupil in a gel lens to occlude vision in a patient with insuperable diplopia.

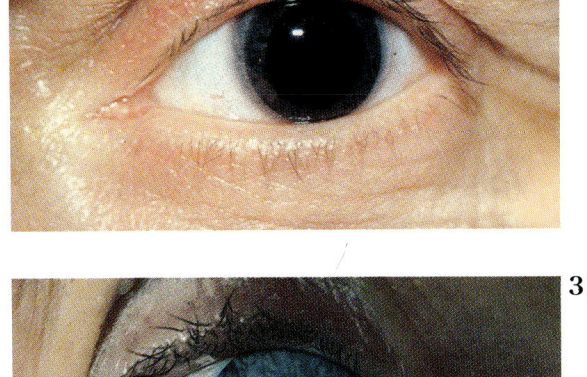

312 Black pupil to occlude vision in a patient with dyslexia of binocular vision aetiology. The iris is coloured and has a blue posterior to it (Weicon).
N.B. Poor gas flow through coloured opaque lenses can make the lenses unsuitable for prolonged periods of wear.

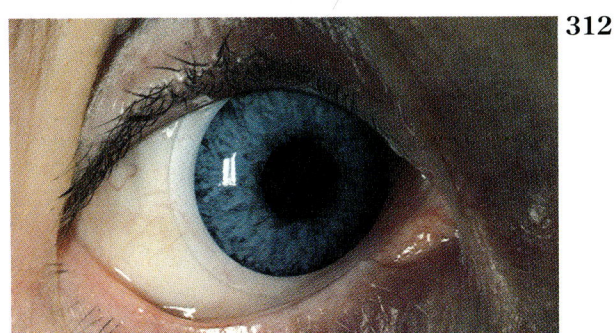

Anisometropia and aniseikonia

The contact lens tends to reduce differences in retinal image size as compared with spectacle correction. Aniseikonia is chiefly a problem when the anisometropia is induced, such as after surgical intervention or trauma to the eye.

313 Unilateral aphakia. Aphakia, when unilateral, is the commonest example of induced anisometropia. The problem is particularly important if the aetiology is a cataract that results from trauma. The retinal image size relative to the position of the correction is shown in the graph (Bennett) with a vertical spread for the pre-aphakic refractive state of the eye (i.e., hypertropia, emmetropia or myopia).

The graph indicates that a pre-operation emmetropic eye with a contact lens can still have a high degree of retinal image size increase (15 per cent) and even the intra-ocular implant if the eye were hyperopic a 10 per cent decrease in image size from the normal emmetropic state. While these figures are entirely theoretical they do relate to the problems that can occur in the use of the contact lens or implant to achieve binocular vision in the unilateral aphakic.

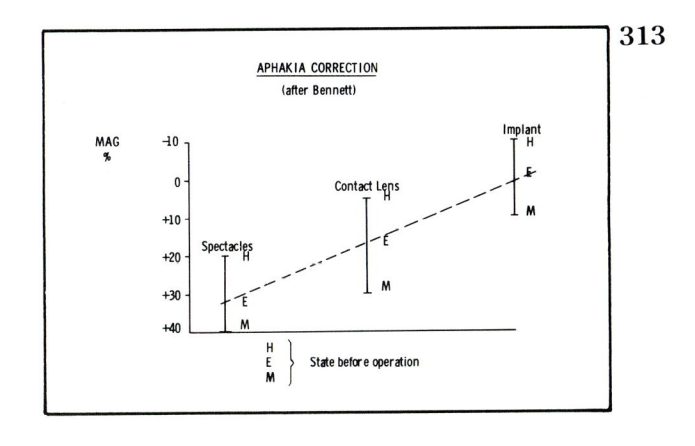

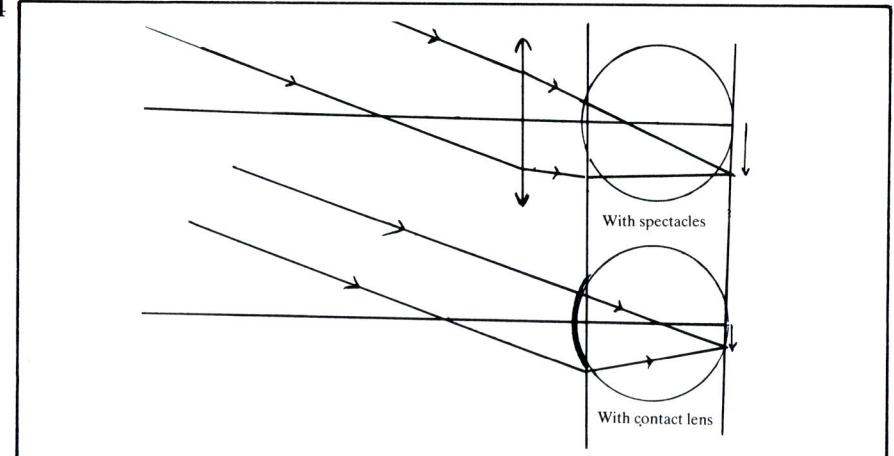

314 Spectacle and contact lens correction. The diagram shows the difference in image size between spectacle and contact lens correction (see **313**).

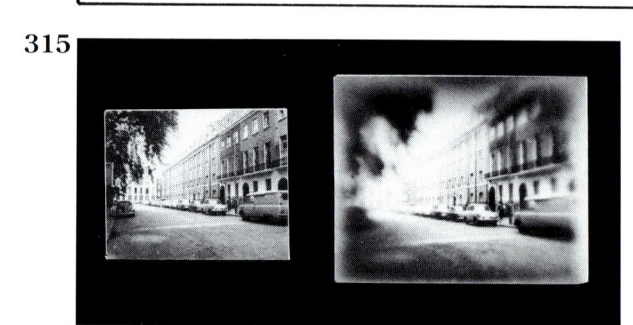

With spectacles

With contact lens

315 The simulation of aphakia and its correction will help the practitioner understand the image distortion and size problem.

A camera was made to have a short focal length equal to +15.0d aphakic state and the image was brought into focus with a spectacle lens. A picture was then taken and also another picture (that on the right) with the correcting lens in the form of a rigid contact lens placed on the lens of the camera.

The image size difference and the peripheral distortion are obvious.

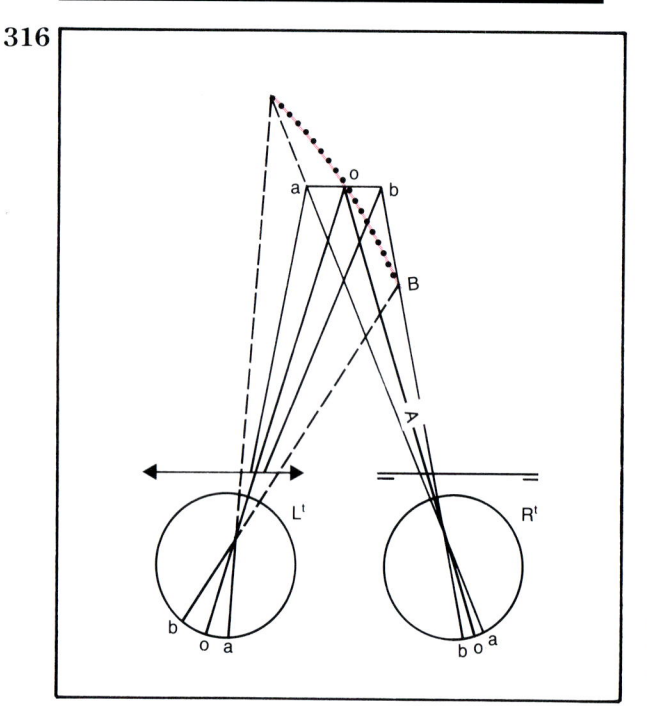

316 Basis of tilted image in aniseikonia. A state of anisometriopia corrected by spectacle lenses. The left eye has a larger image of 'boa' than the right eye. Corresponding retinal areas with similar spatial projection values are consequently not stimulated. In order to maintain binocular vision the compensation of spatial values results in the image appearing in the tilted plane AoB. If this compensation results then the perceptual processes can eventually compensate, reducing the tilt effect and avoiding disorientation. Too large an image difference leads to diplopia and either strabismus and/or suppression of one of the images.

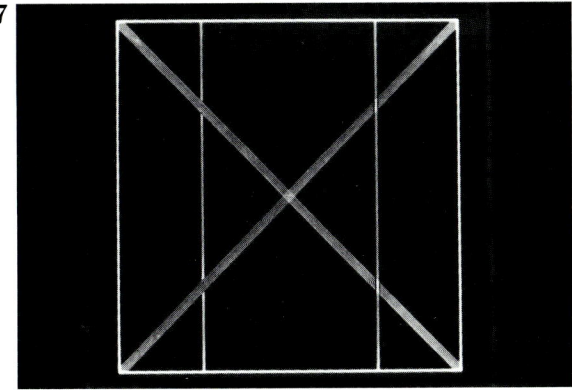

317-319 Measurement of aniseikonia. Using the haploscope or synoptophore and a set of targets based on the Ames-Ogle three-dimensional figure, together with a set of aniseikonic lenses, the aniseikonia can be measured. There are other similar methods e.g. using an aniseikonometer. The slides illustrated used forced duction to break fusion when doubling of the vertical lines occured on one side only. This can be corrected with the aniseikonic trial lenses.

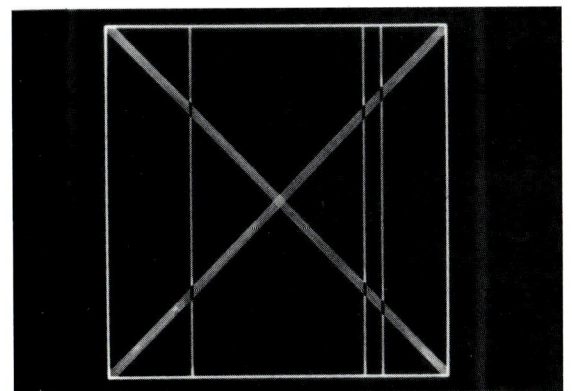

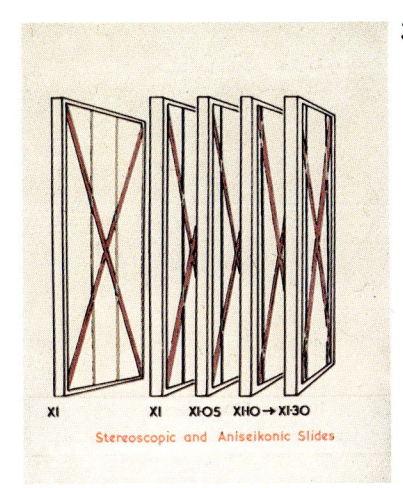

Congenital hyperopia

320 Hereditary form of hyperopia (small eye). Fitted with gel (38 per cent water) lens for daily wear. Rx: 8.60:9.00/9.00:13.0 Power + 18.00 Red. Front optic = 8.50.
$T_c = 0.60$ $T_e = 0.16$
N.B. Because of the high power and thickness this lens has a rigidity that can cause occlusion problems. Consequently a bicurve back surface was prescribed to give peripheral looseness. An aspheric back surface of shape factor +0.6 or less would also suffice (see Chapter 2). Such a lens made of an aspheric front surface design and of a high water content material would be preferable.

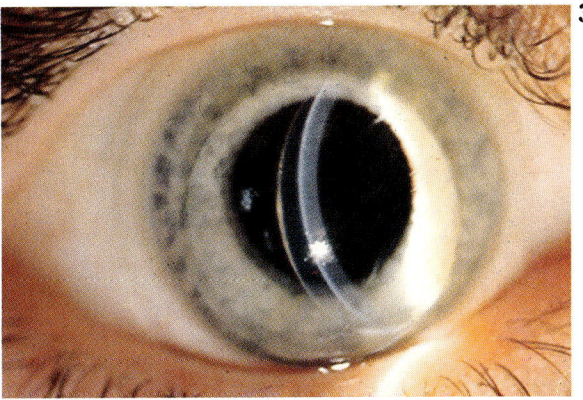

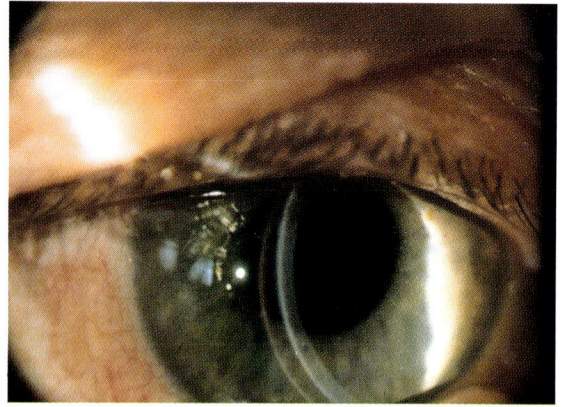

321 Adult hypermetrope wearing a 45 per cent water lens. This lens does not appear to have a reduced front optic and is excessively thick.

Regular and irregular astigmatism

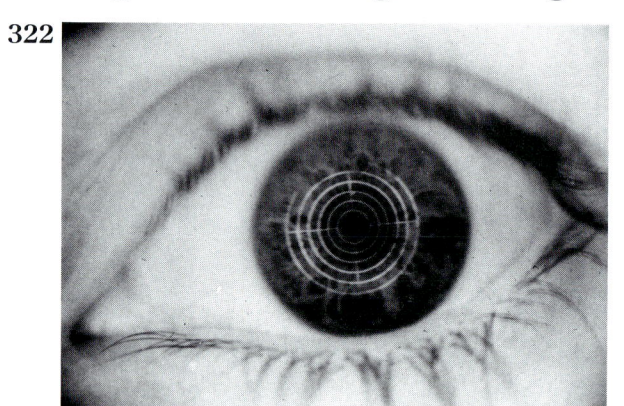

322 Photokeratoscopy of a normal cornea (physiological astigmatism with the rule −0.50d. cyl. 180°).

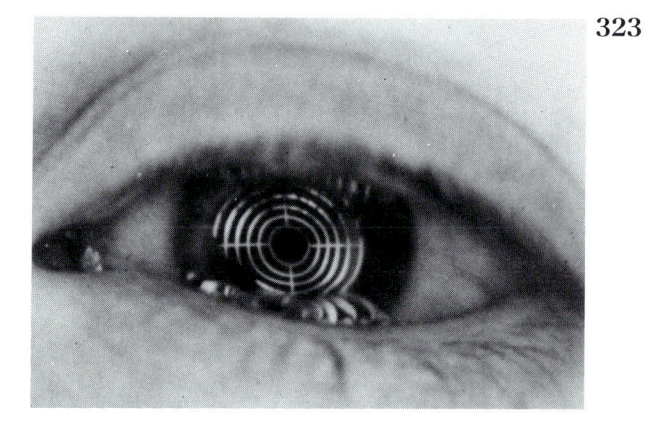

323 Regular astigmatism oblique (after keratoplasty) of 3 dioptres.
  K reading 7.9 at 150° 7.4.

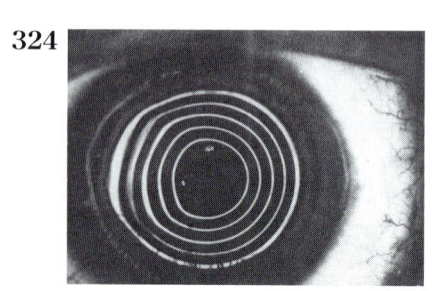

324 & 325 Irregular astigmatism as a result of the scarred healing of suppurative keratitis. Best acuity with a spectacle lens was 6/18 (20/60) which improved to 6/9 (20/30) with a hard contact lens.
  The other normal eye spectacle Rx was: −2.0s. −2.0 cyl. ax. 180°.

Subnormal vision aids

326 The partially sighted. There are now many sophisticated aids for the partially sighted. Even with video and TV equipment the enlargement of the retinal image without hand held magnifiers is worthwhile. The illustration shows the eye made hypermetropic by a contact lens and then corrected by use of a large plus lens (which can be a fresnel lens). The telescopic principle used here will only be effective if there is sufficient distance from the eye to the lens—at least 30 mm is required using extended bridge spectacles.

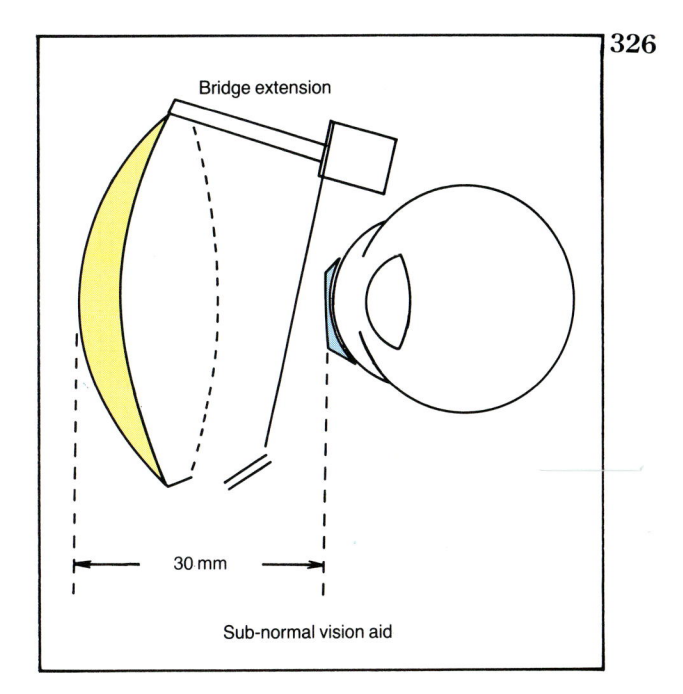

327 Illustration of the powers. Contact lens of −15d corrected by +10.5 spectacle lens at 30 mm.
$M = I/1 - dF$ and therefore $= \times 2$.

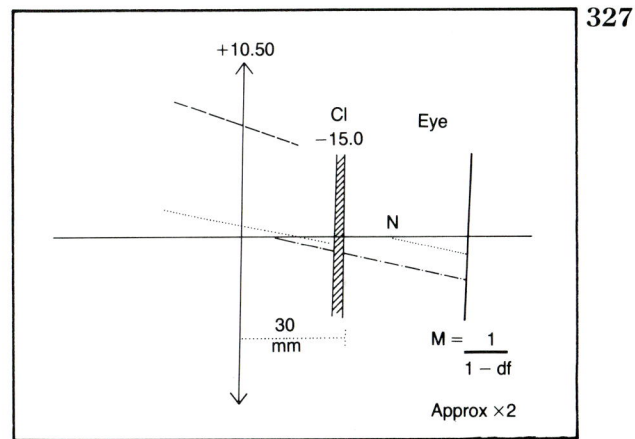

328 A further modification of this is to use a bifocal lens so that near vision is the primary concern in the correction.

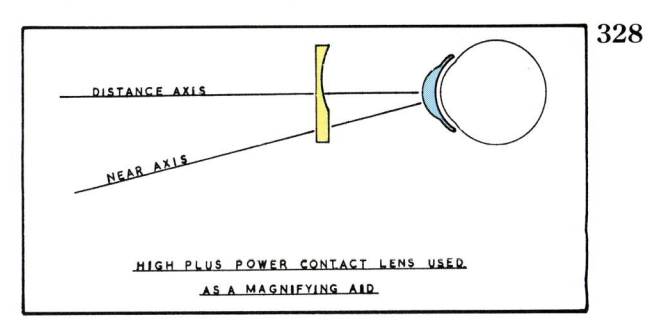

Albinism and aniridia

These conditions require cosmesis as well as light occlusion.

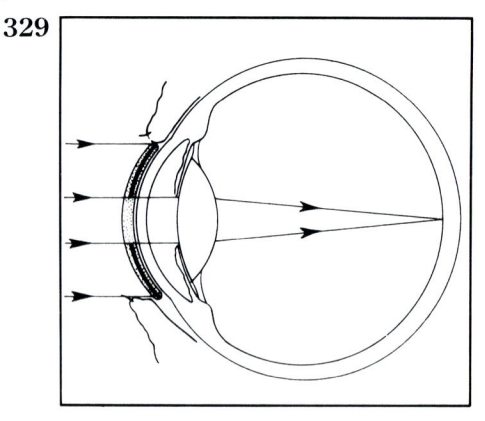

329 Large corneal lens with a clear pupil and an occlusive but coloured iris. The lens can be made in hard or soft materials.

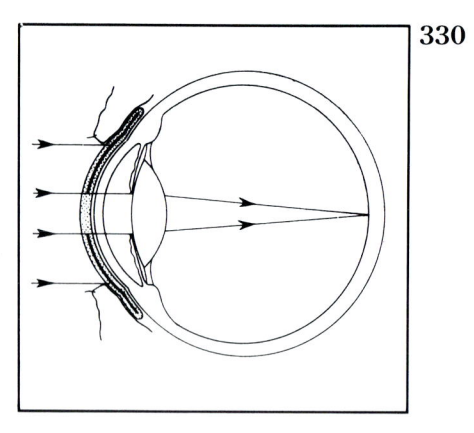

330 Scleral design to achieve the same effect as in **329** but giving a larger area of occlusion. It can be made in hard or soft materials, too.

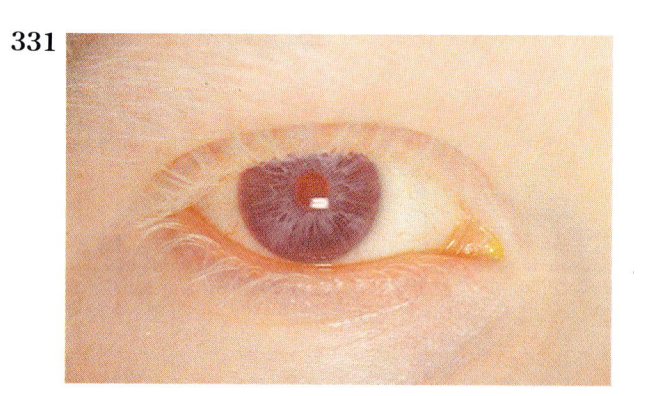

331 Albino eye.

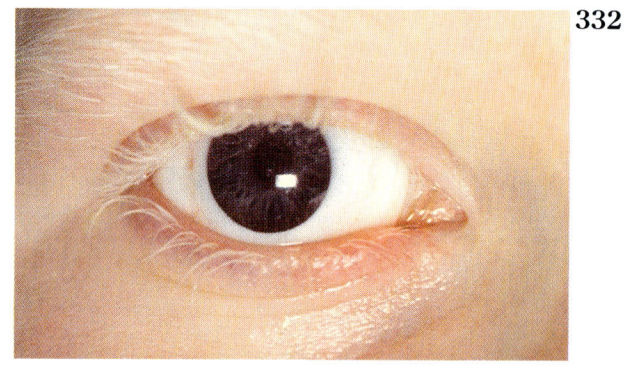

332 The same eye as **331** fitted with a large scleral painted occlusive lens. The pupil is clear.

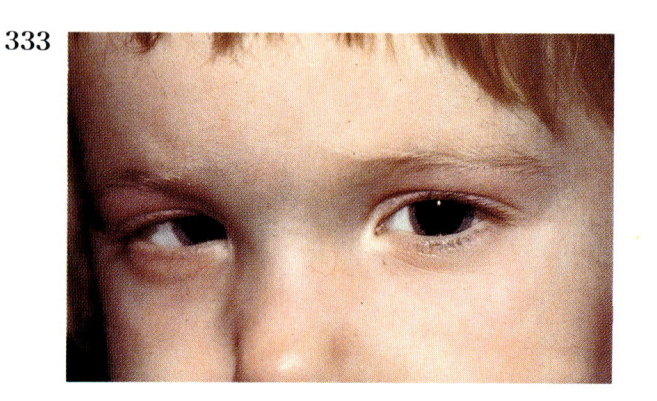

333 Aniridia of congenital aetiology.

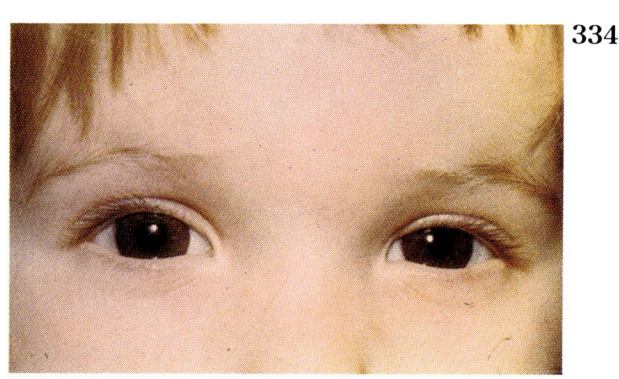

334 Iris gel lenses. The same patient wearing coloured iris gel lenses (Weicon).

112

335 Close-up of the lens fitting.

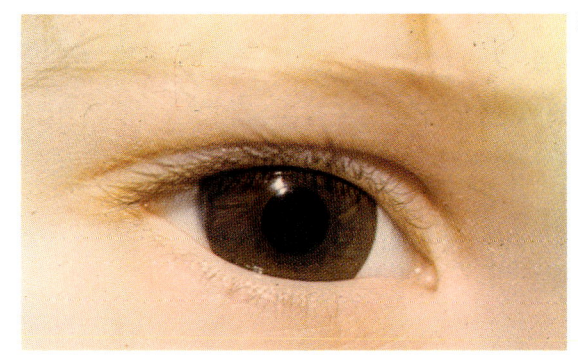

Nystagmus

Some practitioners report a decrease in nystagmus if large hard lenses are worn and especially if a high degree of ametropia is present—even plano power lenses have improved the acuity.

336 Scleral lens with a metal insert below to provide ballast and reduce the nystagmus.

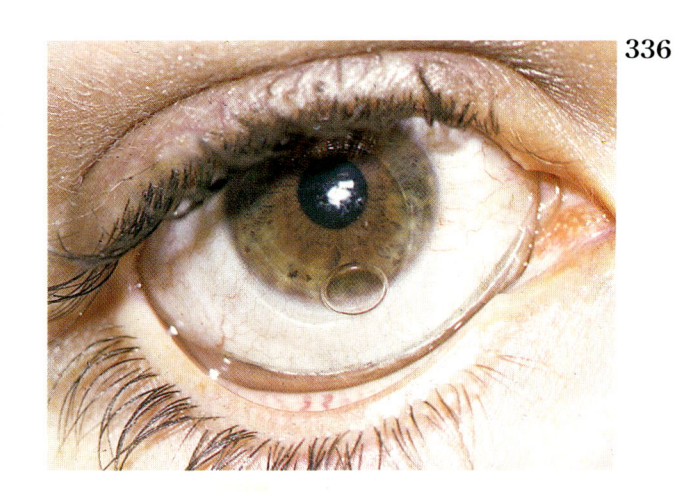

Aphakia

The majority of aphakic patients are fitted with intraocular implants. However, there remain some eyes which do not have implants, chiefly traumatic aphakia and aborted implant cases. Some surgeons avoid implants for infants and children, diabetics, those eyes with a history of uveitis and angle glaucoma and where the first eye had a posterior segment complication. Therefore there is still the need for the best contact lens for aphakia.

Table 11. Optics of aphakia. Ametropia, eye length and keratometry.

Ametrophia - $Ax = K = \dfrac{1.333 \times 10^3}{L} - K$

$K = \dfrac{0.37 \times 10^3}{r}$

Ax = axial power of eye
L = axial length of eye
K = keratometric power in dioptres
r = radius of curvature of corneal optic zone

When $Ax = K$ = pseudo-emetropic state.
This occurs when the eye has high degrees of axial myopia (approximately -18.00d.).

Table 12. Choice of contact lenses for aphakia.

	Corneal hard	Scleral hard	Gel DW	Ew Gel
Acuity	Good	Good	Moderate	Moderate
Near vision	Can be good	Poor	Poor*	Poor*
Irregular astigmatic cornea	Good	Good	Poor	Poor
Senility	Poor	Poor	Poor	Good
Infants	Poor	Poor	With help good	With help good
Tolerance	70% success	20% success	90% success	90% success

*N.B. With the future improvement of multivision simultaneous vision lenses in hard and soft materials, there would be a change for the better.

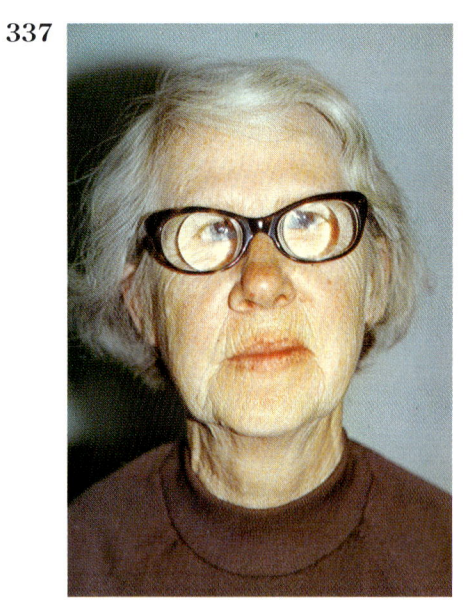

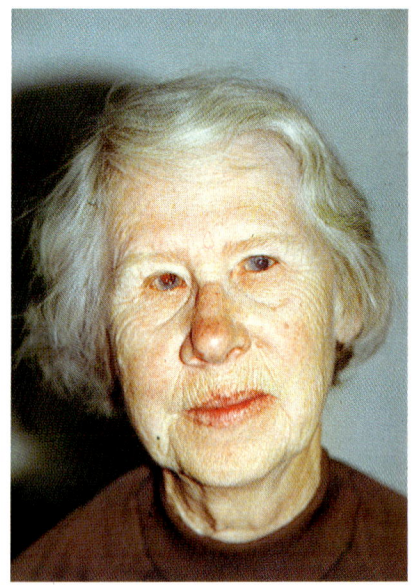

337 & 338 Elderly bilateral aphakic successfully wearing corneal lenses.
Rx example: Av. K 7.45
Back surface: 7.50 : 7.00/9.00 : 8.70/12.00 : 9.20
P = +14.0 Front optic 8.7
  Note that the front optic is bigger in diameter than the back central optic in order to give some near vision.

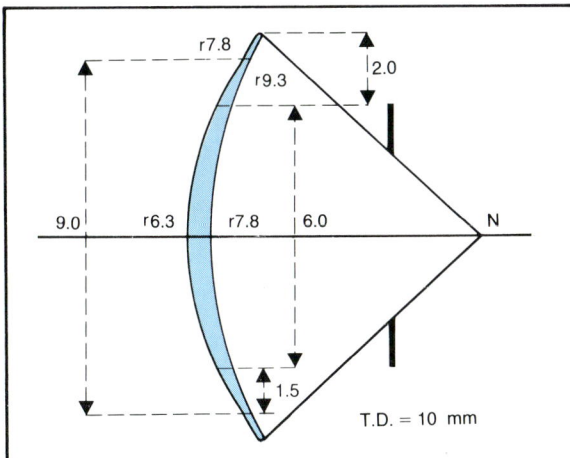

339 Aphakic corneal lens. Design of an aphakic corneal lens to give a concentric bifocal effect. (Total diameter = 10 mm.)

340 Extended wear gel lens (75% water content).
Av.K = 7.6   BC = 8.70 : 14.0   P = +18.0 T_c = 0.54
Front optic = 8.0 T_e = 0.16

341 & 342 The heavy lid displaced the thick optic of this lens. When the lid is pulled away from the eye the fit is satisfactory. This patient achieved satisfactory extended wear. A better result may be possible with a smaller front optic diameter or front aspheric shape.

343 Subluxed contact lens in a patient with arachnodactyly (Marfans syndrome) who elected to have aphakic vision corrected with a contact lens in view of poor aphakic vision.

344 Hard corneal contact lens 9.50 mm in diameter with a steeper than keratometry central fit. Note the good edge lift.
Av. K = 8.3
BC = 7.90 : 7.0/8.50 : 9.20/12.0 : 9.70
 The fluorescein picture is also typical of wide band intermediate back curves such as are likely to be found in pseudo-aspherical back curves.

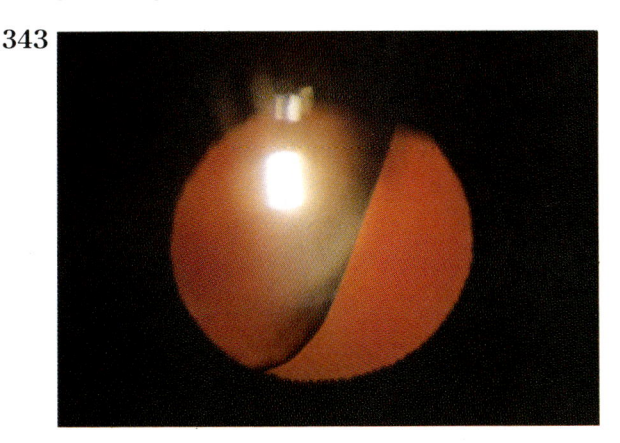

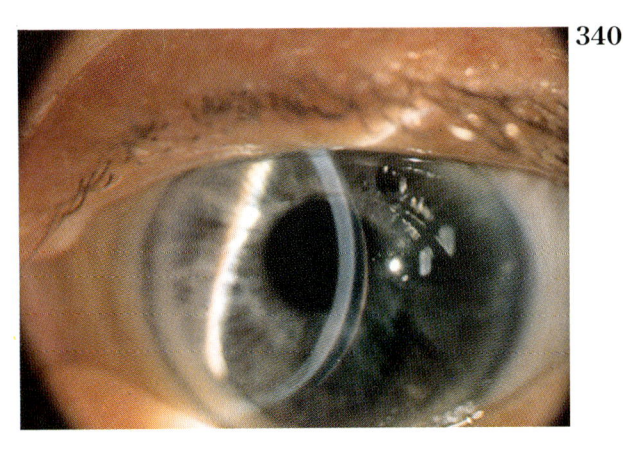

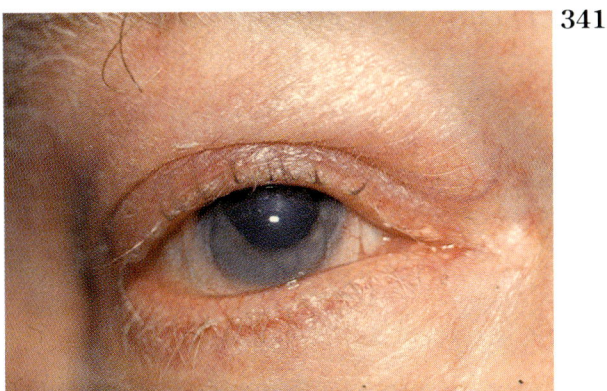

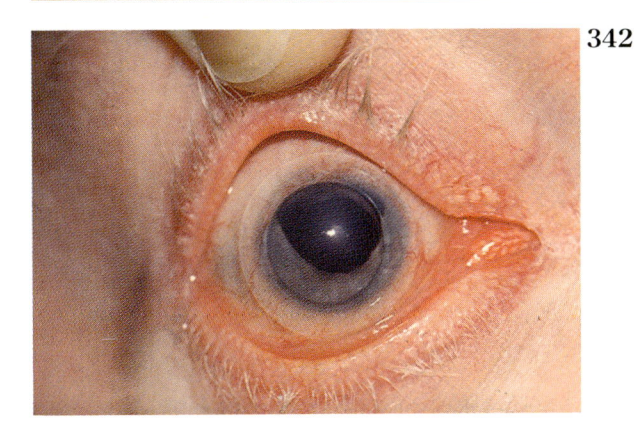

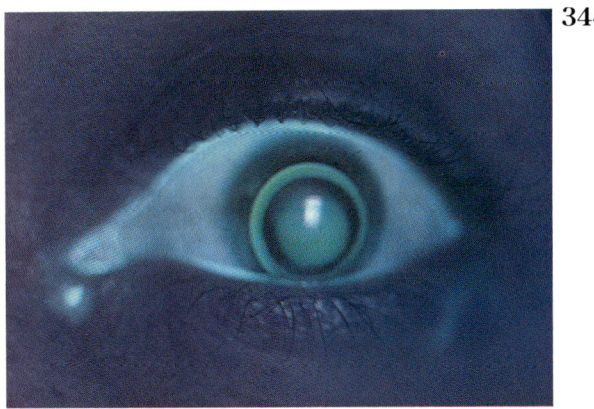

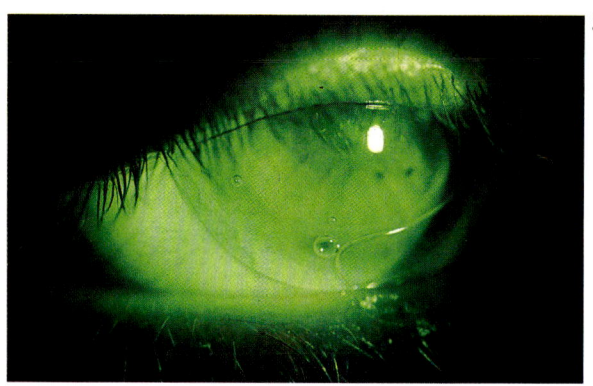

345 & 346 Corneo scleral lens. In the diagram, the interrupted line is the limbus and the large lens rides high to fit the apex of the aphakic cornea which is sometimes displaced superiorly. Note that the upper lid will play an important role in stabilizing this lens. These large, rigid lenses are useful to obtain stability in the aphakic eye with high irregular astigmatism.

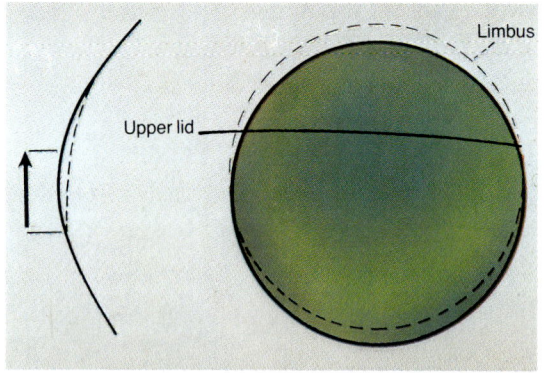

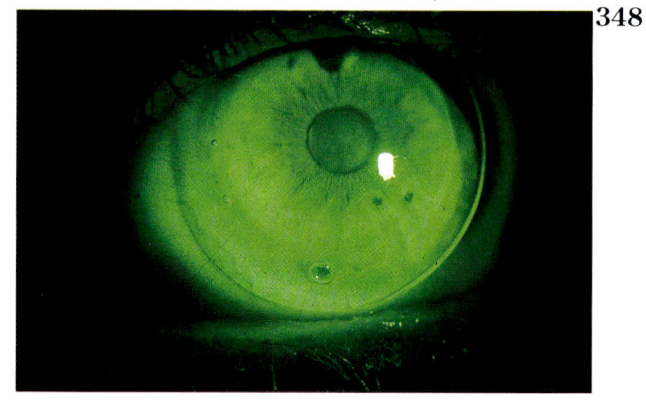

347 Corneo scleral lens on the eye. The high corneal astigmatism in this patient is against the rule (90°).
K = 8.7 at 90° 7.3
Back surface and lens size: 8.60 : 8.20/9.00 : 12.50

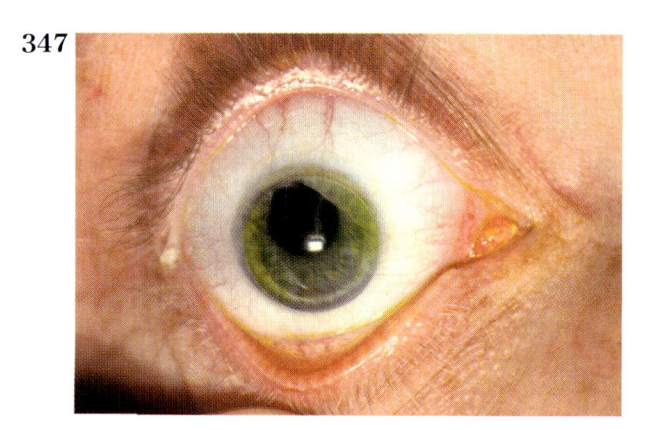

348 Corneo scleral hard lens. TD = 13 mm. Note the fenestration (useful even with GP materials to avoid negative retro-lens pressures).

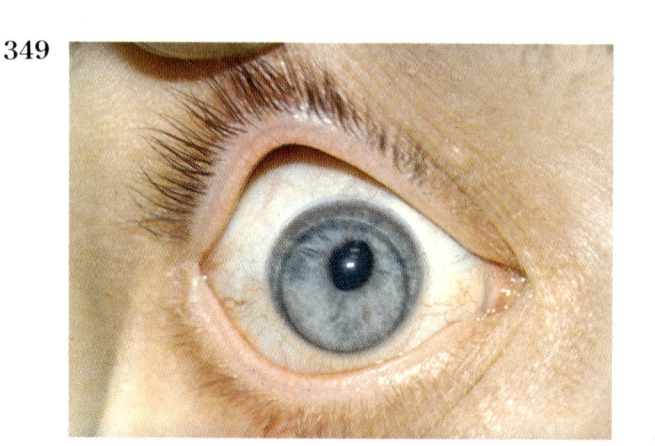

349 Scleral lens. Fitted rarely for an irregular shaped cornea. This picture appears to be of a corneal lens but is in fact the small reduced front optic of a scleral lens.

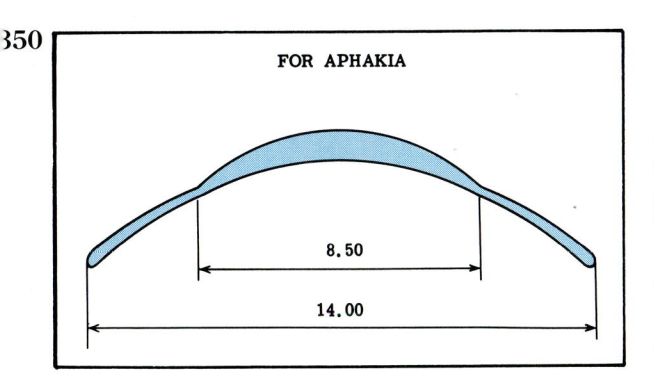

350 Soft lens. Note the slightly thickened edge due to its negative power peripheral profile. This type of edge on a soft lens helps to stabilize it and does not (as in a corneal lens) give lid adhesion.

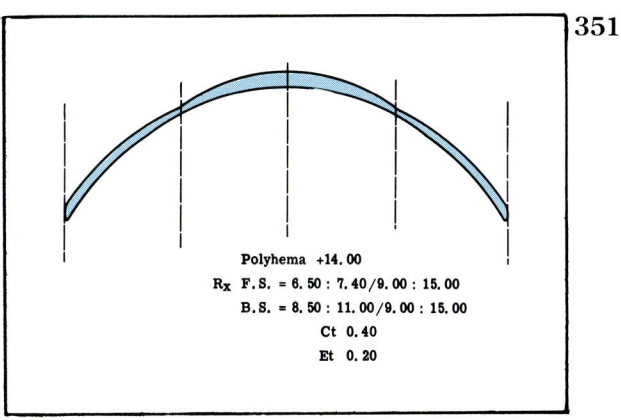

351 Soft lens profile. A much smaller optic than in **350** and a thinner lens with better adhesion properties.

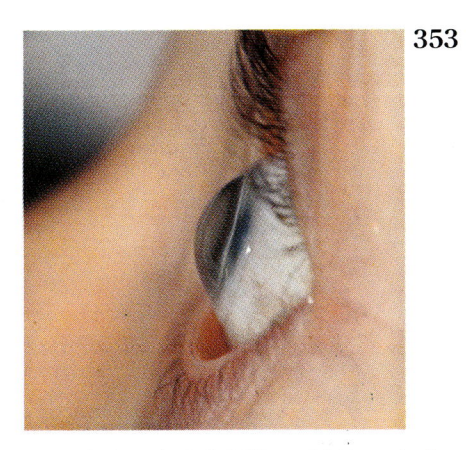

352-354 Spun moulded aphakic contact lenses. Different types of spun moulded aphakic contact lenses of HEMA 42 per cent water. They are usually only available in one fitting. **352 & 353** are 12.5 mm in diameter. These lenses make an ideal stock lens for immediate issue for aphakia.

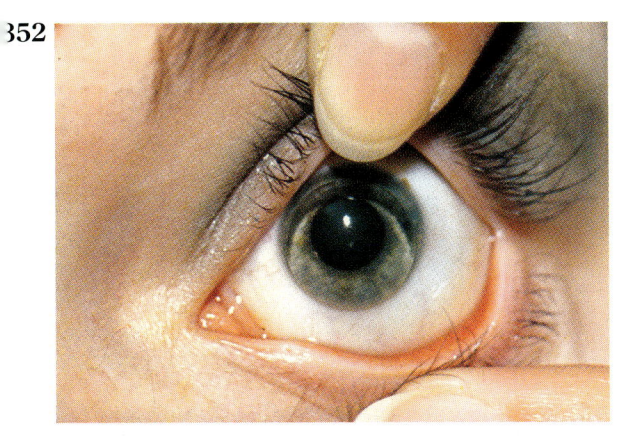

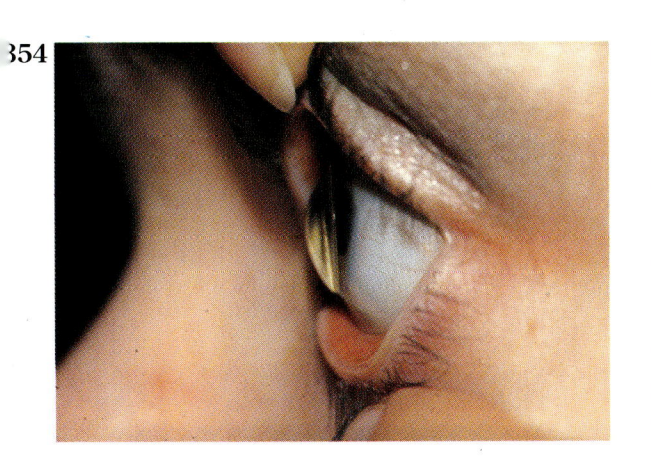

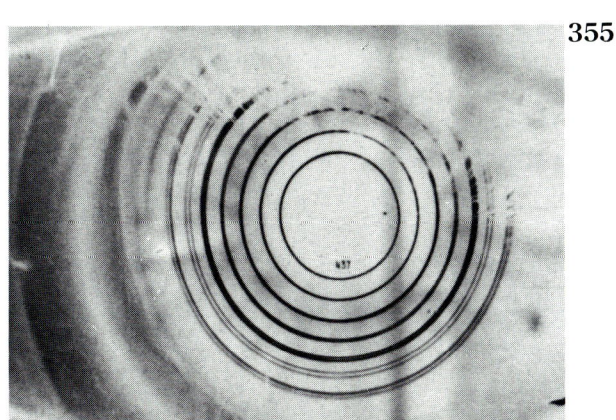

355 Over-lens photokeratograph to show how regular is the spherical soft lens surface.

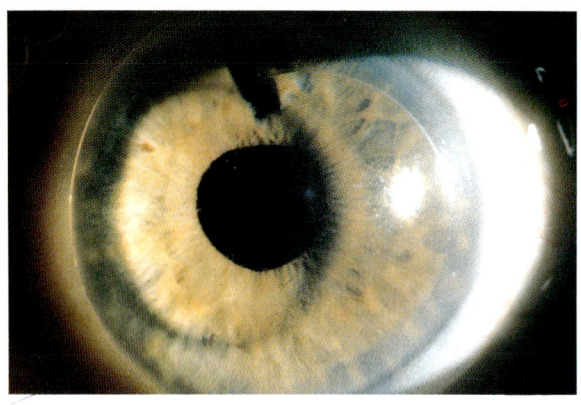

356 & 357 Silicone rubber lenses. Both are 12.5 mm diameter. **356** is a satisfactory fit but it was not possible to obtain a better fit for **357** because of the limited number of fittings.

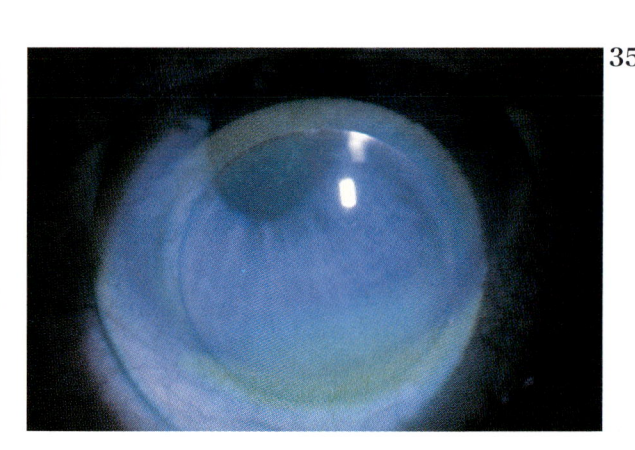

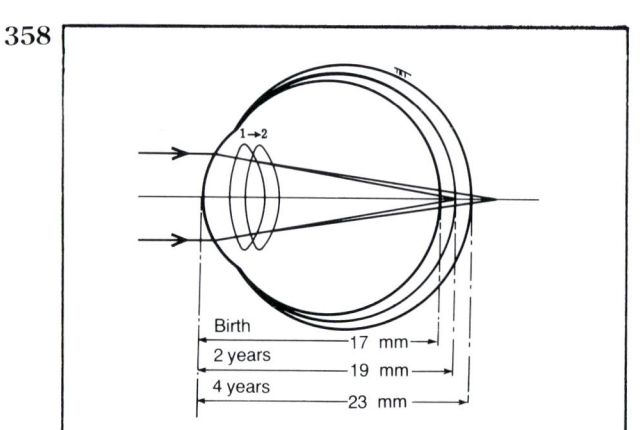

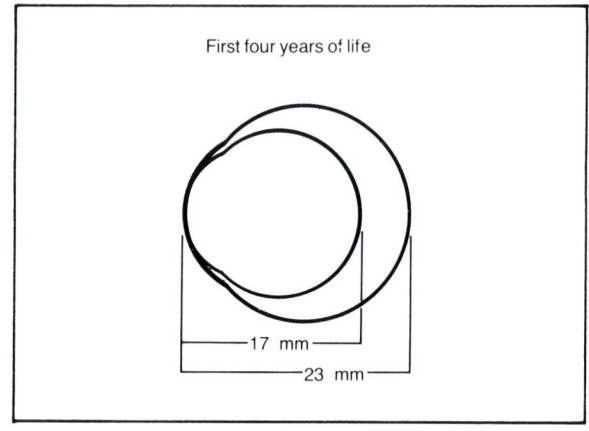

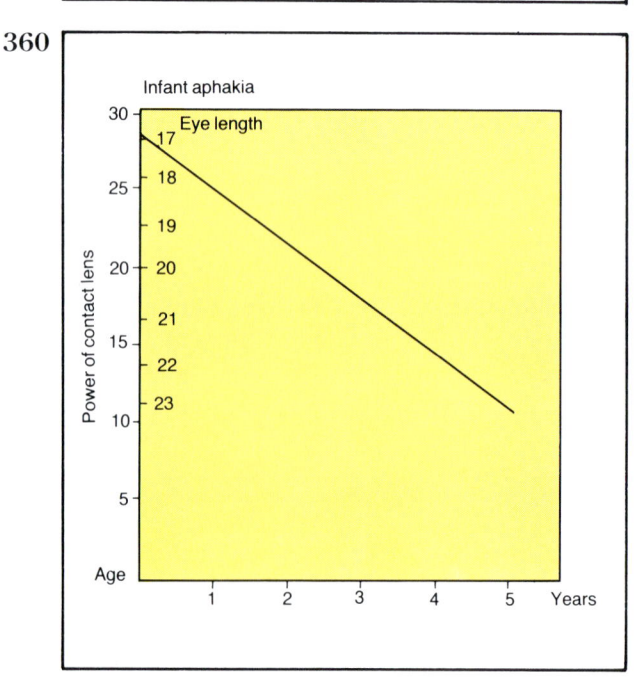

Aphakia in infancy

358 Optical factors in development. Between the age of one and four the eye will grow from 17 mm to 23 mm in length and from then until skeletal growth stops the eye will only grow another 1 mm. Therefore the eye size appears to be more controlled by neurogenic growth factors than skeletal factors (the skeleton doubles in size between the age of 4 years and adulthood).

The infant cornea is just over 10 mm in diameter but the keratometry is similar to the adult. Therefore the peripheral cornea, *not* the central curvature, develops in the skeletal growth period.

359 & 360 Aphakic eye in infancy. The aphakic eye, as it grows, will modify its power almost entirely from axial changes. The power will be over +30d. after birth, decreasing to +12d. after the age of 4 years. Any optical correction for the infant eye must be correct within ±2d. to be of any value to developing foveal vision but such tolerances may not apply to the development of directional sensitivity (it is important to control peripheral BV to avoid strabismus).

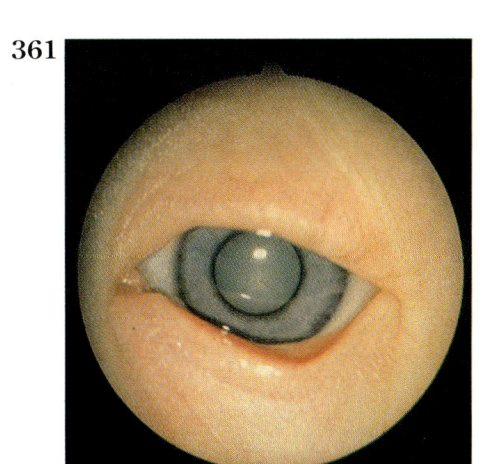

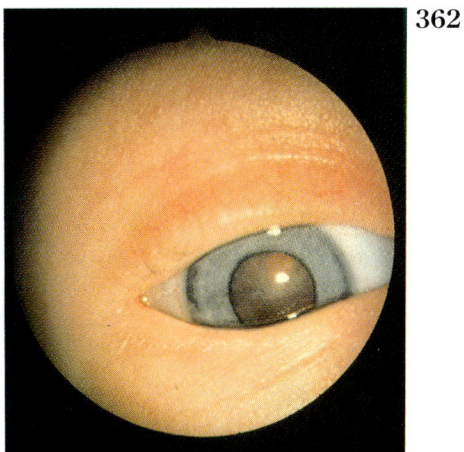

361 & 362 Total cataracts at birth.

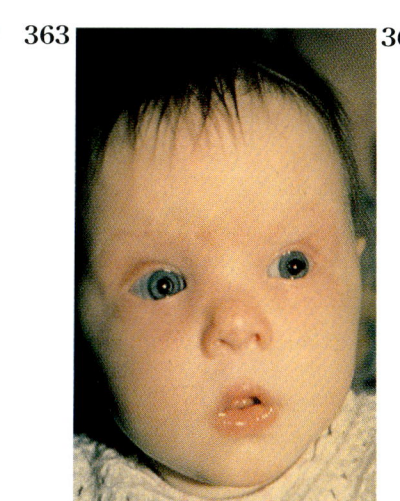

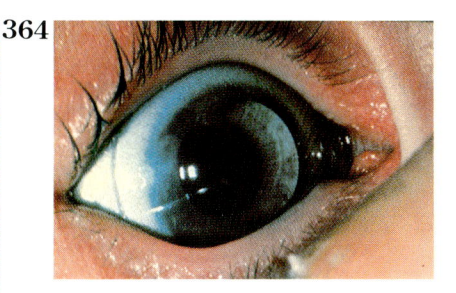

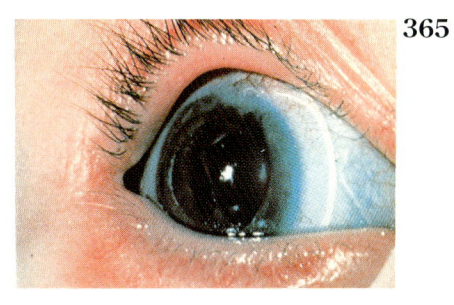

363–365 **With contact lenses.** The cataracts in **361 & 362** were extracted soon after birth and the eyes were fitted with high water contact gel lenses (75 per cent Duragel). (Patients of D. Taylor FRCS.)

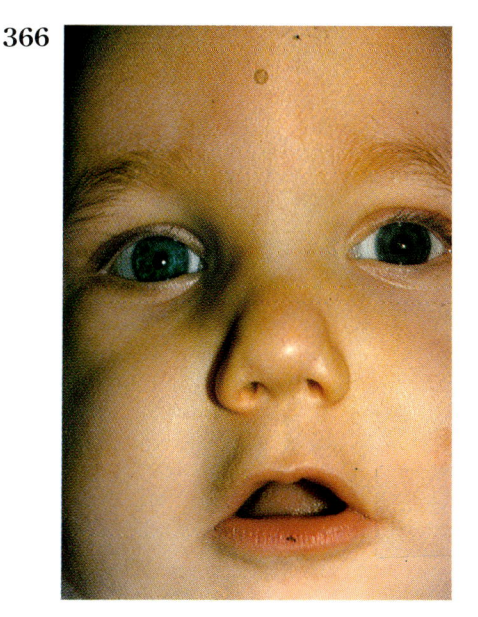

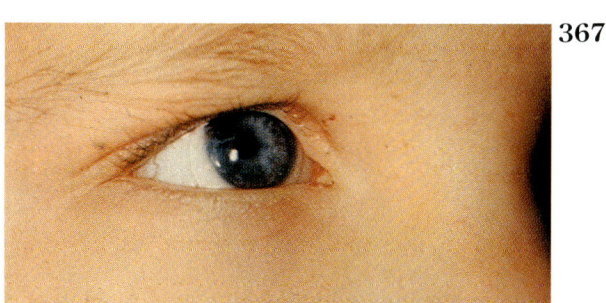

366 & 367 **Extended wear gel lenses.** Other examples of an infant wearing extended wear gel lenses. A fitting and issue set of sterile lenses should be available for this type of patient. Note that steep corneas and small eyes determine the size of the lenses.

Thus the fitting set suggested is as follows:
7.20 : 10.00/8.00 : 13.50
by 0.2 increments to 8.00 : 10.00/8.60 : 13.50.
Powers +20d. to +30d. in 2 dioptre increments.

Fitting procedure for infant aphakia:

- Place the lens on the infant eye, commencing with the flattest fitting lens and power as determined from Chapter 6.
- Study the movement of the lens. If it is not centring, use a lens with a steeper fit.
- Over-refract and reinsert the best-powered lens.
- Wearing periods should be of 1 month duration and then fit a *new* lens.
- Extend the wearing periods to 2 months if the lens is successful.
- Change to a daily wear pattern whenever possible.
- If high astigmatism is present, consider a GP rigid lens for daily wear.

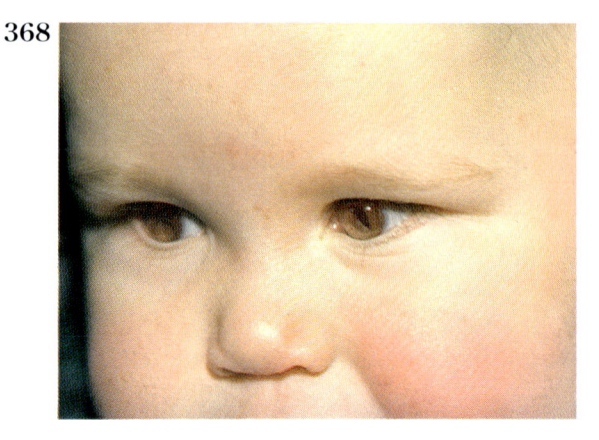

368 Silicone rubber lens. Baby aphakic fitted with silicone rubber lens (10.8 mm diameter). It was fitted with fluorescein and under general anaesthetic.

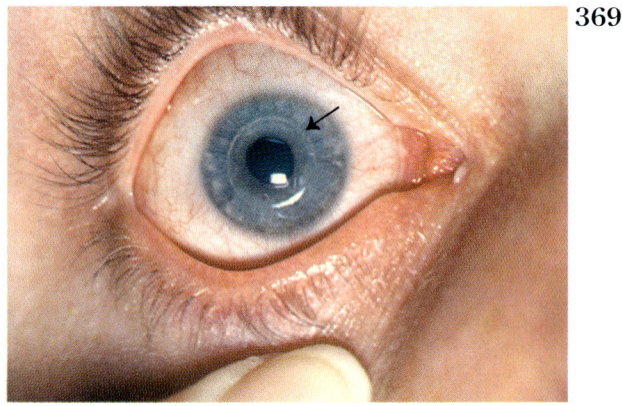

369 Epikerato prosthesis. The picture shows an old procedure of adhering a thin contact lens to Bowman's membrane. This was used to correct aphakia and irregular astigmatism. In the future, advances in bioplastics may result in similar procedures.

The present procedure of epikeratoplasty is, in some ways, similar but uses donor material. This is used where contact lens tolerance fails for aphakia, irregular astigmatism and early keratoconus.

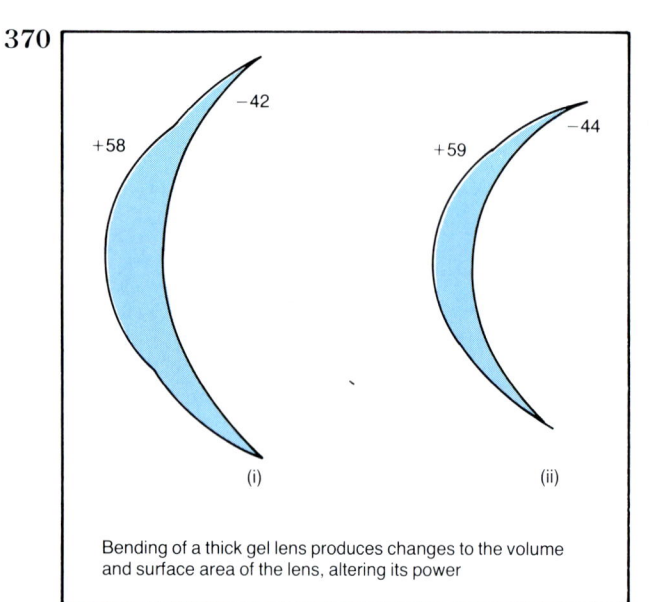

370

Bending of a thick gel lens produces changes to the volume and surface area of the lens, altering its power

370 Thick soft lenses have a degree of rigidity and therefore mould *partially* to the cornea. This is useful to maintain retro-lens tear flow and to correct corneal astigmatism. The moulding (wrap) effect also alters the lens power. In the example given, the left-hand lens (i) is in air and has a power of +16d.; but on the eye (ii) the curvatures bend unequally and then the power is +15d. This effect may take several hours of wear to become apparent.

Keratoconus

371 Keratoconus—1° corneal collagen dystrophy. This text does not detail diagnostic aspects of eye disease. However, there are some aspects of the diagnostic findings that assist the contact lens practitioner and will be illustrated only in that context. The experienced practitioner can, with the lateral view of the cornea, estimate the degree of cone.

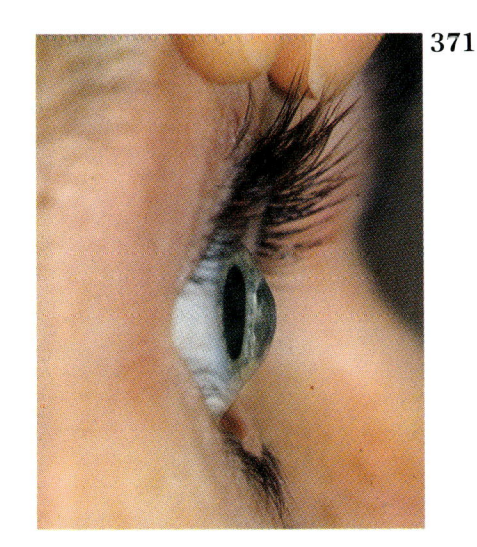

Note the following:

- **Irregular astigmatism:** note that the keratometry (Javal-Schiöty) mires are non-alligned and the size differences of the mires. (372)

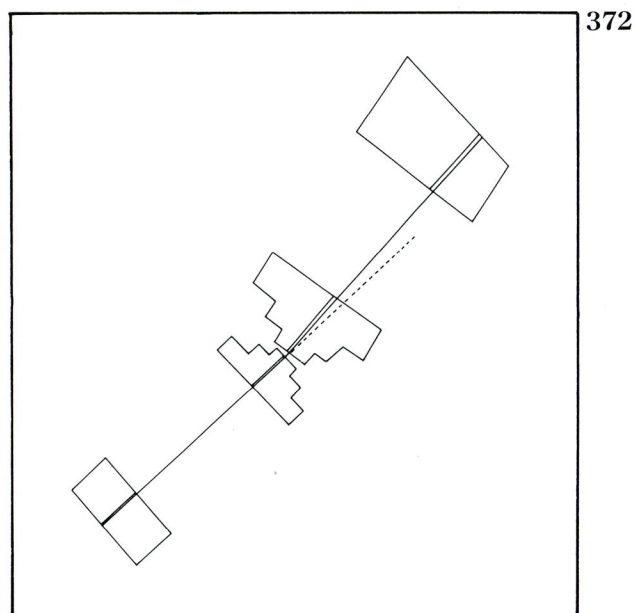

- **Steep anterior keratometry.** Find the position of the apex, central or paracentral with the thinning of the cornea. Do not confuse this with rare posterior conus, or 1° marginal dystrophy. (373)

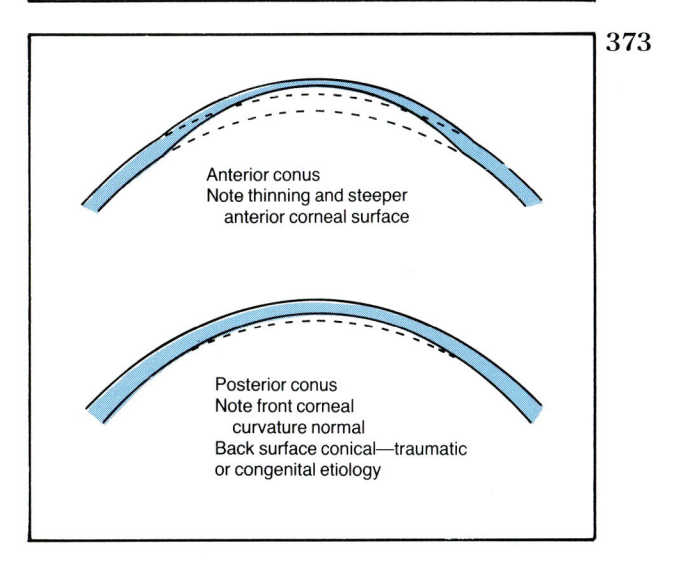

Anterior conus
Note thinning and steeper anterior corneal surface

Posterior conus
Note front corneal curvature normal
Back surface conical—traumatic or congenital etiology

121

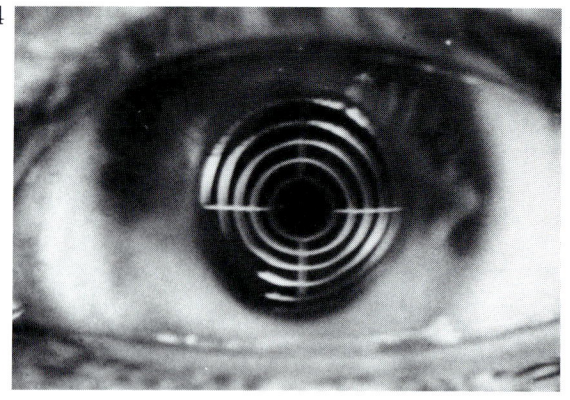

• **Photokeratograms are difficult to focus**, if used for fitting. (374)

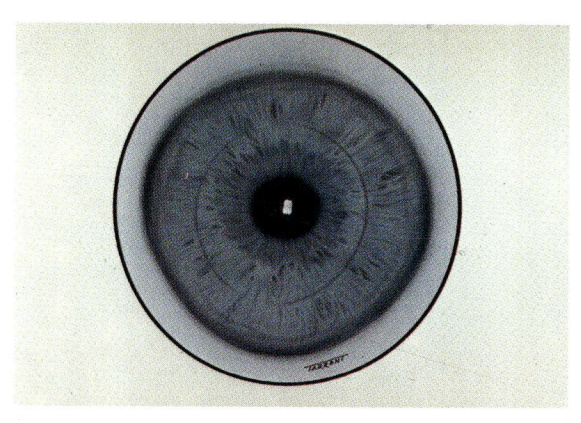

• **Fleischer's ring**, while not always present, does give a guide as to the position of the base of the cone. (375)

Keratoconus contact lens fitting

Keratoconus patients are usually young and eager to have better vision and not with cosmesis as the prime factor. These patients are highly motivated to obtain tolerance, and overcome sensitivity problems which are typical of this condition (vernal catarrh conjunctivitis). Thus, in practice, the fitter sees patients tolerating bizarre fittings and wearing lenses that give subnormal vision.

The corneal rigid lens is best fitted, and if tolerance is poor the spherical types of soft lenses are used. If all else fails, scleral lenses are fitted, even though the wearing times may be limited and the fitting protracted in time. Contact lens intolerance and poor uncorrectable vision is an indication for keratoplasty.

Hard corneal lenses

Types of fit of hard corneal lenses (include gas permeable materials):
  (a) Cone hanging lens with no upper lid support.
  (b) Para-cone fit with upper lid adhesion.
  (c) Cone touch fit, sealed intermediate zone.
  (d) Cone touch fit, bull's eye pattern—vault fit.
  (e) Cone parallel fit.
(See **376**).

Size of lenses:
• Fit small diameter lenses (8.0-9.0 mm) to early cones.
• Fit large diameter lenses (9.0 mm up to scleral) to advanced cones.

Back surface design:
• Multispherical: small base curve diameter (5-6 mm) with three peripheral curves, or
• Aspherical: steep shape factor (steeper than SF = +0.6), or
• Pseudo-aspherical: small, steeper than Av. K base curve and small base curve diameter (5-6 mm) with peripheral cone or offset curves.

The shape factor (see **30-31**) will vary for each cone and modifications will need to be made to the lens to obtain fit from the optic diameter and peripheral curve.

Fit from trial sets:

Multispherical:
5.7 : 5.0/6.7 : 7.0/7.7 : 9.00/8.7 : 9.5
by equal increments of 0.20 to
7.70 : 6.00/8.70 : 7.00/9.70 : 8.20/10.5 : 8.70
P = −12.0d for the smaller lenses decreasing to
P = −4.0d for the larger lenses

N.B. The fitting philosophy is the opposite to that applicable to the normal cornea. Toric back surfaces can be used giving at least 1 mm difference between the meridians of the radius of curvature.

The above fitting set is purely empirical.

Equal increments of the sagitta fitting set:

Examples:
Sagitta = 2.5 then BS = 5.50 : 5.0/6.0 : 9.0/8.0 : 9.50
Sagitta = 2.0 then BS = 6.75 : 5.0/7.25 : 9.0/9.25 : 9.50
Sagitta = 1.7 then BS = 7.50 : 5.0/8.0 : 9.0/10.0 : 9.50

Intermediate sizes can be calculated (see M. Ruben in *Contact Lenses*, Edited by Stensen, Appleton & Lange (Norwalk USA, 1987).

This fitting is for lenses that will *vault* the cornea and are all the same size. Note: without a trial set several fittings may be required.

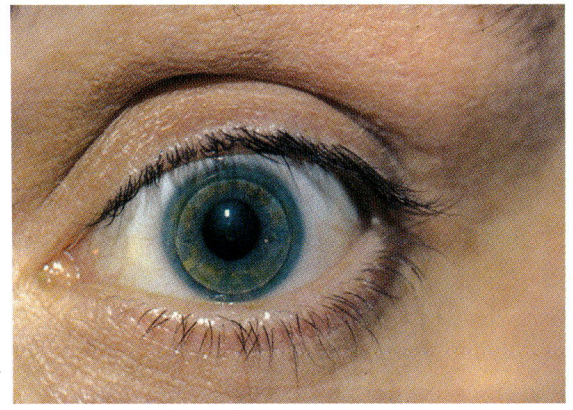

377 Good lens fitting of an early cone—lens size 8.90 mm.

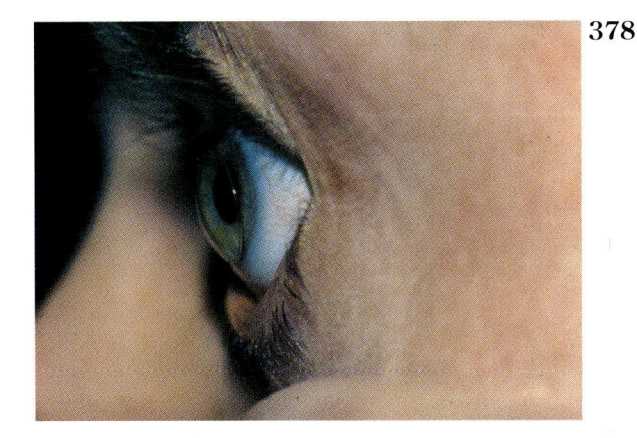

378 Profile of 377.

379 Early keratoconus. A diagrammatic representation of **377** and **378**. Note the upper lid adhesion and good inferior ventilation. Practitioners elect to fit this lens from the para-conal keratometry readings.

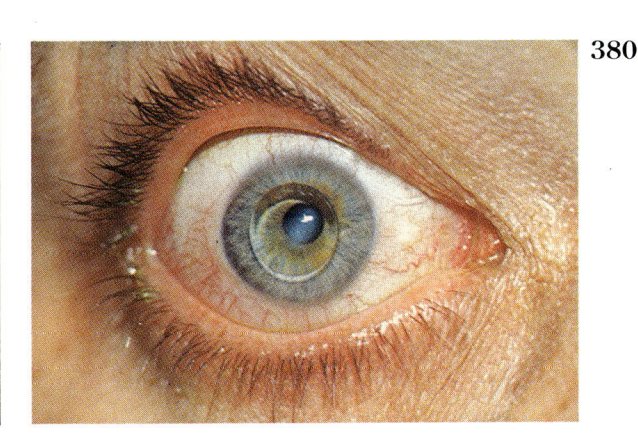

380 Attempted small lens fitting of an advanced cone. Note the stromal scarring.
Back surface: 6.0:5.0/8.0:6.9/9.0:7.2. P = −10.5d.
T_c = 0.08 mm. T_e = 0.13 mm. Reduced optic 5.5 mm.
T_j = 0.35 mm.
This was a vaulted fit but failed because of the very thick junction necessary with the high power. A flatter-fitting, lower power and larger lens succeeded.

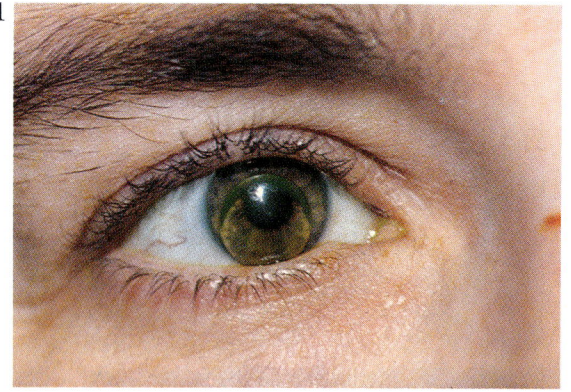

381 Small cone hanging lens. Excessive wearing of such a lens can produce corneal scarring.

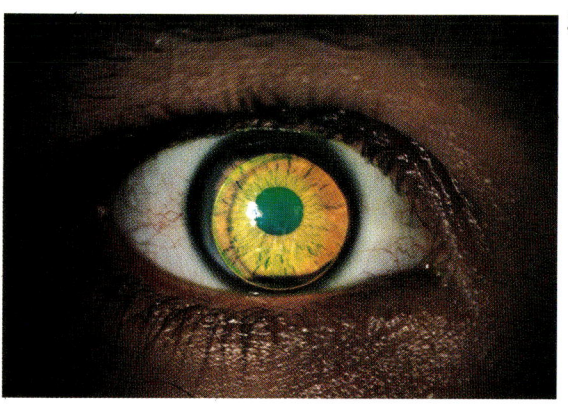

382 Parallel cone touch—9.50 mm lens. Note that, in keratoconus, sealed retro-lens areas are often unavoidable. Even with gas permeable materials if corneal oedema results then fenestrate the lens in the sealed zones.

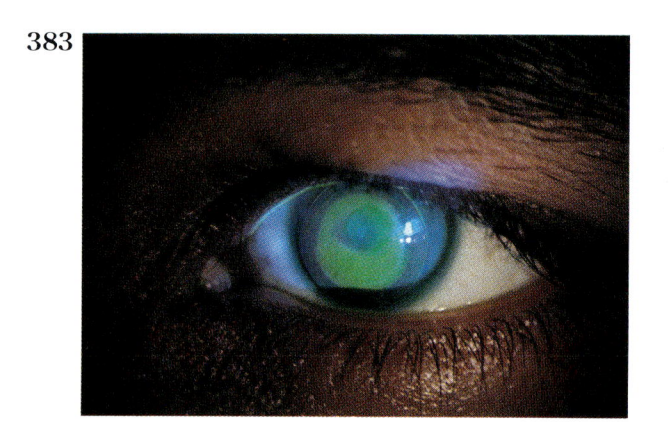

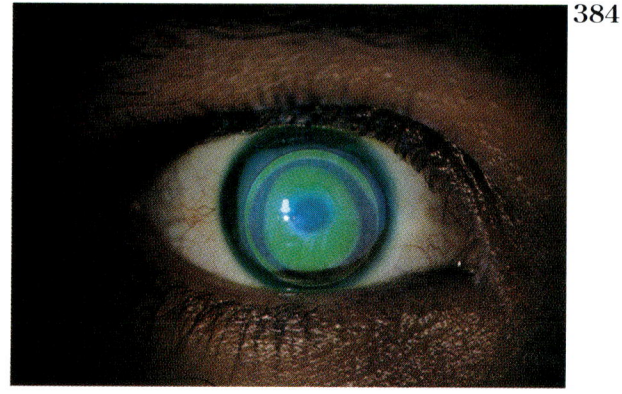

383 & 384 Bull's eye fit. Right and left eyes with a vaulted bull's eye fit.

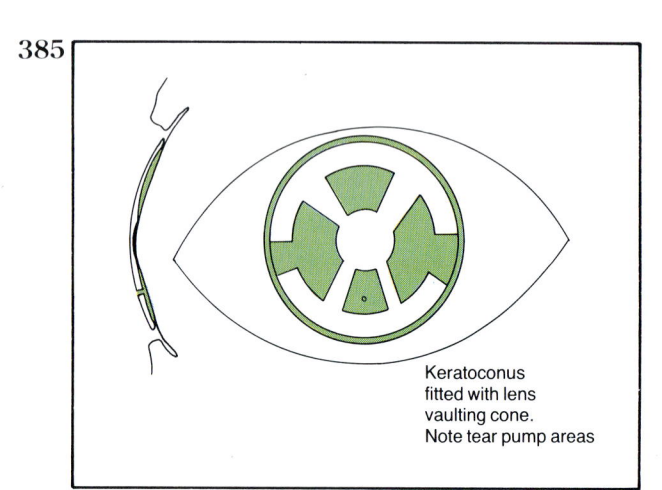

385 A diagrammatic representation of a bull's eye fit with a fenestration.

Keratoconus fitted with lens vaulting cone. Note tear pump areas

386 Fitting keratoconus with large corneal hard lenses. For advanced keratoconus, the large lens can be used as an alternative to the hard scleral lens.

Example: keratometry Rt. eye 5.6 at 90° 5.9 irregular.

The fitting illustrated is as follows and the material is a silicone acrylate of Dk 50.

6.00:7.5/7.00:9.50/7.50:11.50. P = −8.0d.

T_c = 0.13 mm. T_e = 0.11 mm

The fitting commenced with a lens of 12 mm size which was reduced in size to 11.50 mm to give apical touch with minimal movement (a vault type fitting).

387 Combination of hard and soft materials. The harder material is limited to the central zone to give better acuity and the periphery is soft for comfort.

Three types are illustrated:

(a) GP hard corneal lens (10 mm diameter) fitted over a 15 mm bandage lens.
(b) Small hard lens inserted into a gel lens.
(c) Hard material fused with a soft gel (e.g. Saturn).

There are problems of fitting and managing but this method can give good results.

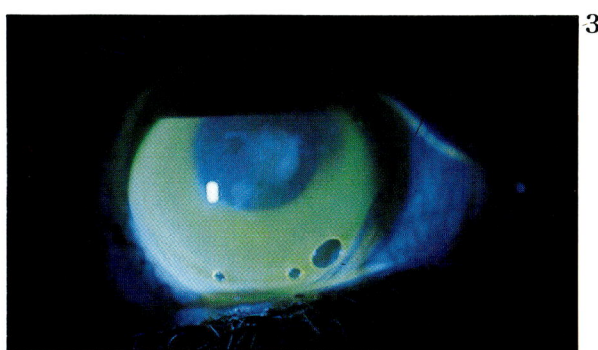

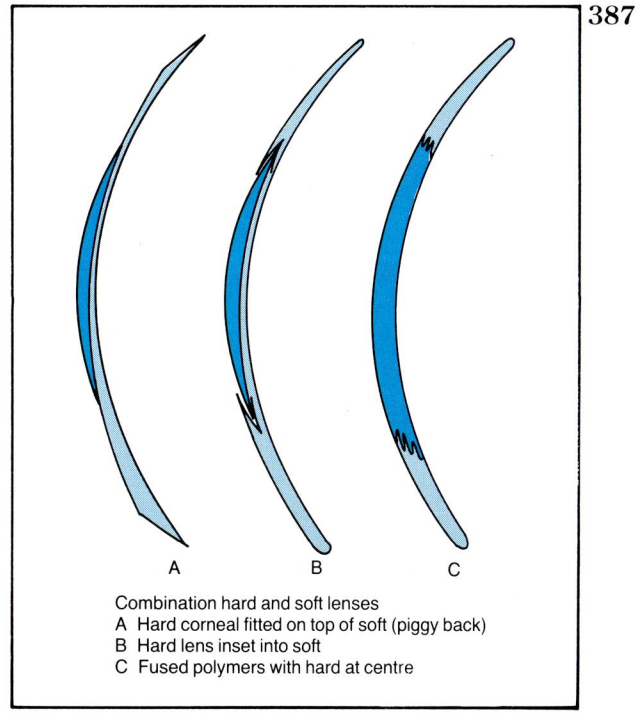

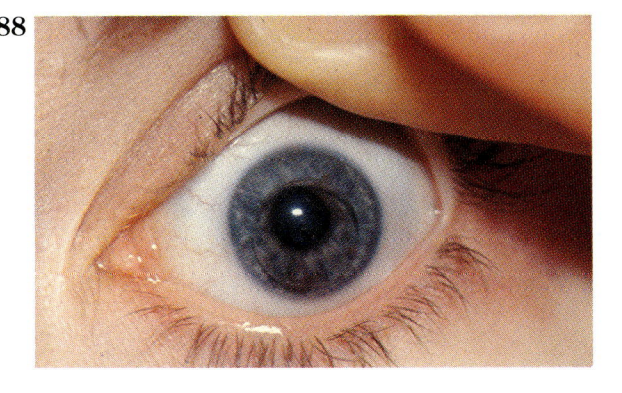

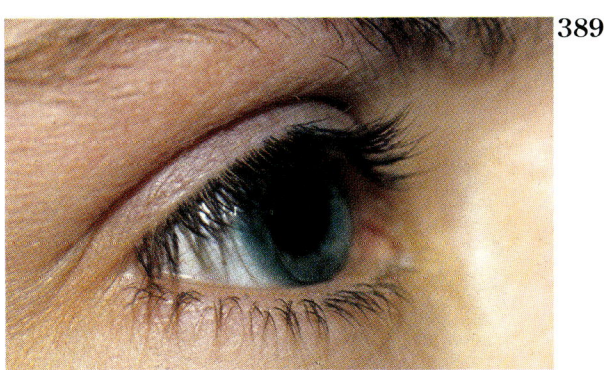

Combination hard and soft lenses
A Hard corneal fitted on top of soft (piggy back)
B Hard lens inset into soft
C Fused polymers with hard at centre

388 & 389 10 mm diameter lens fitted over a gel lens. Centration is difficult unless the hard lens peripheral curves are steep.

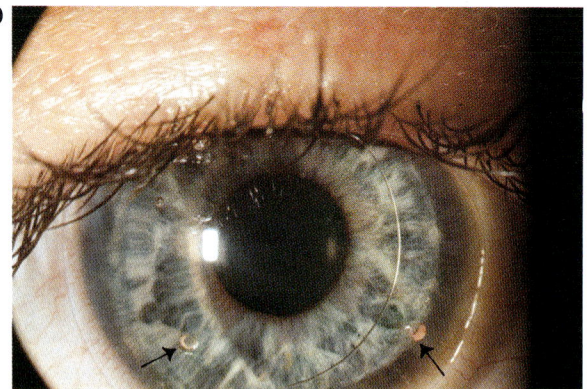

Soft lenses

390 Soft lens and keratoconus. The conventional thin (T_c = 0.03–0.60 mm) centred minus soft lens is not of much use in the correction of moderate to advanced keratoconus. There are exceptions, especially where the cone is central and a spectacle over-correction for a residual cylinder can substantially improve the vision. Very steep back curved gel lenses are often not available.

Thick centre gel lenses can be custom made to individual Rx and some success obtained. When this is not possible then toric soft lenses of prism ballast type often have sufficient central thickness to give vision correction.

The custom-made gel lens illustrated is sufficiently rigid to require fenestrations in the area of clearance from the cornea (arrows), to avoid sealing.

(Note the reduced front optic transition.)

Trial set of thick gel lenses (42 per cent water):
7.0/13.0 to 8.0/14.0
Plano power:
T_c = 0.30 mm over central 5 mm T_e = 0.16 mm

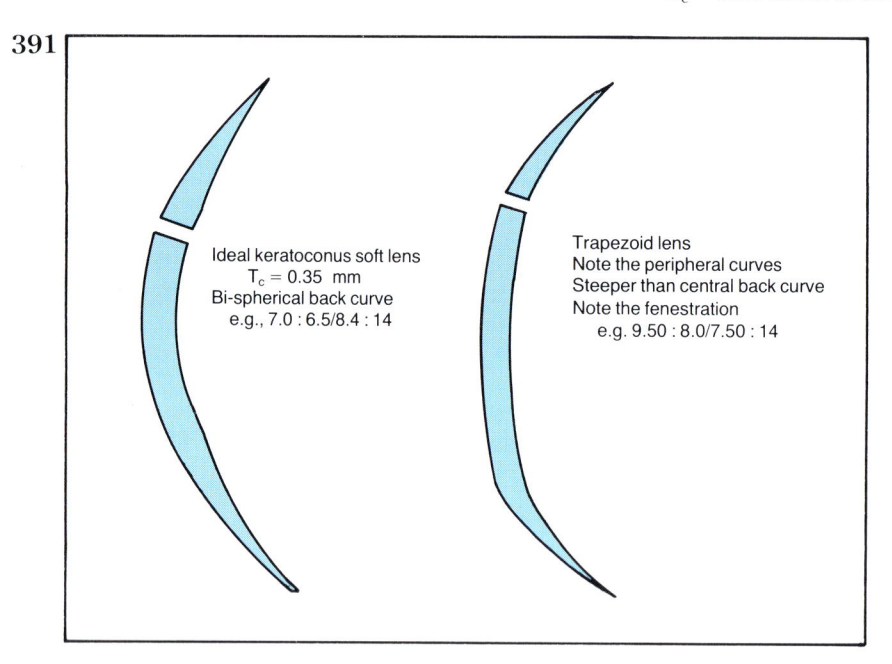

391 Other examples of thick soft lens design. The trapezoid lens has a central zone that is flatter than the periphery. Excessive central touch must be avoided otherwise pulsation of vision occurs.

Ideal keratoconus soft lens
T_c = 0.35 mm
Bi-spherical back curve
e.g., 7.0 : 6.5/8.4 : 14

Trapezoid lens
Note the peripheral curves
Steeper than central back curve
Note the fenestration
e.g. 9.50 : 8.0/7.50 : 14

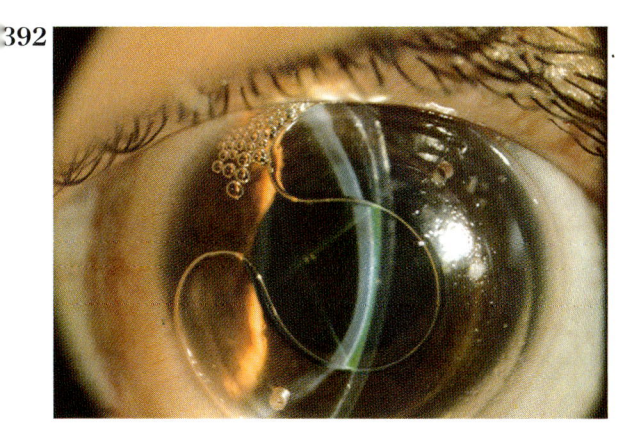

392 & 393 Keratoconus fitted with a trapezoid type back surface. Note the fenestrations and air bubbles which give the appearance of a scleral lens. The

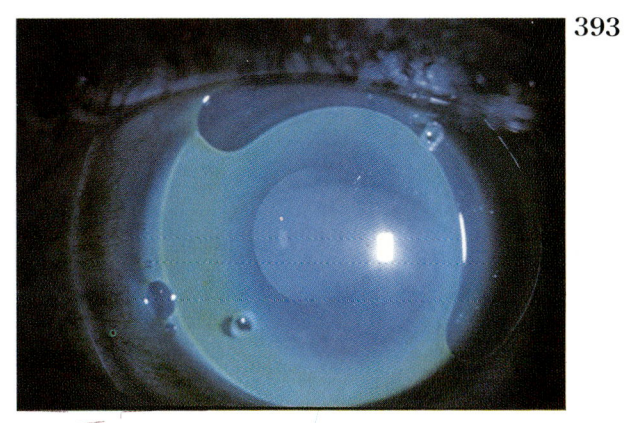

Rx of a trapezoid back surface:
K readings 5.80 at 160° irregular 6.40 for
10.0:6.50/9.0:13.50. $T_c = 0.30$ mm. $P = -4.0$
The front optic is reduced to 6 mm and there are two intermediate fenestrations.

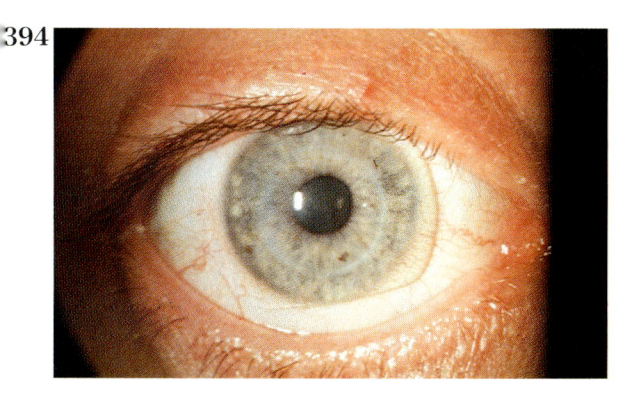

394 & 395 Use of a toric soft prism ballast lens to correct keratoconus. Note: the centre thickness was specified to be 0.25 mm. (See page 93 for toric soft lens details).

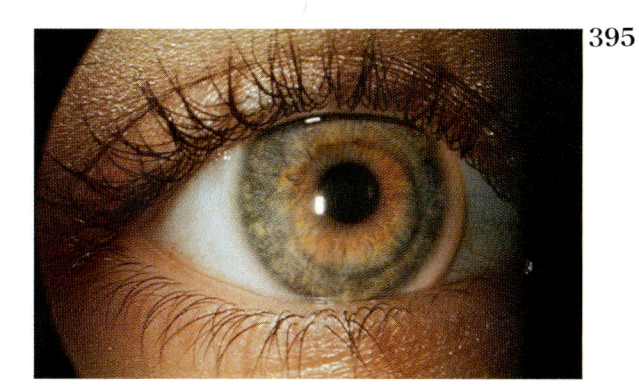

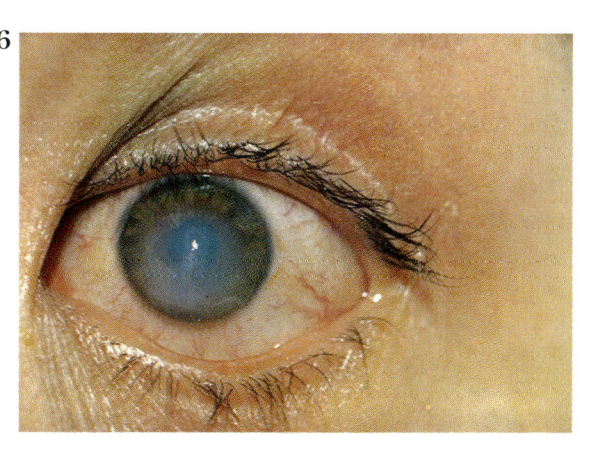

396 & 397 Hydrops. A not uncommon complication of the advanced cone is hydrops (unfortunately this is sometimes called acute keratoconus). If painful, a gel lens can be used of therapeutic type (see page 135).

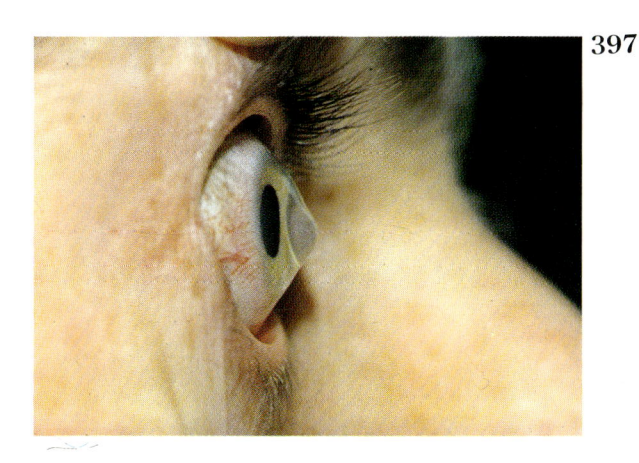

Keratoglobus

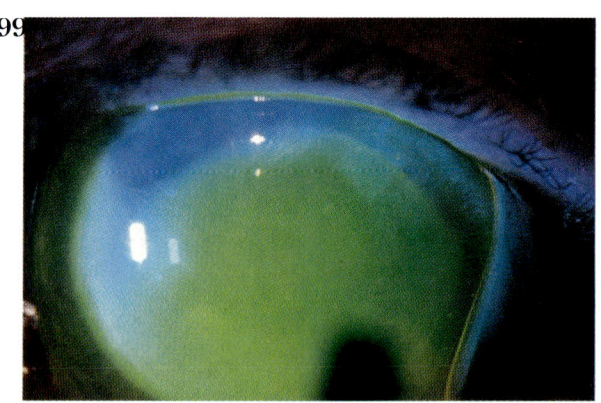

398 & 399 Keratoglobus is a corneal collagen dystrophy affecting the whole cornea. This condition is best fitted with a scleral hard contact lens.

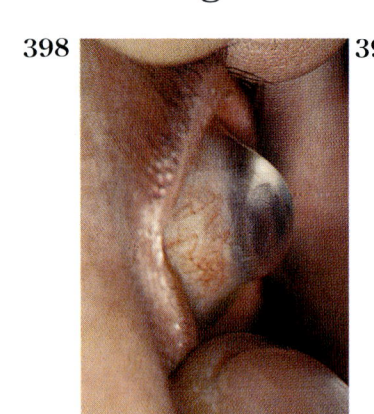

Marginal dystrophy

400 & 401 Corneal collagen dystrophy—marginal type—Terriens dystrophy (synonym). The corneal central zone has a normal thickness and has irregular astigmatism with *flat* curvatures. The thin area is covered by a noninflammatory pannus. In advanced states only a rigid scleral lens will fit satisfactorily. Note the multiple fenestrations at the limbal clearance zone.

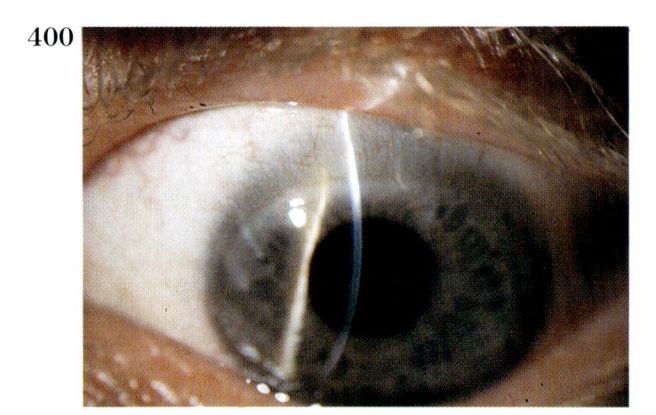

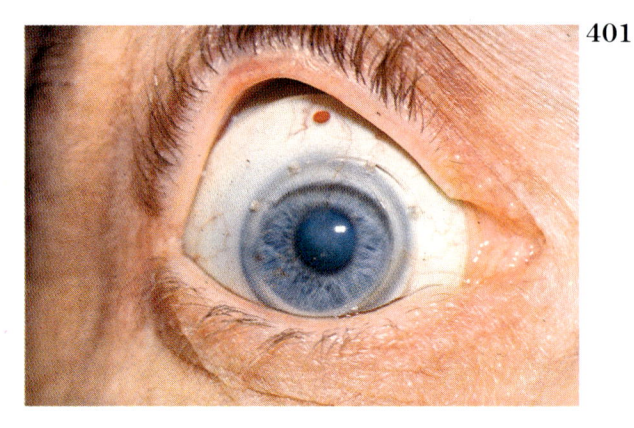

Heredokeratodystrophies

402 & 403 Heredokeratodystrophies. Patients who have anterior corneal pathology can achieve better vision with rigid contact lenses, but with deep corneal pathology only keratoplasty will help. In the Reis-Buckler dystrophy illustrated, a hard corneal lens was subsequently fitted to the grafted eye.

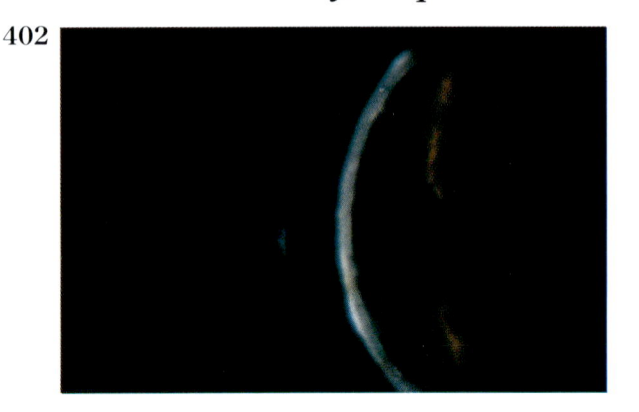

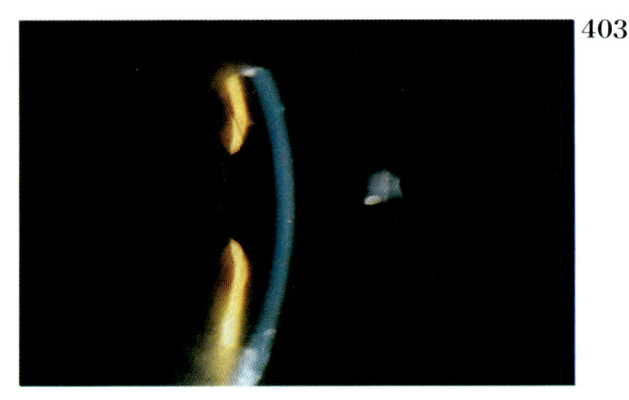

Keratoplasty

There are several ways in which the contact lens can be of assistance to the keratoplastic eye. Commencing with the operation, either a therapeutic extended wear lens can be applied immediately at the end of the operation or a temporary collagen bandage lens that will disintegrate. Later, if the graft is not tolerated, a protective bandage lens can be used. If the graft becomes oedematous, the sutures come loose or it elevates from its bed again, a large bandage lens can be fitted either as a temporary or long-term device until further surgical intervention is planned.

After several months, if the graft is clear, a hard GPR lens can be fitted for daily wear to give vision, especially if spectacle correction will cause binocular vision problems.

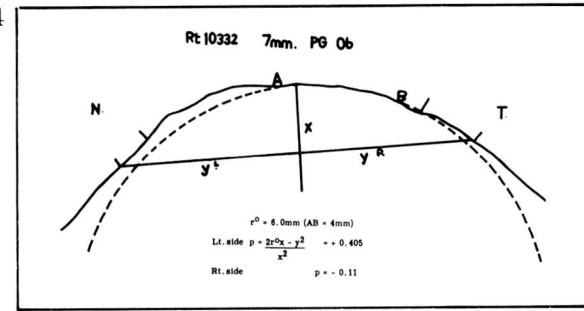

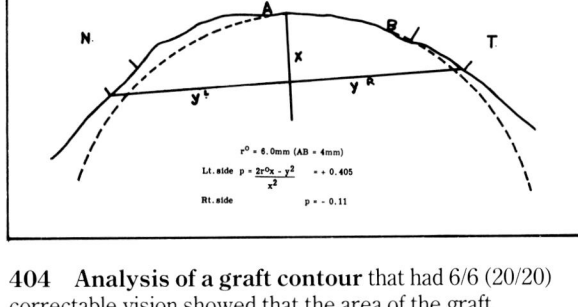

404   Analysis of a graft contour that had 6/6 (20/20) correctable vision showed that the area of the graft responsible for the good result was only a few mm (AB) in chord. Comparison of the nasal and temporal areas of the graft showed extremes of shape factor of -0.11 and $+0.405$ respectively and $r_o = 6$ mm (very eccentric curves).

405   Follow-up of keratoplasty over 2 years showed a decrease in the astigmatism and in the degree (axis).

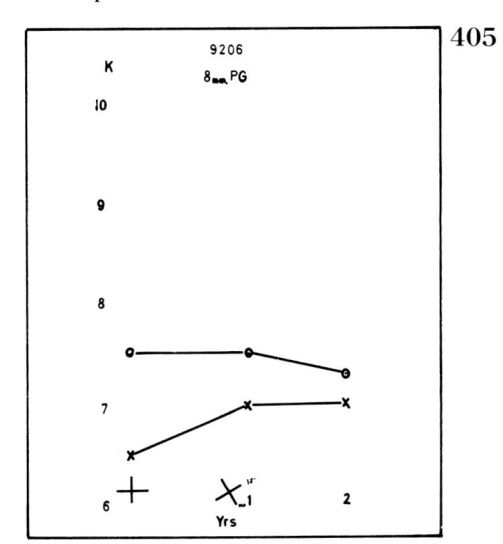

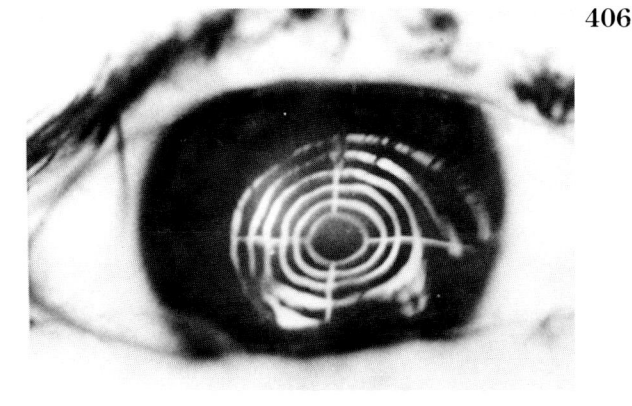

406-408   Photokeratographs to show curvatures of a large therapeutic lammelar graft (**406**), inferior graft elevation (**407**), and finally a good penetrating graft with 6/6 (20/20) vision unaided (**408**).

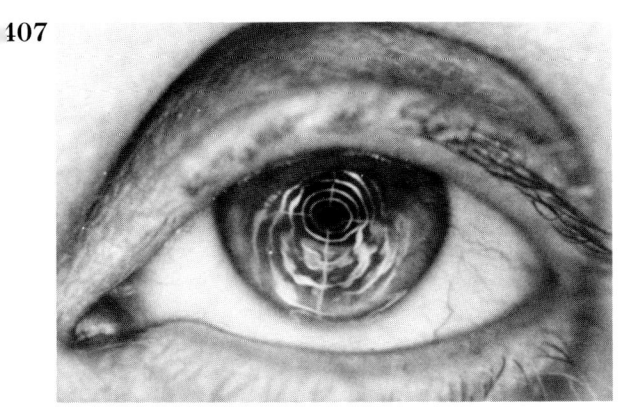

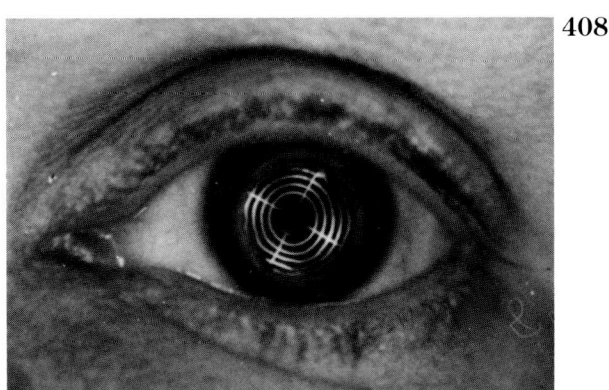

Keratoplasty eye fit

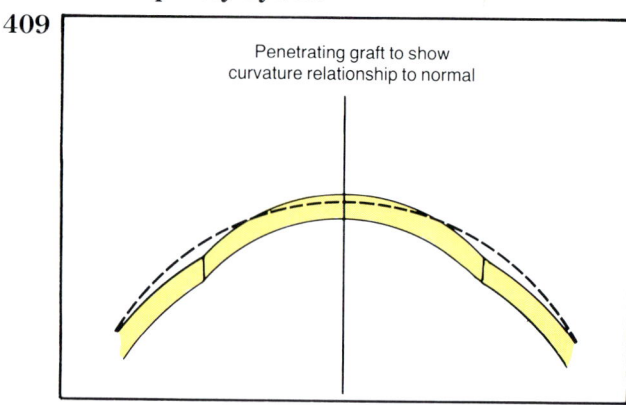

409 The curve of the PG are often similar in contour to the shape of the keratoconus cornea.

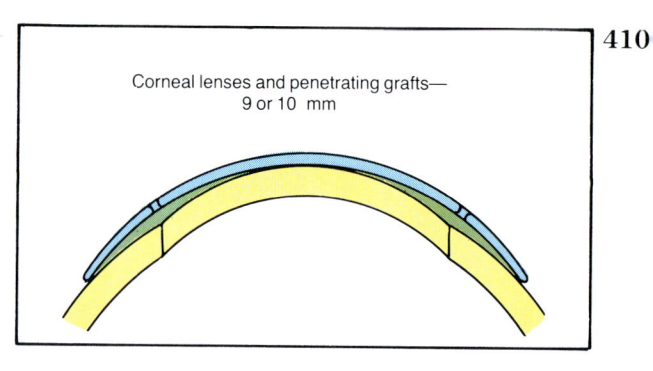

410 If the graft is sufficiently large then a small corneal lens can be fitted within the graft diameter. However, in most cases the graft has a steeper than normal curvature and can be a difficult fitting. Thus lenses between 9 mm and 10 mm and in difficult cases even corneoscleral or scleral lenses are required.

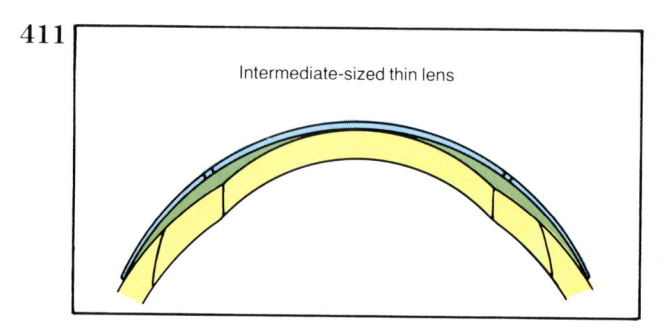

411 Corneoscleral lens diameter 12-13 mm.

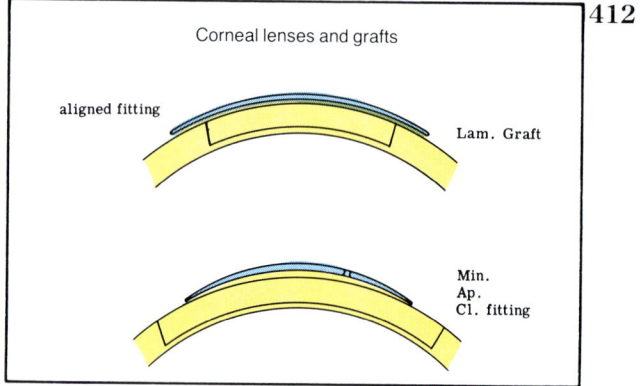

412 The lamellar graft presents the same problems as to size of lens as the PG.

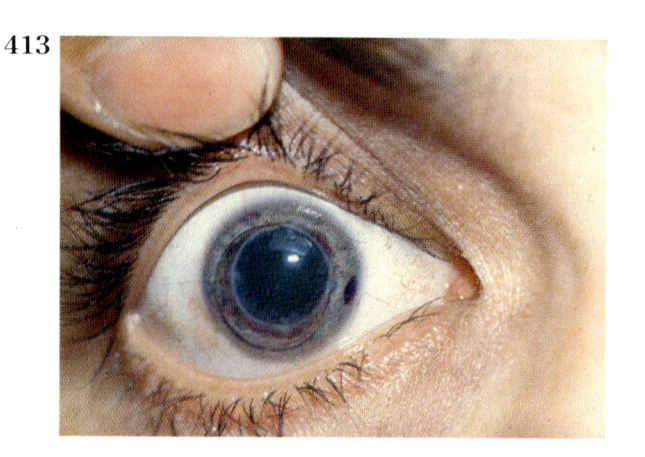

413 A penetrating keratoplasty fitted with a 9.3 mm diameter lens (8 mm graft).

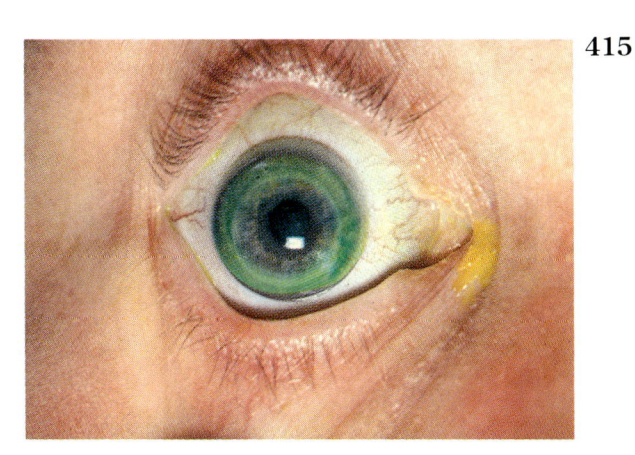

414-416 Highly irregular post-graft eye shapes that could only be fitted with 12-13 mm diameter lenses (gas permeable materials). (**416** also shows fenestrations).

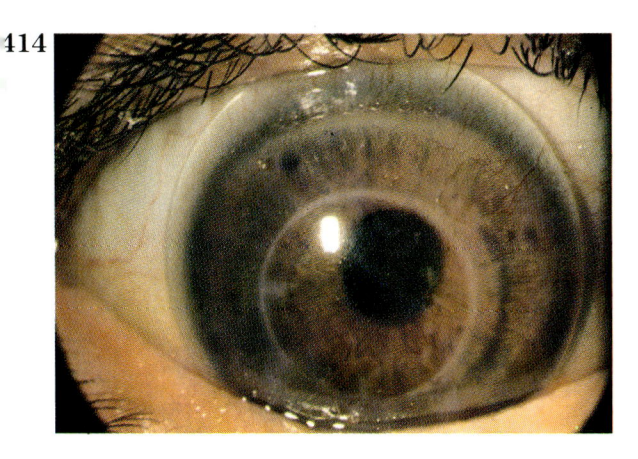

Example: PG size 8 mm K reading = $6.95 \times 100°\ 7.4$
Back surface fit 7.9:8.0/8.5:11/9.0:13.0
$T_c = 0.1$ $T_e = 0.18$ $P = -4.0$

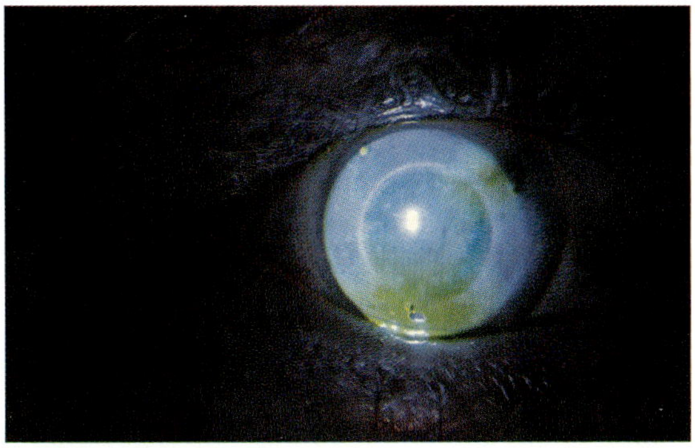

417 Corneoscleral fit where a back tricurve or an aspheric curve would have given less intermediate clearance.

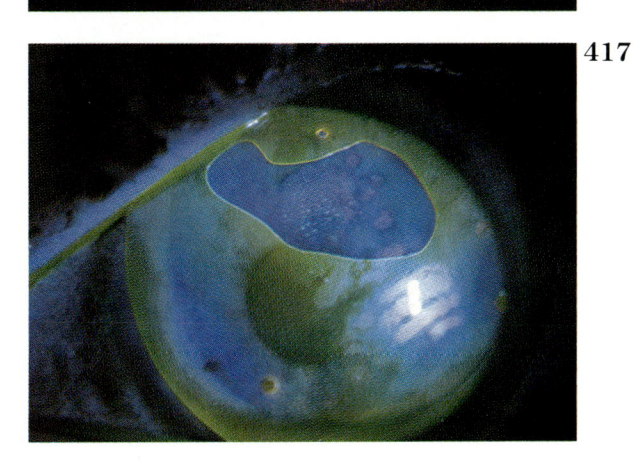

418 Moulded fit scleral hard lens for a PG.

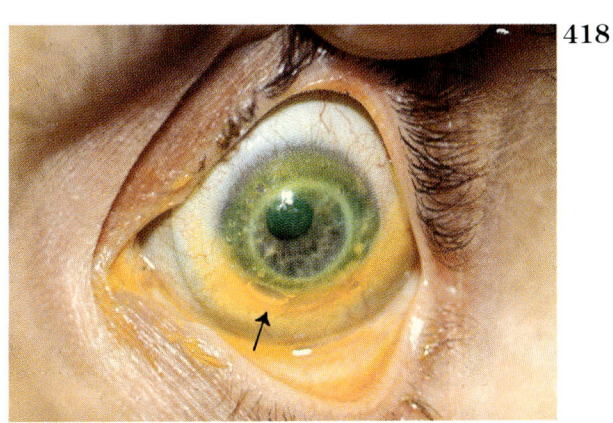

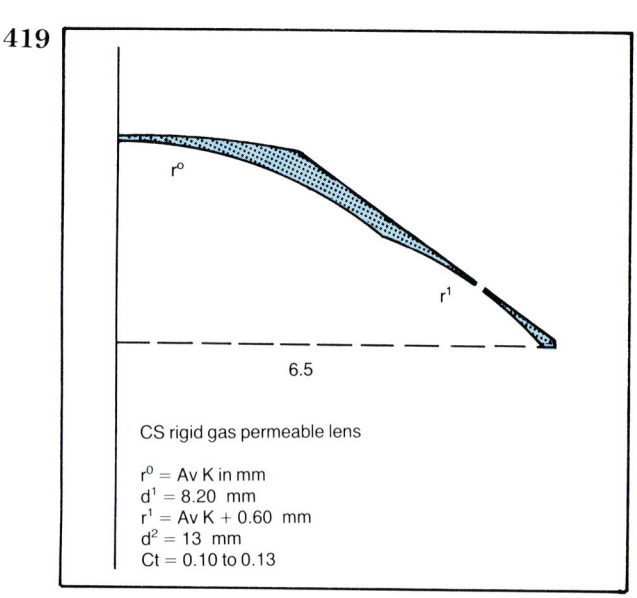

419 The formula for the design of a corneoscleral lens is given. Note the thin areas for gas flow and the thick areas to give lens rigidity. Note also the fenestration.

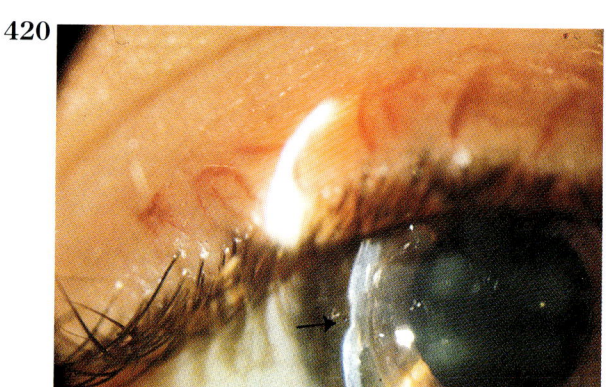

CS rigid gas permeable lens

r^0 = Av K in mm
d^1 = 8.20 mm
r^1 = Av K + 0.60 mm
d^2 = 13 mm
Ct = 0.10 to 0.13

Bandage lenses in keratoplasty

The forms are described on page 134. Temporary materials that eventually dissolve could include alginates or collagen, which must be sterile and can be impregnated with antimicrobial medications.

The use of gels of high or low water content is permissible providing the thicknesses are consistent with good gas flow.

420 Bandage lens over a graft elevation and juxta Dellen formation (dessication). (See arrow.)

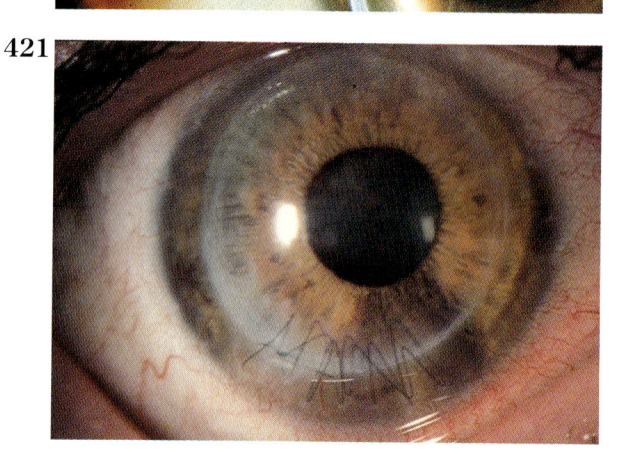

421 Bandage lens over a graft after a segment section to reduce astigmatism and re-suturing.

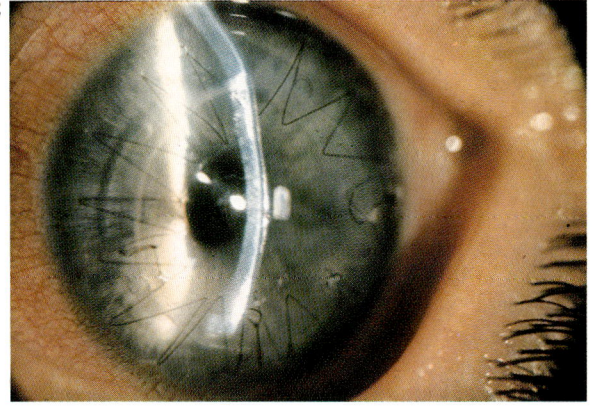

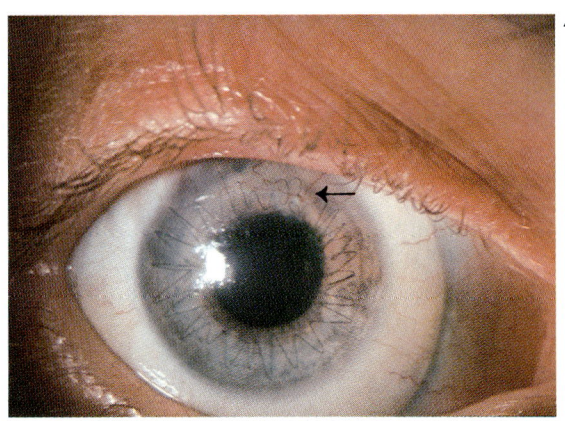

422 & 423 Bandage lenses placed after an operation. Note the thinness of the lens in the section of the beam.

Radiokeratotomy

The procedure may not be followed by a complete refraction correction; in some instances corneal irregularity can also result (this also applies to the other refractive surgery procedures such as epikeratoplasty, keratomileusis and keratophakia).

The following examples are illustrative of how contact lenses are used after the procedure. The case reports and photos are from Dr Joseph A Janes OD, of Bellaire Eye Associates, Houston.

424 History: 3 years post-operation examination.
Pre-op, refraction: Rt. −4.5s. −2.75c × 180°.
Lt. −5.5s. −2.0c × 180° E.E = 20/20 (6/6).
Pre-op K's: Rt. 8.89/8.27 at 93° Lt. 8.58/8.31 at 85°
Post-op refraction: Rt. + 0.75s. = 20/20 Lt. + 1.50s. −2.0c. × 100° = 20/40.
Post-op. K's: Rt. 10.89/9.52 at 72° Lt. 10.53/12.43 at 88°
Fitted with contact lenses 8.15/9.50-4.75d. (left eye only)
With lens of Polycon II = 20/30

Comment:
- The contact lens fitting corrected the anisometropia. The fitting produced a central clearance which could be fenestrated if corneal oedema was a problem.
- The fit and power of the lens used does appear to be within the range of a minimal apical clearance fit that may have been advised pre-operation.
- Smaller diameter lenses will not fit such a flat RK cornea and the only alternatives to consider are corneoscleral lenses or theoretically trapezoid back surface lenses.

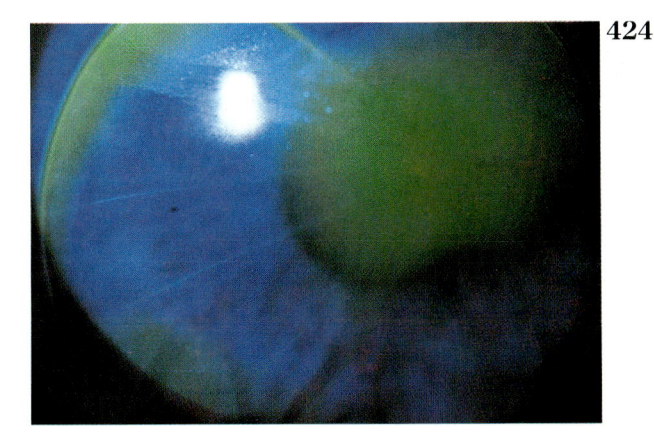

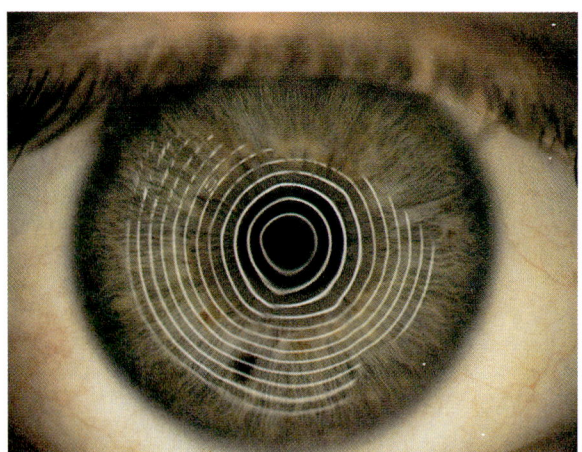

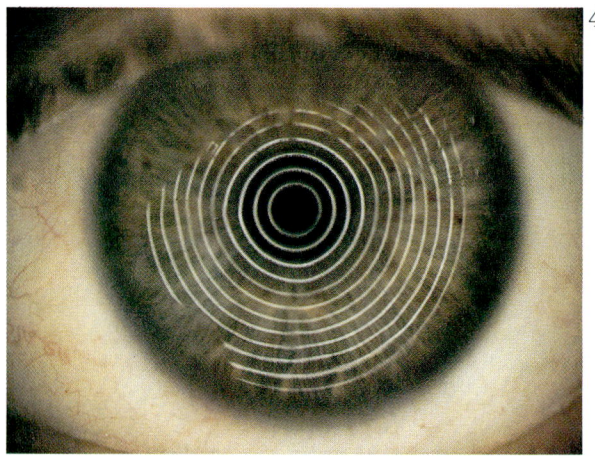

425 & 426 PEK of the eyes 3 years post-operation shows distortion in the right eye and therefore irregular astigmatism. The right eye was fitted with Paraperm EW 8.0/10.5 and the acuity was 20/25.
Specs. Pre-op: Rt. $-3.75 = 20/20$. Lt. $-0.75 -1.75 \times 103° = 20/20$.
Post-op: Rt. $+2.50s - 2.50c. \times 90° = 20/30$. Lt. $+0.50s -1.50 c.x 105° = 20/20$.

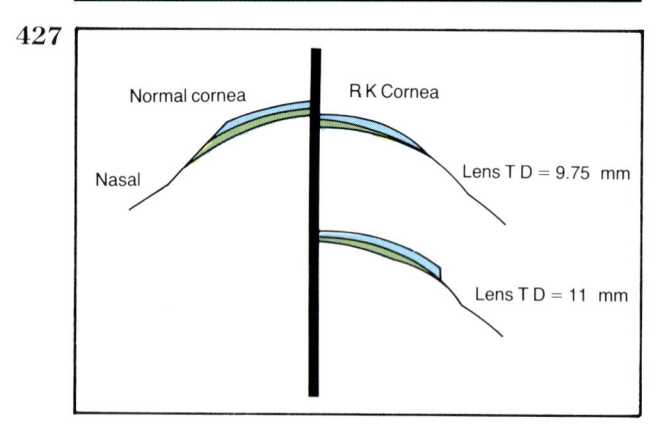

427 Normal and RK cornea and hard lens fits.
The schematic diagram compares the normal and RK cornea and hard lens fits. Note that the spherical back curves for lens sizes up to 10 mm will give central clearance unless the lens is larger or of trapezoid design. A corneoscleral lens with a flat back curve will also give a good central fit.
   Data for the schematic normal corneal shape:
$r_o = 8.0$ $d_o = 6$ mm Sagitta = 3 mm for chord of 12.50
Temporal corneal periphery offset r = 15 mm
Nasal corneal periphery offset r = 10 mm

N.B. After RK the sagitta has decreased over the same chord.

Therapeutic bandage lenses

Hereafter these lenses will be called either bandage lenses or protective lenses to distinguish their function from other lenses which have a therapeutic function in a wider sense.

Collagen therapeutic lenses (B&L) can be applied to the diseased cornea when protection is required—preferably for a limited period. At present, three types are available and they have different solubilty properties (with dissolving times of 12, 24 and 72 hours).

As with the hydrophilic lenses (see page 146) there is the potential to charge the material with drugs, thus giving a delivery system to the cornea and limbal areas.

Data of B&L collagen shield:
  Material: Porcine scleral collagen
  Rapid, intermediate and slow absorption lenses
  Design: Back radii 9mm   Total diameter 14.5
  $T_c = 0.127$ mm
  Rate of hydration: 5 minutes.
  Gas flow = Dk = 27×10^{-11} ATVP
  Dk/L = 21×10^{-9} ATVP
  Water content = 63%

It is important to note that the gas flow properties of some of the lenses are low, and this can be a possible occlusion problem for their long term use. Furthermore, the material will require sufficiency of tears or artificially administered substitute to avoid rapid evaporation.

Historically the first protective lenses were hard scleral lenses fitted flush to the cornea and were introduced in the early 1950s (by Frederick Ridley). The historical precursors of such lenses were conjunctival grafts and flaps, vitelline and placental membranes.

Basic requirements of a bandage lens:
- Thin, soft, with a low evaporation rate if a gel, high Dk/L, large diameter, flat curves, and an ellipsoid shape is preferred.
- For long-term use as an EW lens, or as a short-term degradable lens or made from soluble materials.
- Can be impregnated with medications.
- Can be stored in a sterile state for long periods.

Table 13. Examples of bandage gel lenses

		Thickness	O_2* Dk	Dk/l	Hardness
Sauflon	85% water polyvinyl acrylate	0.12	68	56	1.50
Hoya	75% water polyvinyl acrylate	0.10	55	55	2.00
Bausch & Lomb	38% water HEMA	0.03	10	33	2.50

*Dk Units.
Hardness is relative to PMMA at 100.

Bullous keratopathy

Bullous keratopathy - 1° or 2° endothelial dystrophies. Note:
- The aetiology of BK following surgical procedures such as cataract extraction is well known but a small proportion may have an *inherent* endothelial dysfunction.
- There is a paradox. Thus, all contact lenses have the potential to cause endothelial dysfunction and therefore secondary corneal oedema. Their use in the treatment of corneal oedema of a transient and reversible nature would appear therefore to be contra indicated unless they have a high Dk/L.
- The progenitor of the endothelial dysfunction, when contact lens induced, is the epithelium. Therefore, where the epithelium is already abnormal the contact lens only serves to protect and to reduce painful bleb episodes.
- Many BK eyes respond well to PG surgery.

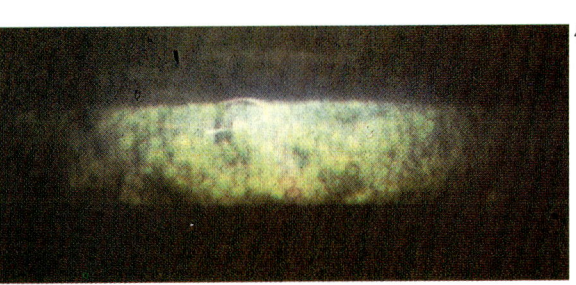

428 Endothelium of aphakic with BK. Note the loss of endothelium.

429 Aphakic BK with a soft bandage lens.

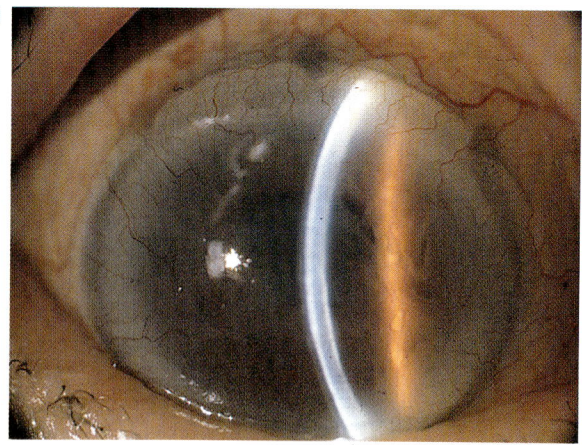

430 BK following anterior chamber IOL implant. Treated with a bandage lens to alleviate pain.

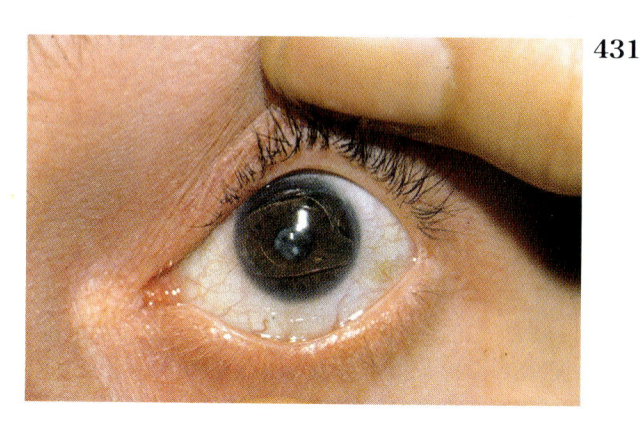

431 The other eye without BK complication.

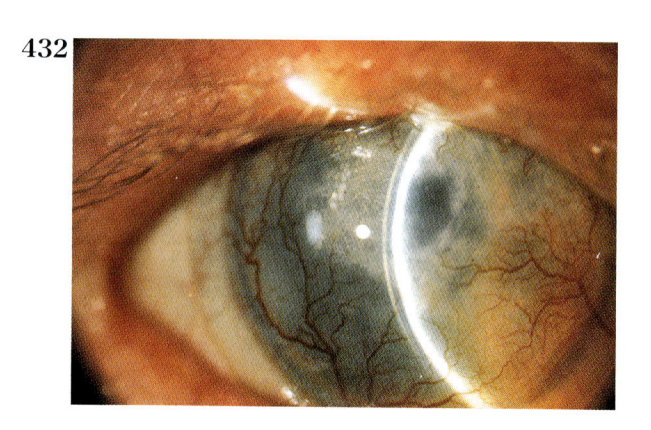

432 Corneal vascularization of BK cornea after the use of a thick gel lens (not a bandage lens).

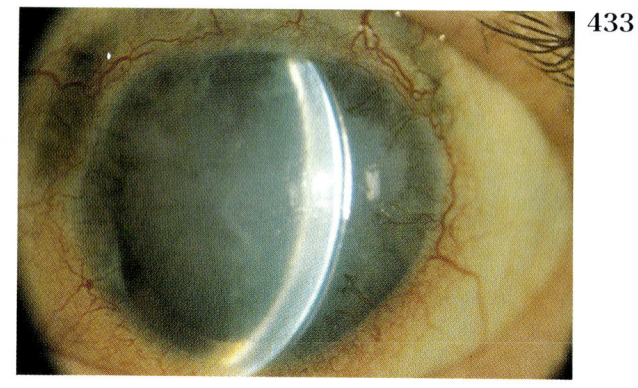

433 Severe BK post-cataract operation subsequently grafted.

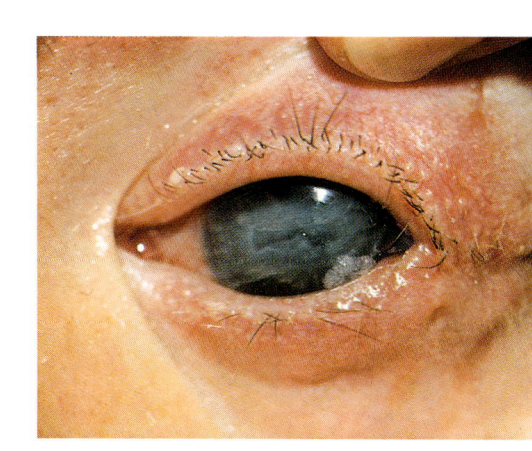

434 Eye with BK combination of a soft and hard corneal lens to give some acuity.

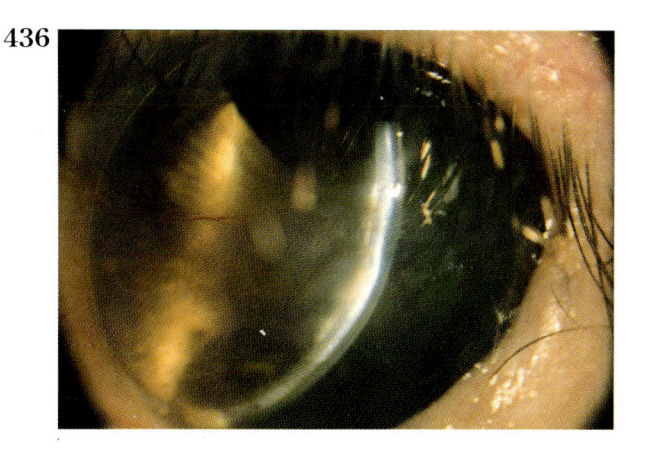

435 Buphthalmos with BK. This adult had severe episodes of suppurative keratitis in an only eye and responded to bandage lens treatment and antibiotics.

436 One year later, still wearing a bandage lens. *N.B.* Some ophthalmologists prefer to use a thicker lens to induce corneal vascularization and therefore rapid healing.

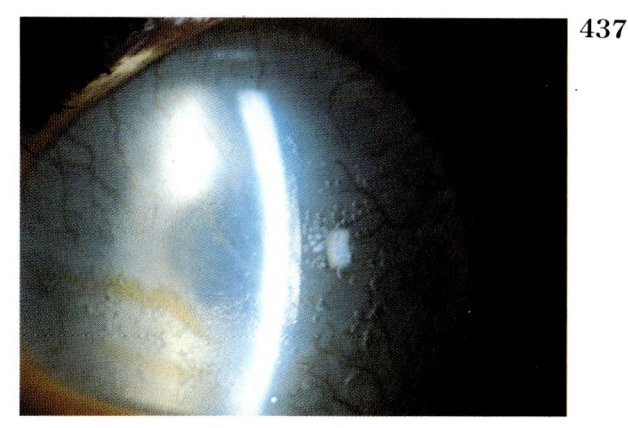

437 Buphthalmos with BK. This adult preferred scleral hard lenses to gel lenses because of the better acuity.

Recurrent erosions

438 Basement membrane disease—recurrent erosions. The bandage lens can give comfort during painful episodes and in those cases where recurrent episodes are frequent.
Paradox. Contact lenses themselves can cause corneal basement membrane injury from over-wear or hard lens trauma and then this can be treated with the gel lens.

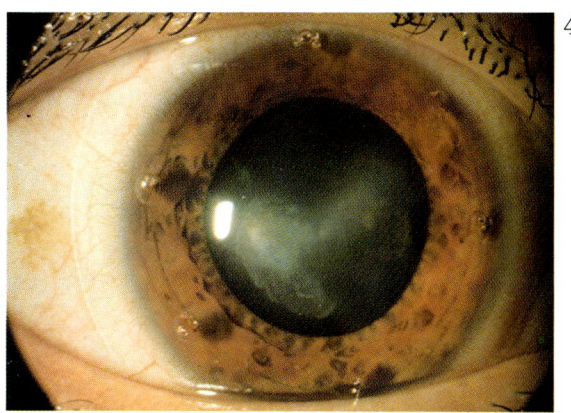

Mesodermal dysplasia

439

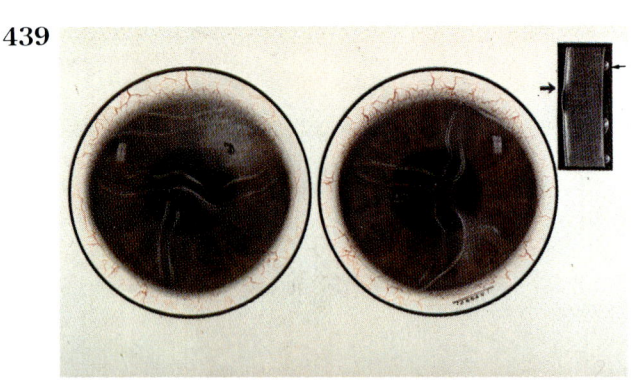

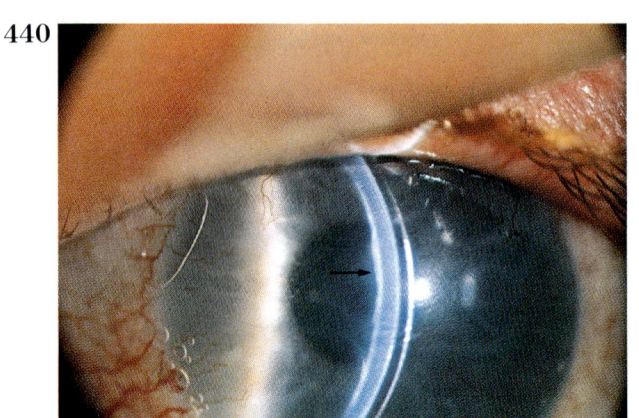

439 & 440 Mesodermal dysplasia and endothelial dysfunction—congenital. In this patient subsequent keratoplasty failed and the remaining eye preferred hard scleral lens wear to gel for reasons of better acuity. The arrows in both illustrations show the abnormal endothelial infolding.

441 Inflammatory kerato conjunctivitis. (Dermatokeratitis, possibly of immune aetiology.)

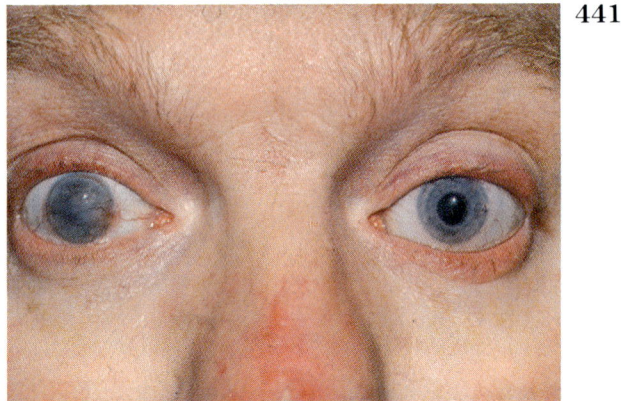

440

441

Acne rosacea

Marginal inflammatory ulceration

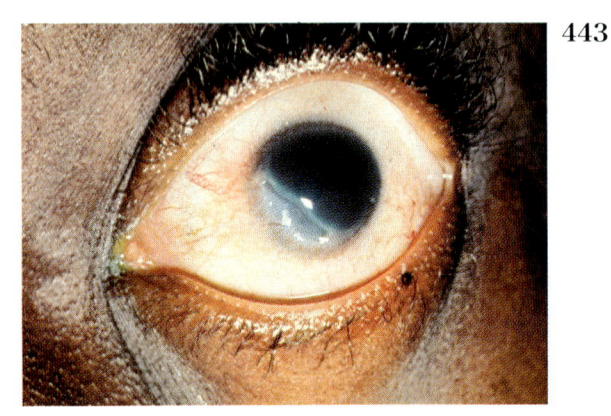

442

443

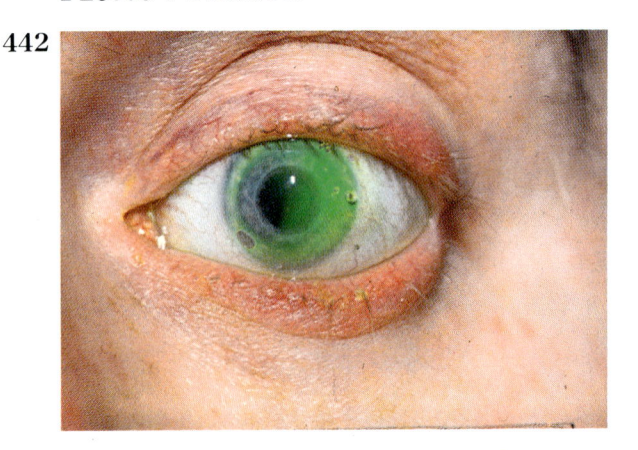

442 Acne rosacea. Contact lenses are used to give better acuity. The grafted left cornea responded best to scleral lens wear (periodic, 4 hours × 3 daily). Other types of lenses were tried.

443 Marginal ulceration (possibly Mooren's ulcer). Treated with a soft lens and steroids during the active phase. Eventually it became quiescent and the patient changed to spectacles.

Pathological dry eye

Dessication of the cornea and conjunctivae can be of several and diverse aetiologies. From the contact lens practitioner's viewpoint, it is necessary to have some classification so that the lens management can be effective. The related dessication problems induced by cosmetic visual contact lenses are not included here.

Causes of pathological dry eye:
- lacrimal gland and accessory glands: atrophy of involutional, latrogenic (toxic), inflammatory or immune reactions.
- Lipid deficiency, e.g. Meibomian gland dysfunction or loss.
- Mucopolysaccharide loss and anomalies due to goblet cell loss, from inflammatory, chemical and radiation trauma, for example.
- Thus, any or all of the three tear film components (lipid, aqueous and mucin), if absent or abnormal, will result in eye disease and only with expert management can the contact lens be of any value.
- Abnormal lid closure (exposure keratitis).

By itself—without adjuvant medications—the lens can be a complication and not a treatment.

Use and function of the contact lens in pathological dry eye:
- To protect dry areas, by the retention and non-evaporation of water.
- To provide artificial tears on a continuous basis.

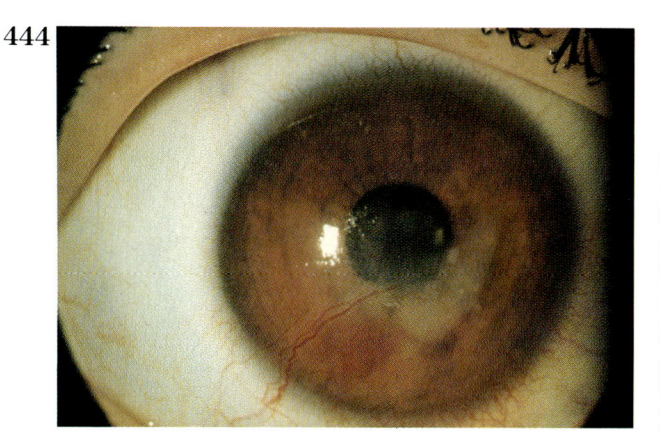

444 & 445 Familial dysautonomia (Riley-Day syndrome). Use of high water content (75 per cent) gel lenses combined with artificial tears and systemic cholinergic drugs. The use of paraffin (medicinal) oils at night with the lenses *in situ*.

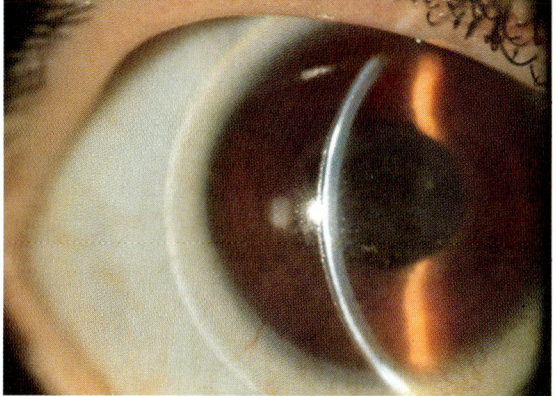

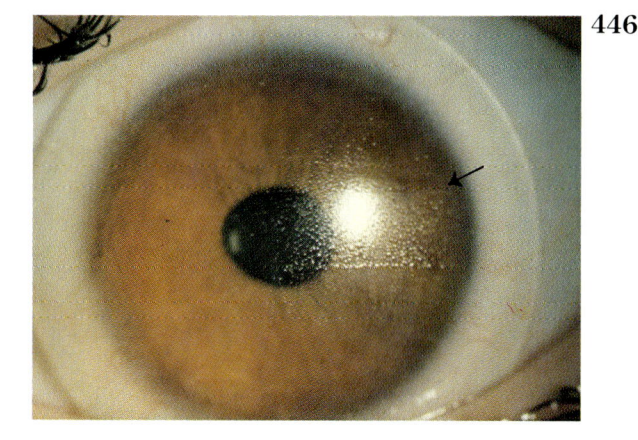

446 After 6 years' wear. The patient then preferred the daily use of paraffin oil drops. The oily haze can be seen on the lens surface.

447 & 448 Neuropathic keratitis (5th cranial nerve ganglion ablation). Both are of young patients referred for contact lens treatment one year after brain surgery and who refused tarsorraphy. Both were treated with daily wear gel lenses and 'Blenderm' strapping of the lids at night.

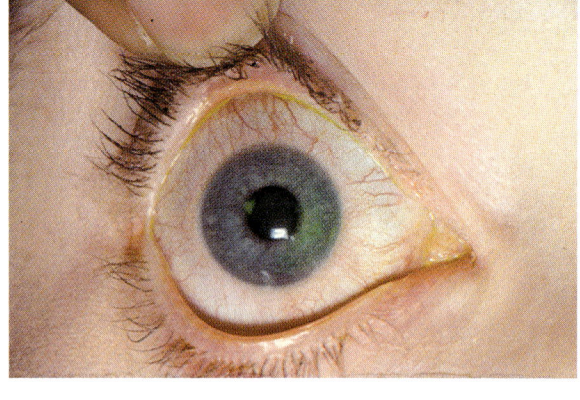

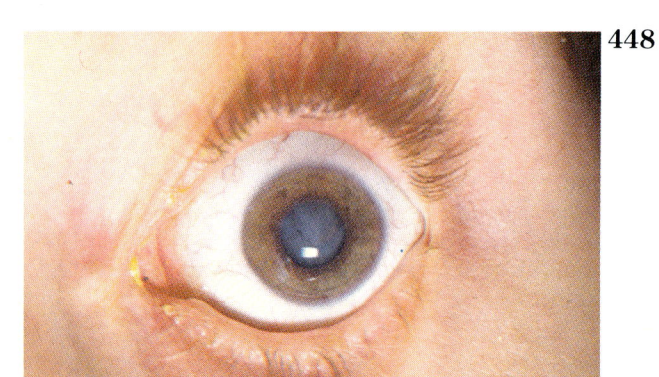

449 & 450 Exposure keratitis—pityriasis rubra. The patient was unable to close his lids because of skin contraction and recurrent corneal erosions. The cornea was protected by scieral lenses—gel lenses dried and fell off the eye.

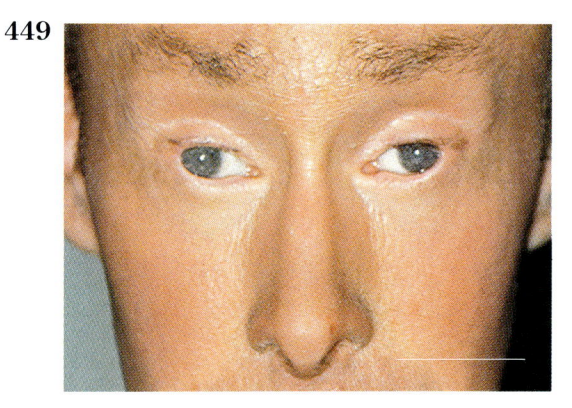

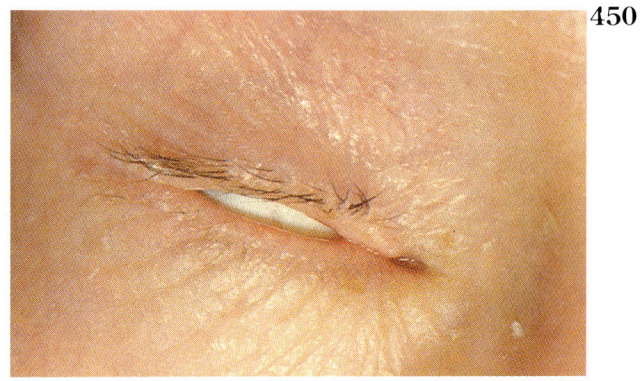

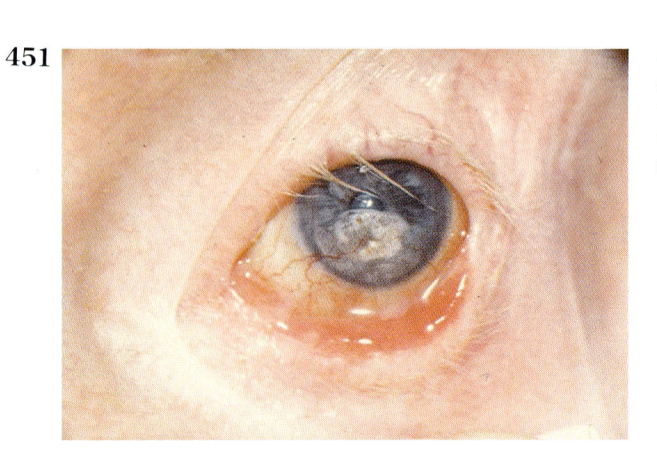

451 Exposure keratitis. Exposure due to chronic ectropia resulting in dessication keratinization, corneal vascularization and eventually lipid infiltration. Surgical treatment was refused and contact lens treatment was not advised after fitting because of the patient's senility.

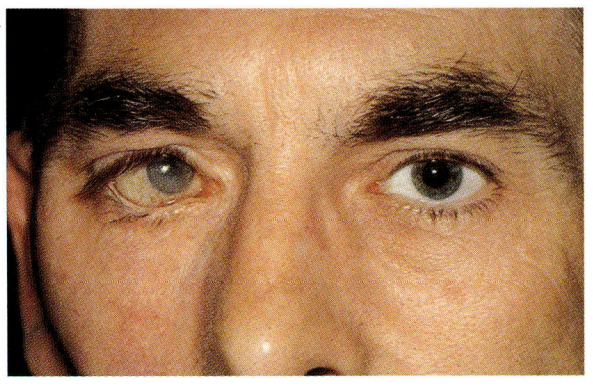

452 **VII cranial nerve paralysis** leading to exposure keratitis. Scleral lenses were worn night and day with periods of rest and lens cleaning.

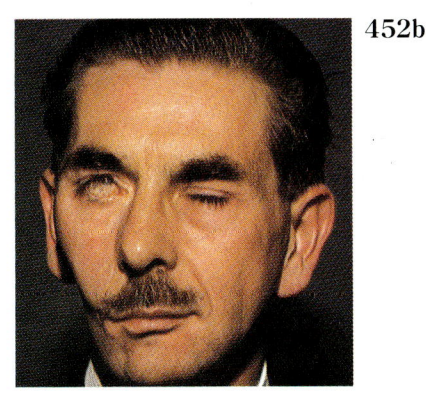

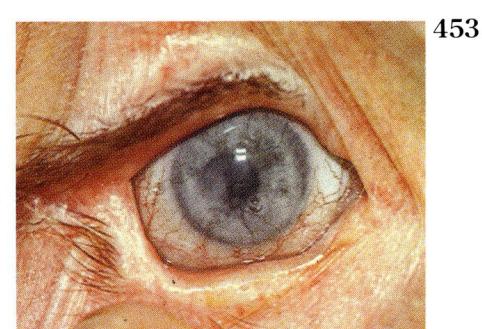

453 **Fenestrations and Bell's reflex**, which is useful to cause tear fluid circulation.

Stevens-Johnson syndrome

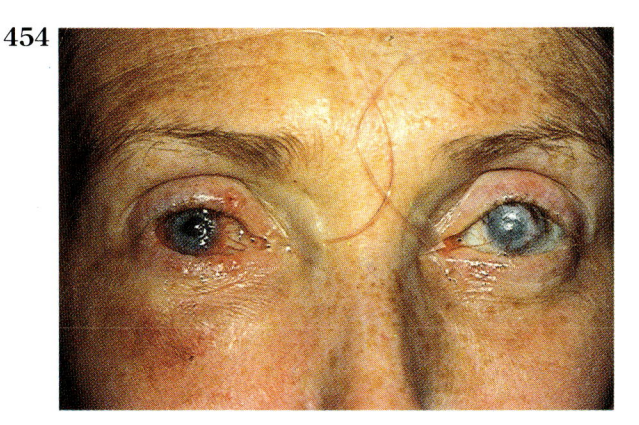

454 **Stevens-Johnson syndrome—erythema multiforme.** Adverse drug reaction. Treated with scleral lenses and continuous wetting by capillary perfusion from a plastic tank.

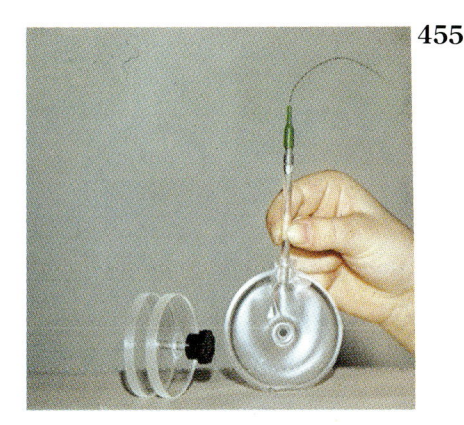

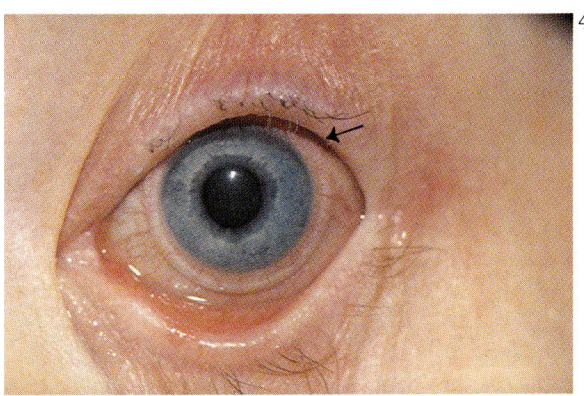

455 **Perfusion tank** taken out of its plastic pressure container.

456 **Stevens-Johnson syndrome.** Mild case treated with daily wear gel lens and periodic use of artificial tears.

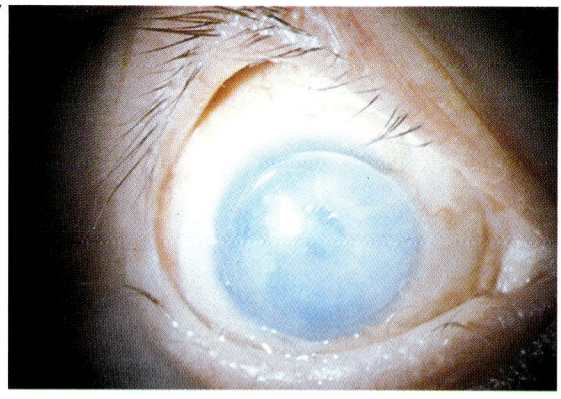

457 & 458 Stevens-Johnson syndrome. Right eye fitted with a clear hard scleral lens and the other, blind eye with a prosthetic lens.

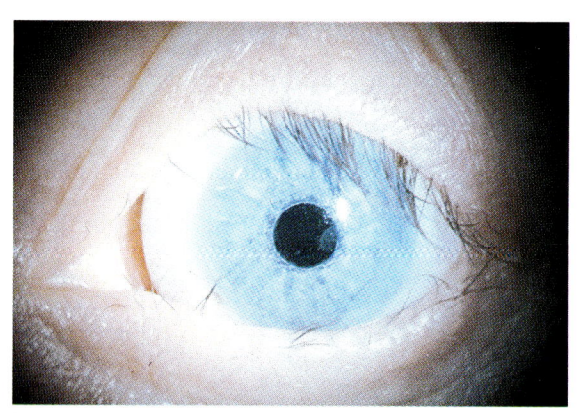

Benign mucus membrane atrophy (BMMA)

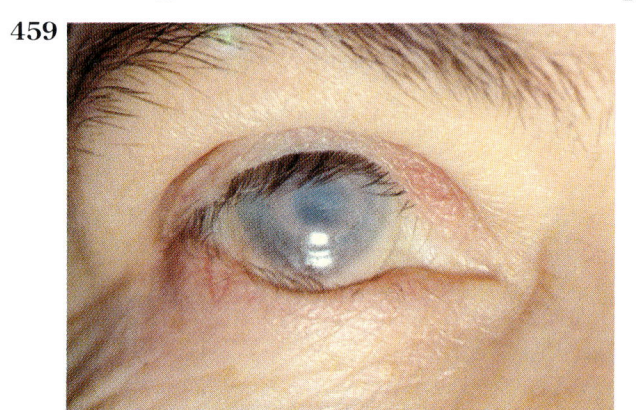

459 BMMA treated with a hard 13 mm diameter contact lens, plus artificial tear drops. High Dk/L, fenestration and plano $T_c = 0.1$ mm.

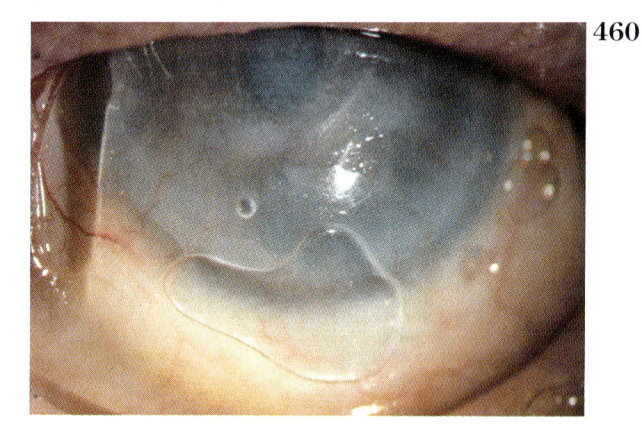

460 BMMA treated with a scleral hard lens.

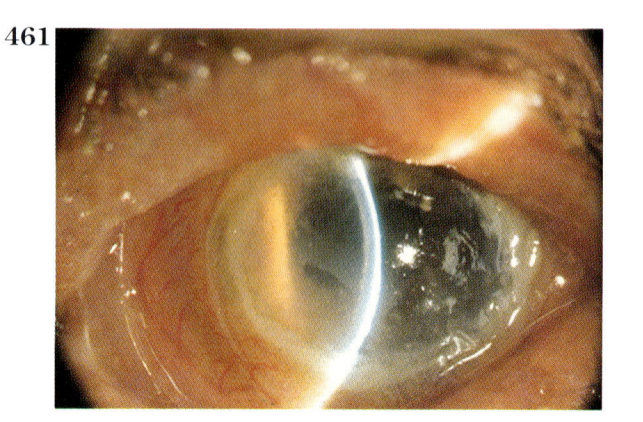

461 BMMA lower fornix—surgically opened and a 2 mm plastic ring inserted for 6 weeks. Treated with steroid local drops until the fornix had epithelialized. The patient was then fitted with a small scleral hard lens.

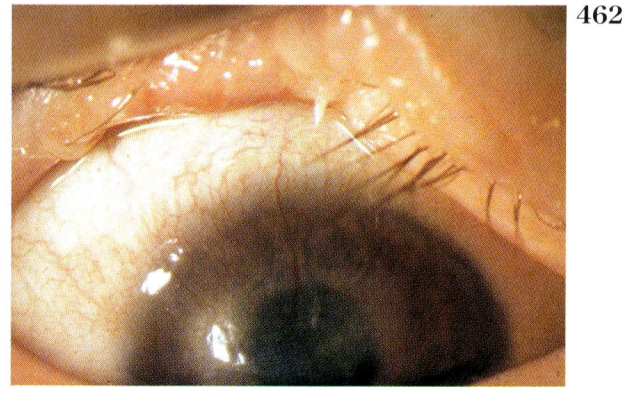

462 Severe trichiasis unsuccessfully treated with surgery. Interim treatment was with a gel bandage lens subsequent to further plastic surgery.

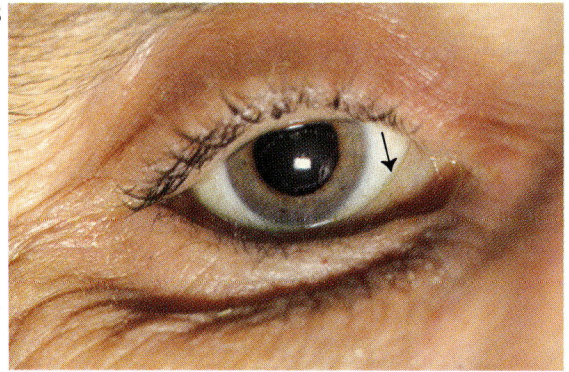

463 & 464   Facial hemiatrophy. Chronic keratitis due to poor lid coverage. The patient is fitted with a scleral ring to hold the lid tear meniscus in place.

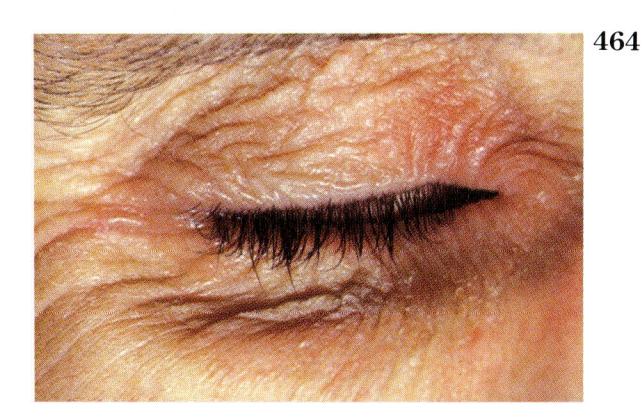

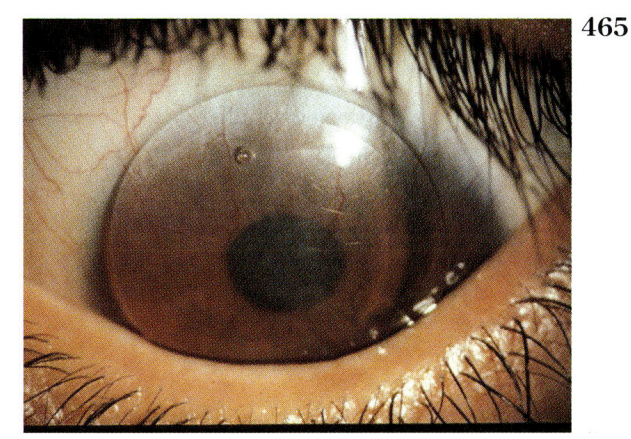

465   Mucous membrane atrophy secondary to trachoma. A silicone rubber lens used with artificial tears. *N.B.* This type of lens is softer than hard materials and does not require water to maintain its form. It must be a loose fitting.

Ocular burns

Ocular burns are mostly of chemical or heat aetiology.

- The principles of contact lens treatment are to prevent symblepharon and protect the cornea.
- If symblepharon is a complication then division and reformation of the fornices is necessary.
- In the instances of the eye permanently blinded by burns there is subsequent plastic surgery and the prosthesis to consider.

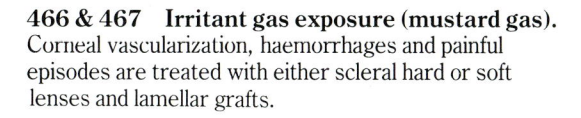

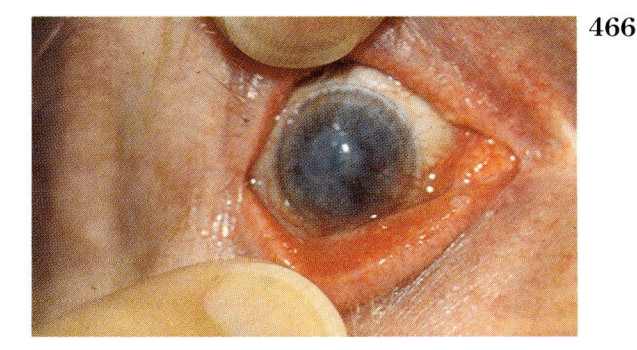

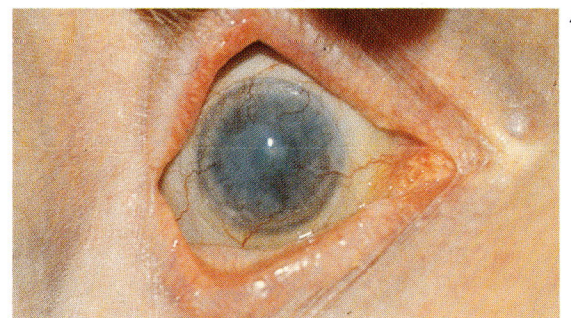

466 & 467   Irritant gas exposure (mustard gas). Corneal vascularization, haemorrhages and painful episodes are treated with either scleral hard or soft lenses and lamellar grafts.

468 & 469 Chemical burns (lye). This eye was treated by early grafting; it showed graft rejection and 2° glaucoma. A soft bandage lens and local steroids resolved the eye for a period of one year before further keratoplasty was undertaken.

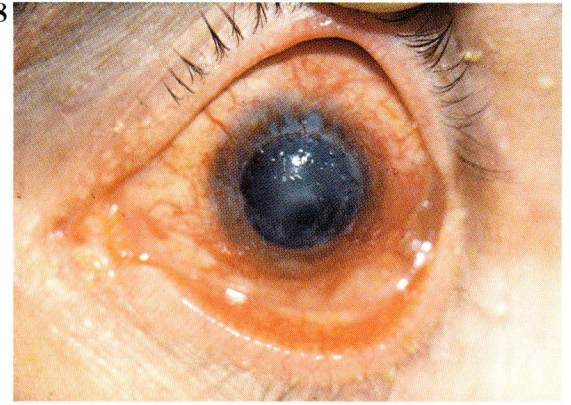

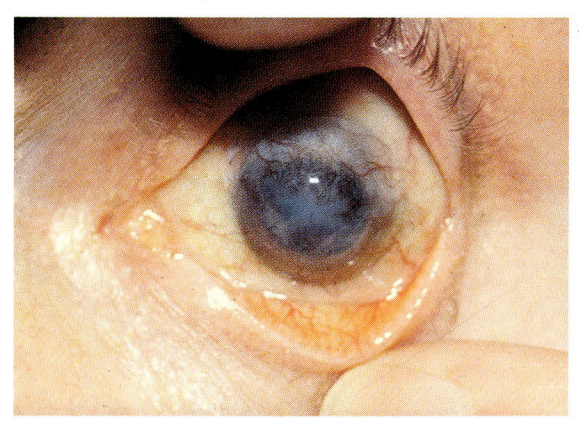

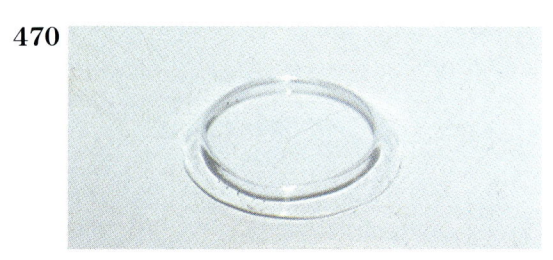

Symblepharon

470 Symblepharon prevention. One of a set of rings of PMMA material 23-26 mm in diameter, 1 mm thick and 2-3 mm width.

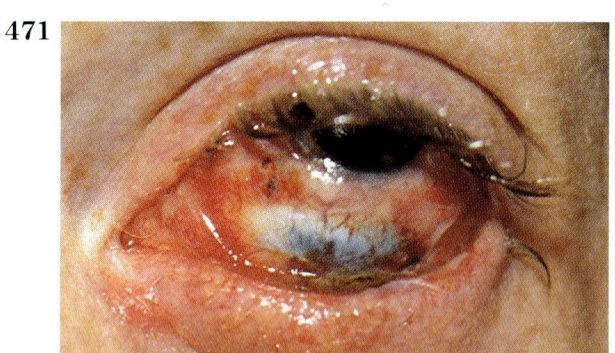

471 Ring *in situ* after molten metal burn.

472 Ring *in situ* after molten metal burn.

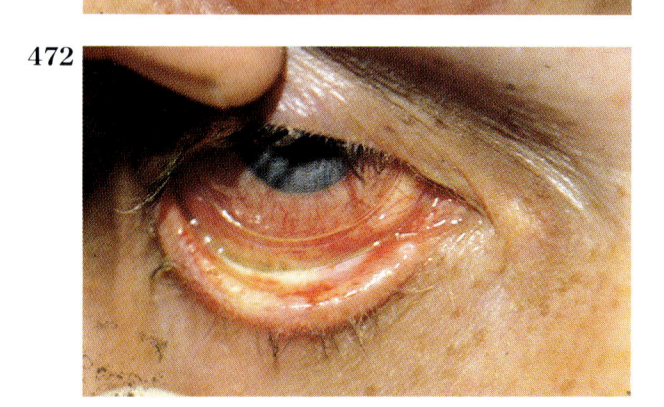

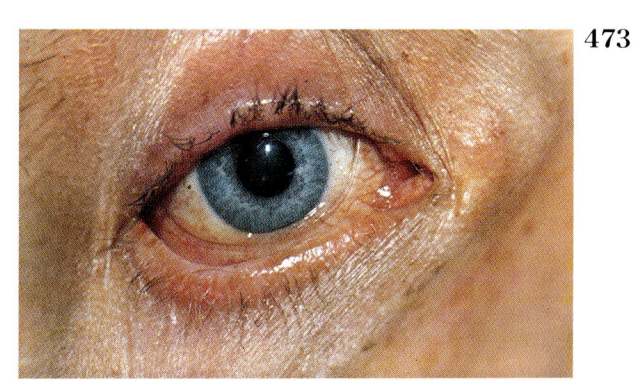

473 Several weeks later, the ring is still *in situ* and there is no symblepharon.

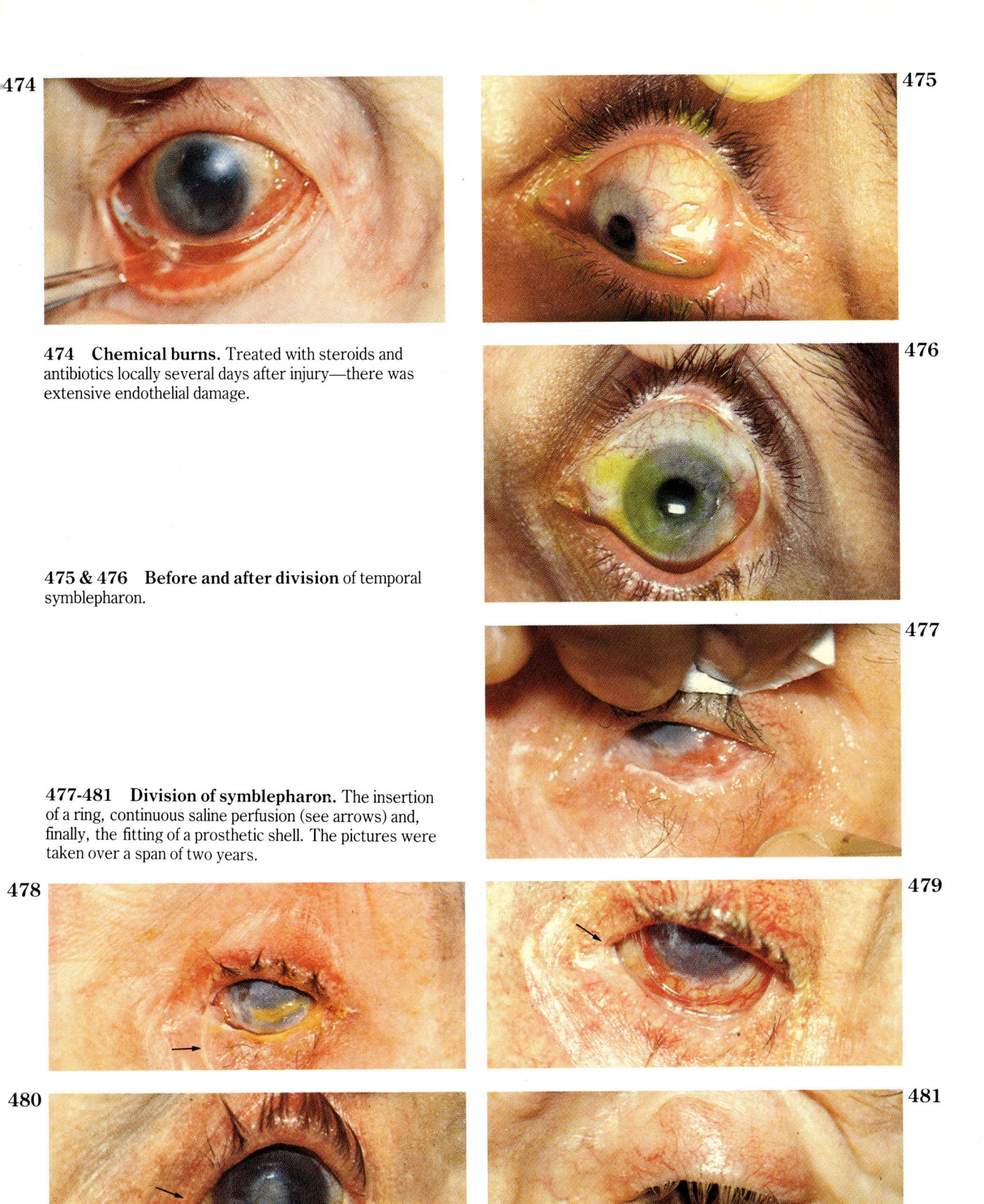

474 Chemical burns. Treated with steroids and antibiotics locally several days after injury—there was extensive endothelial damage.

475 & 476 Before and after division of temporal symblepharon.

477-481 Division of symblepharon. The insertion of a ring, continuous saline perfusion (see arrows) and, finally, the fitting of a prosthetic shell. The pictures were taken over a span of two years.

145

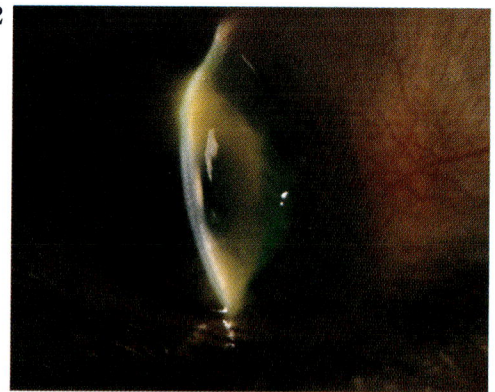

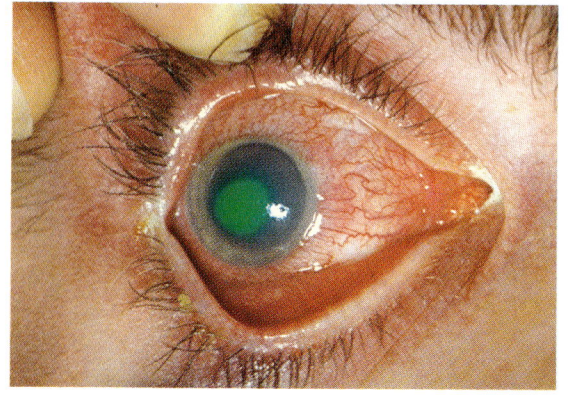

482 **Ammonia burn** (from a criminal attack). A bandage lens is used to alleviate pain.

483 **Ammonia burn.** A bandage lens plus irrigation are used.

484 **Metal burn.** The ring was removed 3 months after injury. Note plaque formation (arrowed) but elsewhere the fornix has epithelialized.

Note: In instances of sealed therapeutic scleral and corneoscleral lenses, Refojo and Rosenthal suggest O_2 retention fluids in the tear-lens space (e.g. halocarbon oil).

Drug dispensing gel lenses

- Hydrophilic gel lenses can be selective in the absorption of drugs.

- The higher the water content, the larger the molecule absorbed and the more rapid the elution.

- Among the many drugs that have been experimented with but never commercialized are pilocarpine, atropine, IDU and steroids. Their use by the practitioner is likely to be limited to the need of the individual case.

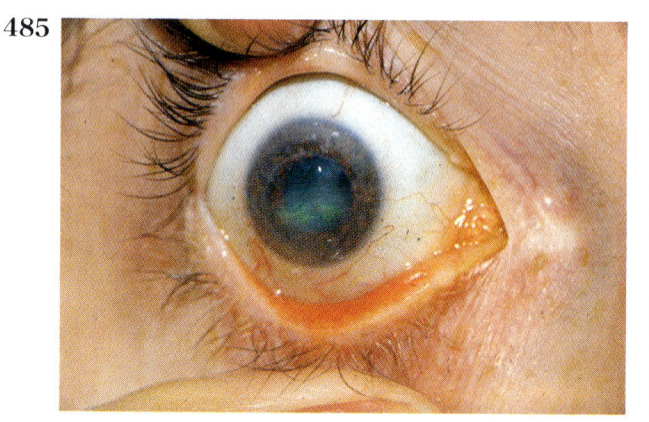

485 & 486 **Herpes simplex.** Antiviral therapy for herpes simplex in a patient who did not respond to drop therapy.

487 & 488 Metaherpetic ulceration The gel lenses have large fenestrations so that additional drug therapy can be administered. Note that the cornea will not be exposed to drugs instilled over an *in situ* gel lens. Only if the lens is pre-charged can it allow a retro-lens flow of the active agent.

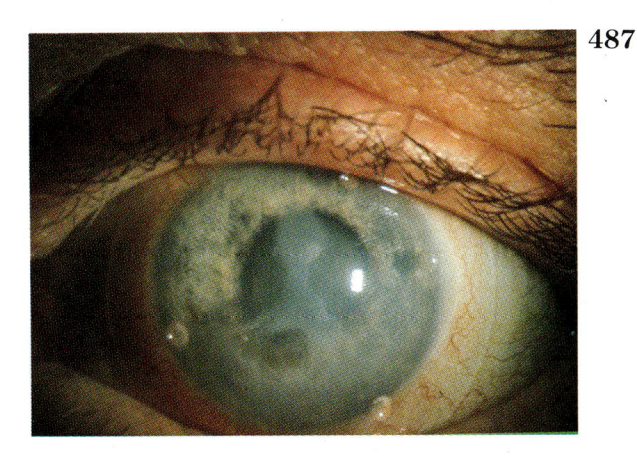

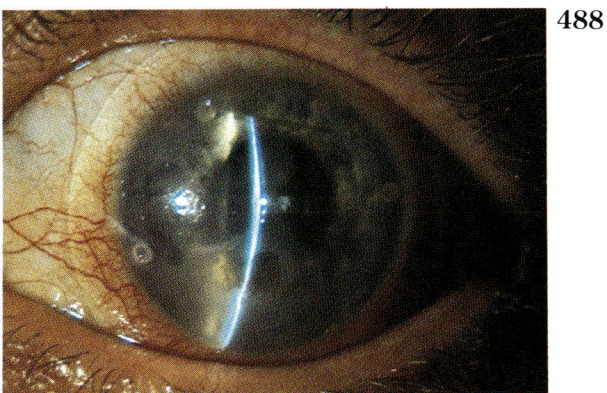

489 Rates of pilocarpine release from different gel materials.

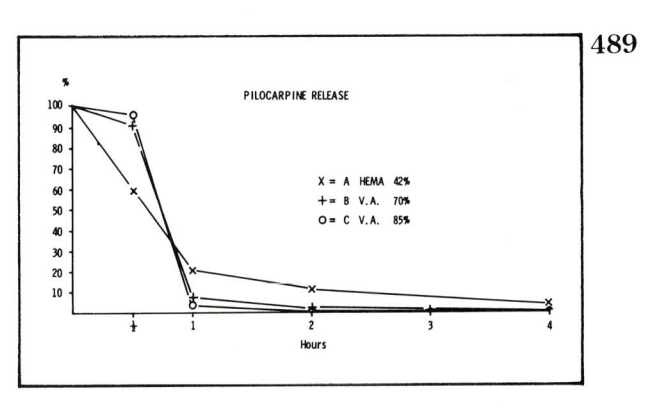

490 HEMA lens charged with pilocarpine 4 per cent without preservative. Good miosis was still present 10 hours later.

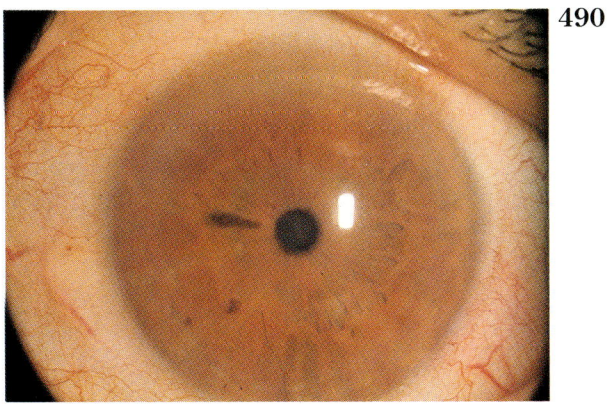

147

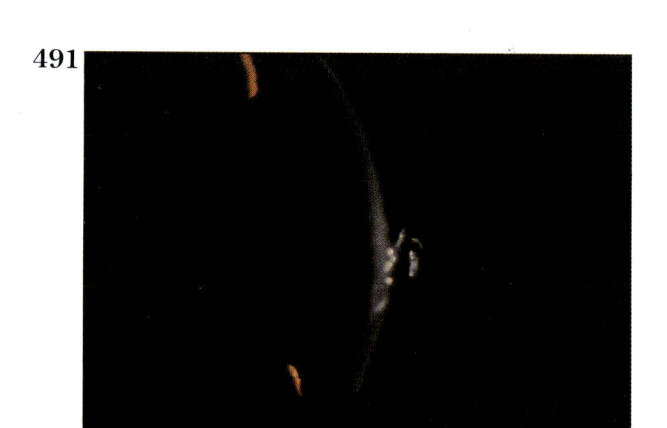

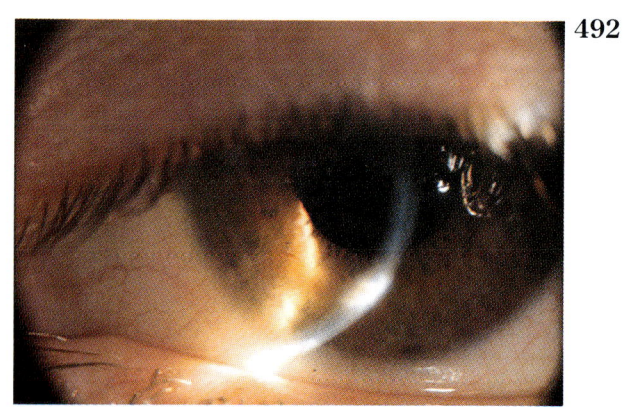

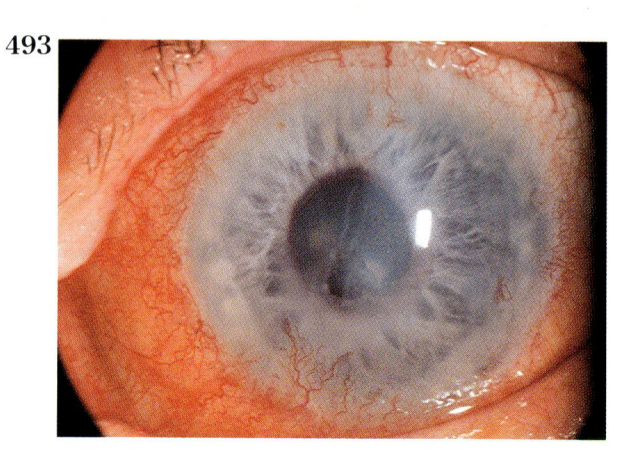

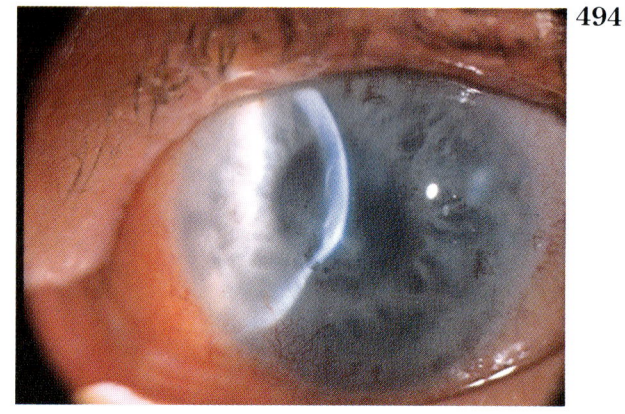

491-494 Anterior chamber reformation using large therapeutic bandage lenses. Such lenses will help those conditions where stromal healing is deficient; it will not necessarily increase the rate of epithelialization. (Figs. 491 & 492 are of puncture wounds of the cornea; Figs 493 & 494 are front and slit-lamp views of corneal perforation.)

Ocular myopathies

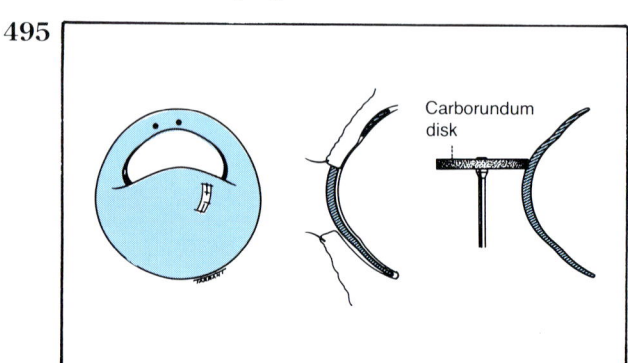

The examples shown are of scleral lenses fitted either with ledges or made with a slot with a thickened centre (Trodd type).

495 Method of manufacture.

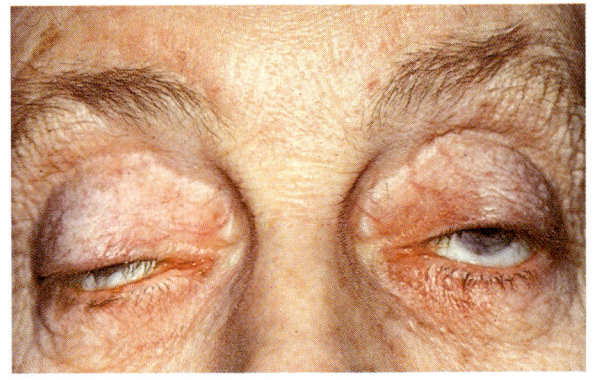

496 & 497 Ocular myopathy patient wearing the lenses.

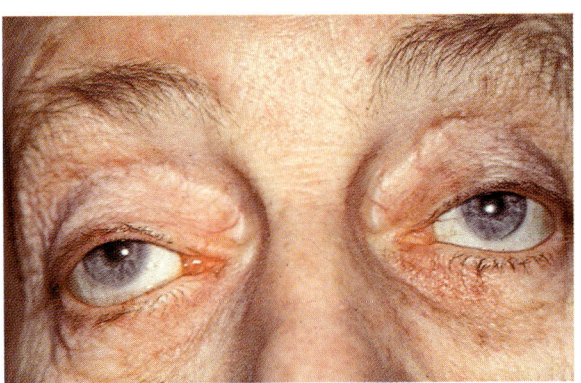

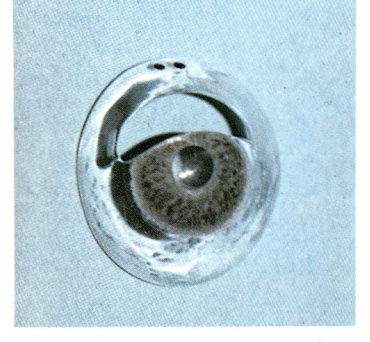

498 Occlusive coloured ptosis—scleral lens.

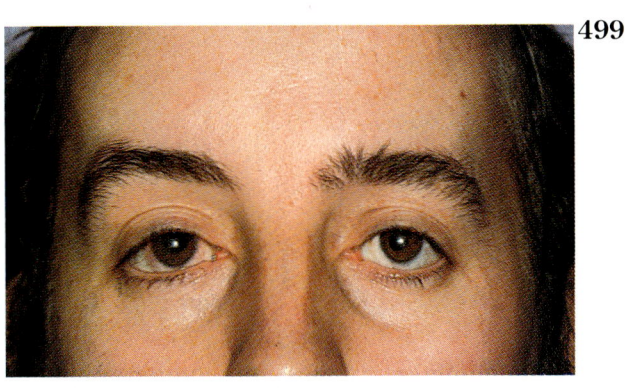

499 & 500 Myotonic dystrophy patient wearing the lenses. Note the collection of coagulated mucin (arrow) due to *no* tear circulation. Myasthenia gravis with myopathy may also benefit from these devices.

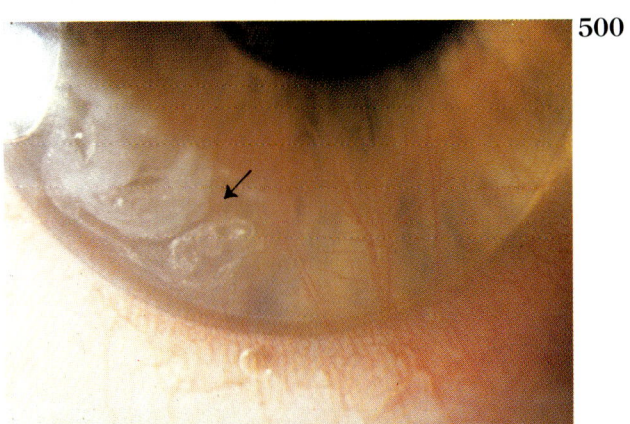

8 Adverse reactions to contact lens wear

During the early years of contact lens development (1900-1950), the chief interest was to obtain a scleral lens that did not produce corneal oedema, and to obtain better tolerance in the fit. Wearing time before problems arose was normally 4 hours. However, every fitter had all-day wearers even with what by modern standards would be considered totally occlusive lenses.

With the advent of the corneal lens (1950 onwards) and later the gel lens (1960 onwards) the fitting and demand for lenses became a commercial venture. At the same time, because many thousands (and later millions) were wearing lenses, health authorities in some countries decided to set standards of safety and quality.

This section illustrates the adverse reactions seen over a 20-year period. Irrespective of the lens worn they follow a pattern. Some animal and laboratory studies are included to illustrate various points.

The eye, more than any other organ in the body, is amenable to diverse and minute quantitative measurements. Thus literature is more than replete

Table 14. Pathological response to contact lens wear

Tissue	Cause	Effect
Epithelium	Pressure	Squamous cell membrane breakdown
	Hypoxia	Cell separation and oedema cysts
	Dessication	Basal cell flattening Cell loss: ulceration, infection Pannus formation
Basement membrane	Trauma	Recurrent erosion of basement membrane
Stroma	Water retention 2° Hypoxia Immune response Inflammatory response Micro-organisms Dessication	Oedema and collagen separation Keratocyte degeneration Infiltration: white cells 　　　　　　　fibroblasts 　　　　　　　new vessels Collagen lysis
Endothelium & Descemet's membrane	pH imbalance 2° to hypoxia	Cell vacuolation Cell separation Cell morphology changes
Lids	Trauma Infection Immune response	Squamous belepharitis Exudative belepharitis Meibominitis Papillary and follicular conjunctivitis
Anterior chamber	Inflammatory response and infection	Anterior uveitis and cells

with data on contact lens research.

The real problem is to know what is of clinical significance to the patient and practitioner. Research into new products is now mostly in the hands of the R&D departments of the large manufacturers and it is important they consider the best interests of the patient as a basis for their work.

Causes of the pathological response to lenses

The basic causes are:
- Trauma
- Cell membrane and metabolic disturbance due to hypoxia and toxic effects
- Immune responses
- Inflammation
- Infection

The eye tissue responds by cellular hypertrophy, atrophy and infiltration of inflammatory and repair cells and agents. Depending upon the individual, the responses may be reversible hypersensitivity or, at the other extreme, chronic and insidious pathological tissue changes.

Gaseous exchange

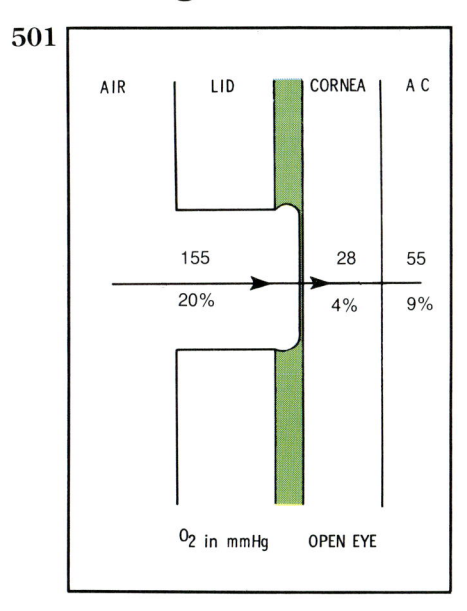

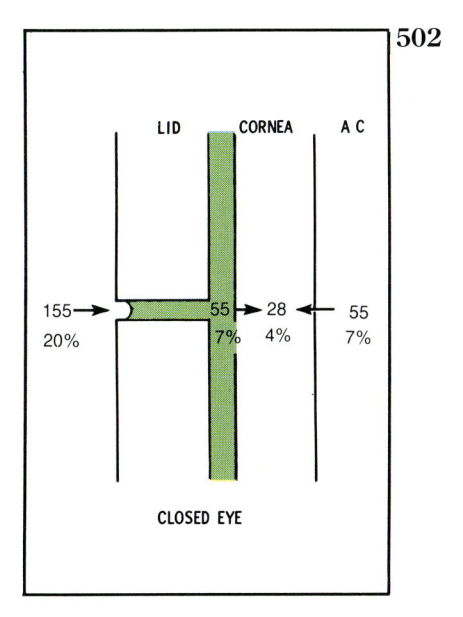

501 Atmospheric O_2 pressure and the open eye state (at sea level). Above sea level or in artificial atmospheres, a lower O_2 pressure can exist and this will reduce these figures.

502 Normal closure of the lids even for several years (tarsorrhaphy) does not produce extreme pathological changes in the cornea. Therefore the corneal epithelium can sustain normal metabolism at corneal tear surface O_2 uptake pressures of 7 per cent (approx 50mmHg, which is one-third of the normal atmospheric pressure). The anterior chamber is at the level of the iris capillaries and is also about O_2 50mmHg, likewise the lid capillaries O_2 pressure. The eye lids are never absolutely sealed in normal sleep or tarsorraphy. Evidence exists to show that *absolute* lid seal does produce corneal epithelial pathological changes.

503

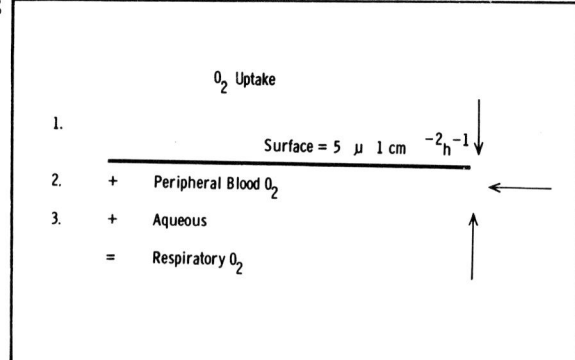

```
                    O₂ Uptake
1.    ──────────────────────────────────  ↓
              Surface = 5 μ 1 cm⁻²h⁻¹
2.    +   Peripheral Blood O₂          ←
3.    +   Aqueous
      =   Respiratory O₂               ↑
```

503 The O₂ uptake of the cornea has individual variations but is between 2 and 5 μ $1cm^2/h$. Most of the O_2 is related to cellular activity and the squamous epithelium takes most of the uptake. Depletion of O_2 decreases the rate of cell reproduction (mitosis) and reduces the reserves of glycogen in the cells. The glycolytic anoxic cycles then become more active but produce less energy and decrease the nucleotide production of the basal cells. The oxygenation cycles required to break down pyruvates and lactates to carbon dioxide and water are deficient and, therefore, corneal hypoxia sees increased lactates in the stroma and AC. The upset in the balance of ions reduces the flow of 'water carrying' molecules such as bicarbonate and chlorine and therefore the stroma becomes oedematous.

504

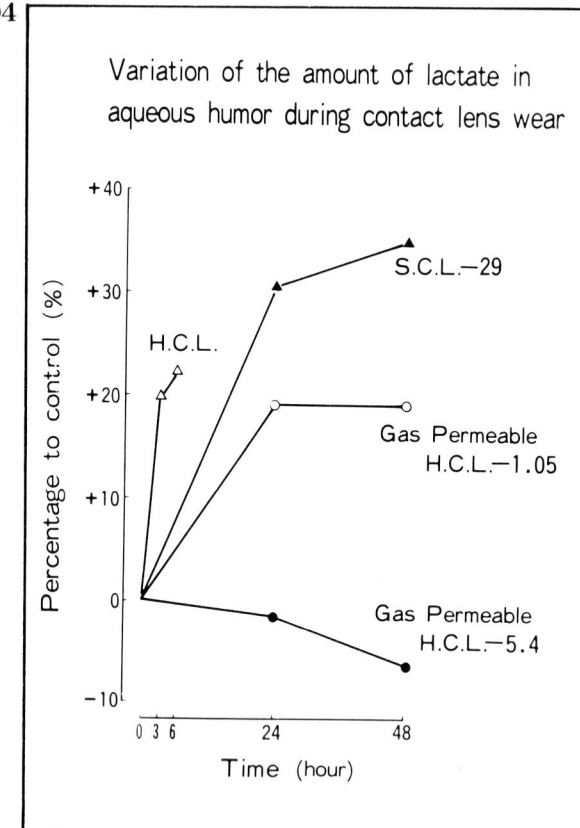

Variation of the amount of lactate in aqueous humor during contact lens wear

(Graph: Percentage to control (%) vs Time (hour); curves labeled S.C.L.–29, H.C.L., Gas Permeable H.C.L.–1.05, Gas Permeable H.C.L.–5.4)

505

Variation of the number of cell division in corneal epithelium during contact lens wear

(Graph: Percentage to control (%) vs Time (hour); curves labeled Gas Permeable H.C.L.–5.4, H.C.L., Gas Permeable H.C.L.–1.05, S.C.L.–29)

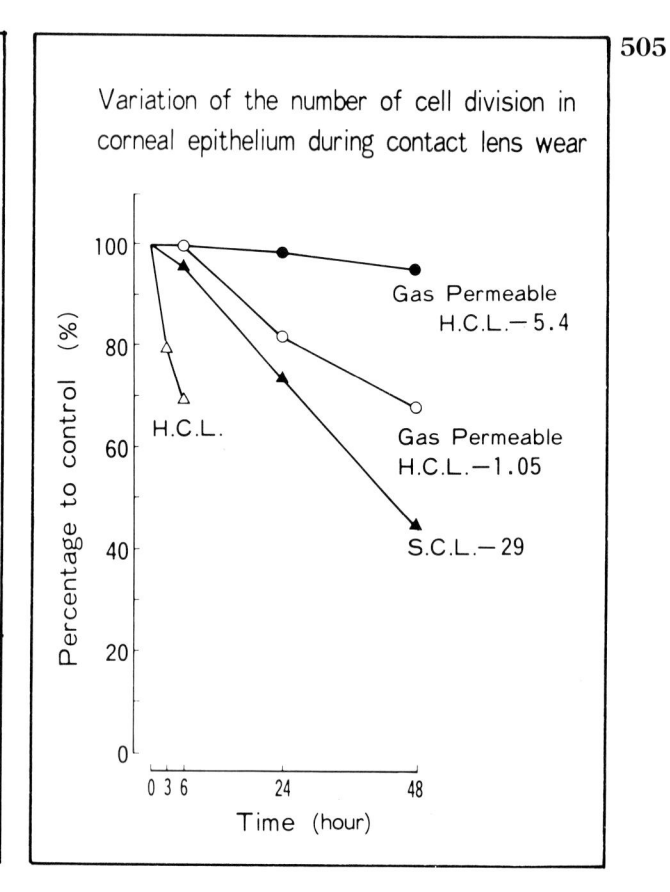

504 & 505 Gas permeability and epithelial cell mitosis. These graphs (Hamano) indicate almost a direct relationship of lenses of different gas permeability to the rate of epithelial cell mitosis and also the level of lactic acid in the anterior chamber. They are only relative and do not take into account the flow of gases possible *under* small hard lenses and furthermore they are for the rabbit eye.

506 Rabbit contact lens wear showing loss of squamous cells. (Bermanson, Ruben, Chu). Synonymous with SPK in humans.

507 Intracellular cyst of a squamous cell. Indicative of membrane transference of water due to the loss of K^+ ions and exchanged for Na^+ ions with water retention properties.

508 EW on the rabbit—a hard lens produced surface sloughing, cell separation and nuclear break-up and increased lysozymes.

Epithelium and lens wear

Adverse effects of CL wear on the rabbit and monkey eye—histology

Epithelial pathology from CL wear—human eye

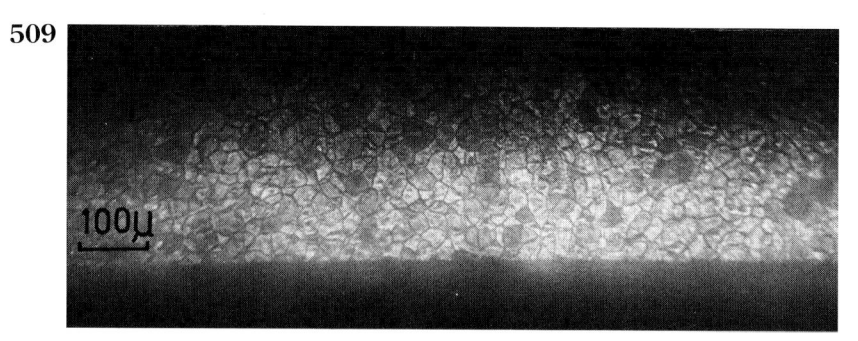

509 Almost normal appearance. Specular microscopy can show a very variable response after contact lens wear. The changes to the cells are not related to the type of lens. The illustration shows an almost normal appearance, with well-defined cell borders and normal pleomorphism.

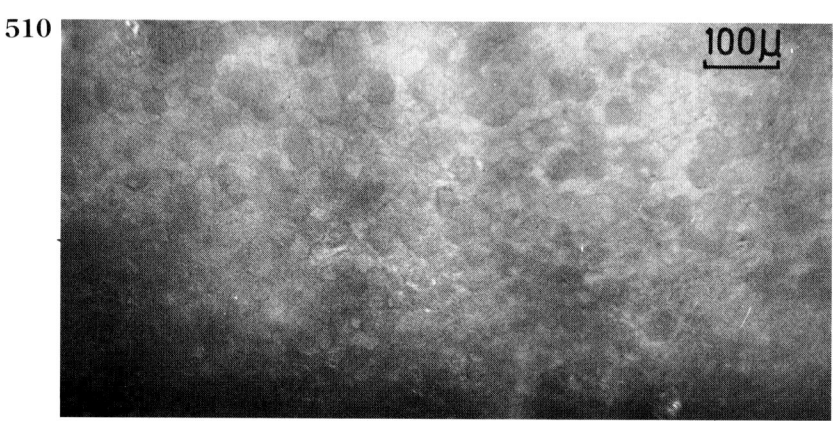

510 Cell separation is more evident because of oedema but there is minimal cell loss.

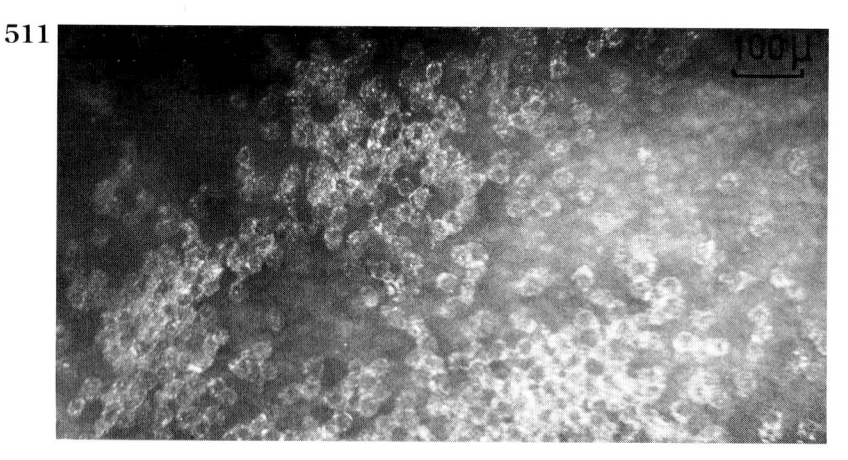

511 Typical fluorescein punctate staining. Specular microscopy shows cell loss; the loose cells are refractile.

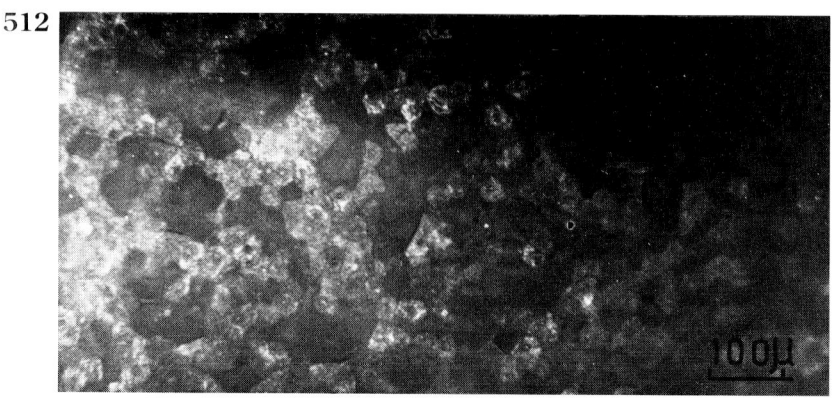

512 Larger basal cell borders. A similar picture to **511** but also showing basal cell borders larger than normal, suggesting oedema.

(Figures **509-512** are courtesy of Ch. Marechal-Courtois and J. Cl. Delcourt—CLAO Journal.)

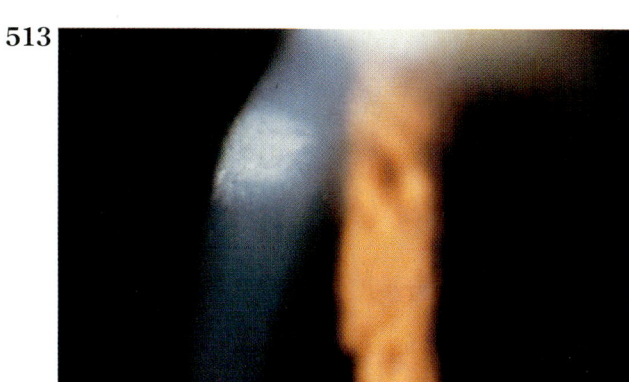

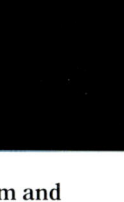

513 & 514 Dessication of the epithelium and erosion below the edge of a hard lens (with and without fluorescein).

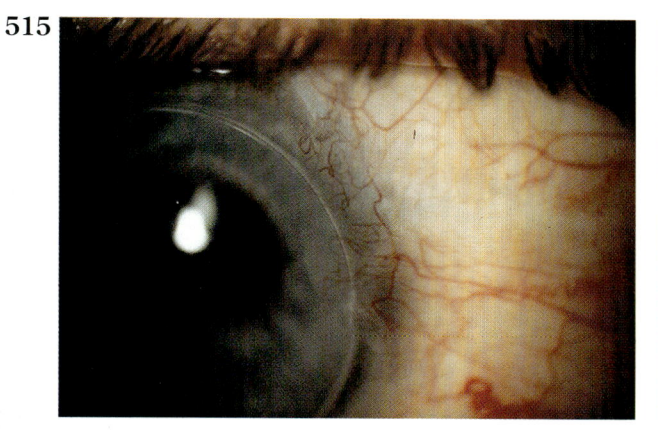

515 Formation of pterygium following contact lens wear (hard). The case is possibly a conjunctival inflammatory reaction growing into a dessication area adjacent to the conjunctiva.

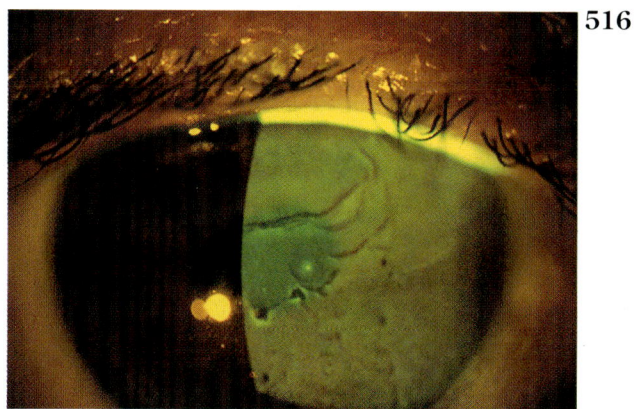

516 Linear cellular hypertrophy seen behind a hard (GP) contact lens.

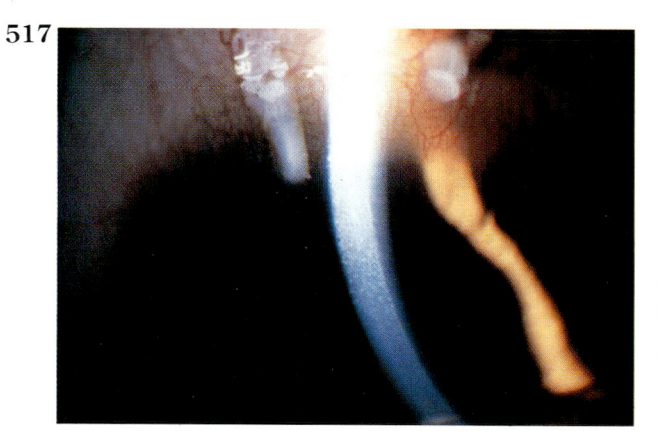

517 & 518 Superior limbal keratitis secondary to papillary conjunctivitis which was contact lens induced. A similar keratitis is seen with vernal catarrhal conjunctivitis.

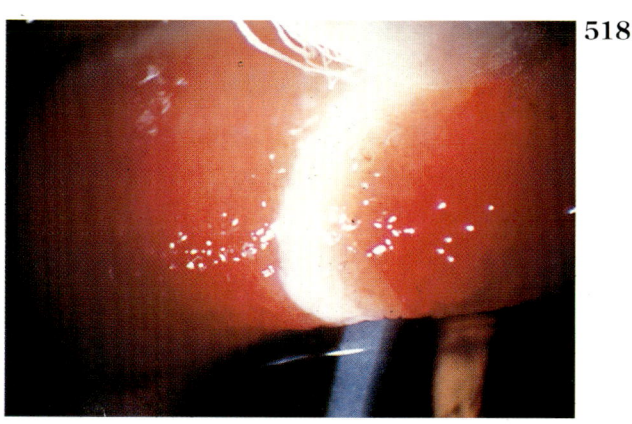

(Figures **513-518** are courtesy of W.J. Benjamin.)

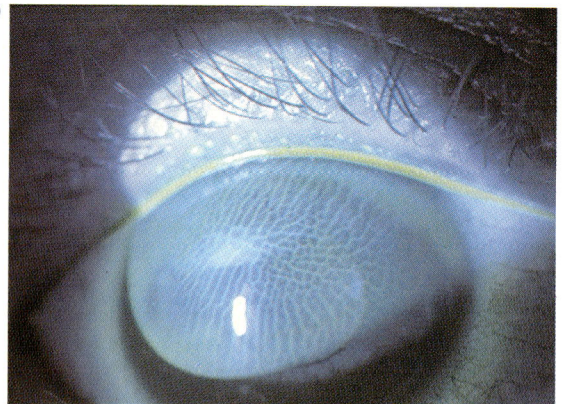

519 Superficial corneal mosaic as seen in a normal cornea after lid massage (with a finger) or sometimes with lens wear. It disappears after a few minutes. (A. Bron)

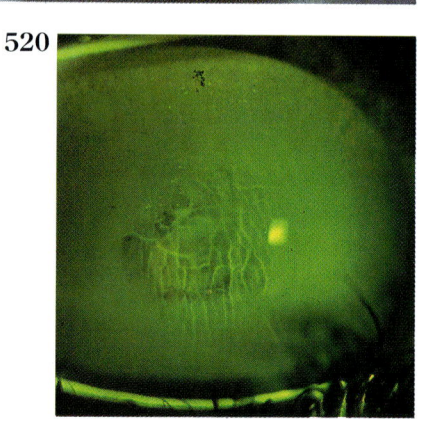

520 Superficial corneal mosaic in keratoconus. This pattern is most likely due to the pressure applied to the loose epithelium onto the basement membrane ridge pattern and at the same time the removal of the deep tear mucous layer which permits the fluorescein aqueous to run in the mosaic channels. Note that the keratoconus ridges are more prominent in the vertical. The pressure of a contact lens can produce this pattern. (Hans Bleshoy)

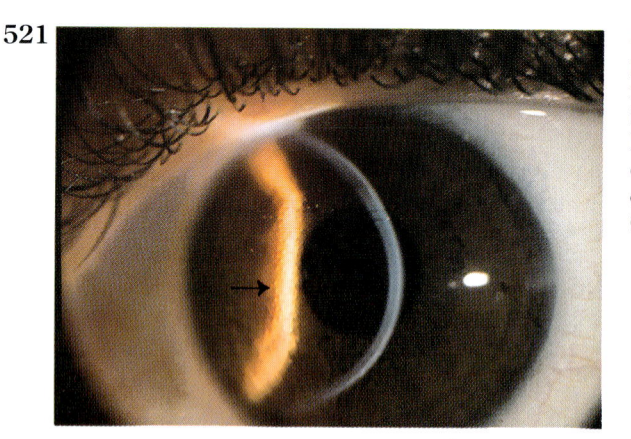

521 & 522 Oedema of the corneal epithelium can produce a negative picture of the mosaic so that fluorescein pools in the depressions where greater intermembrane tension hold cells to the basement ridges. Micro-bubbles trapped under a contact lens will lie in the depressions. Retro-illumination of the cornea with epithelial oedema has a micro 'peau d'orange' appearance (**521**).

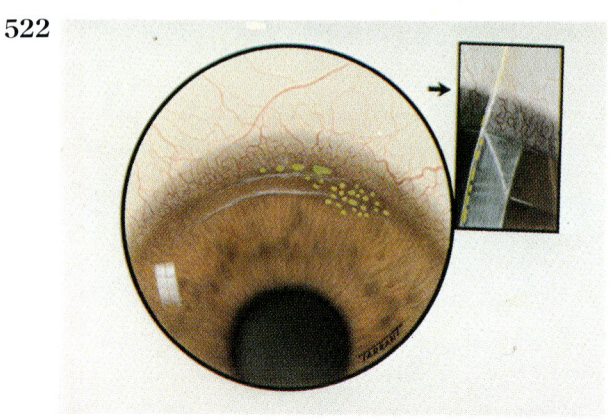

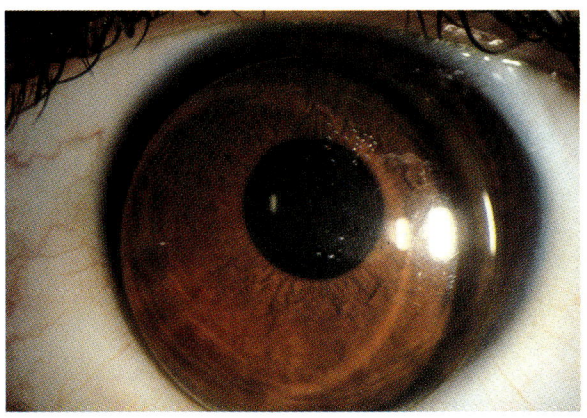

523-525 Epithelial oedema, as described in 521 & 522. Associated with blurred vision (Sattler's veiling). This type of oedema disappears within a few hours when it is contact lens induced. **524** & **525** are of the same eye immediately after the contact lens is removed and then after a few blinks.

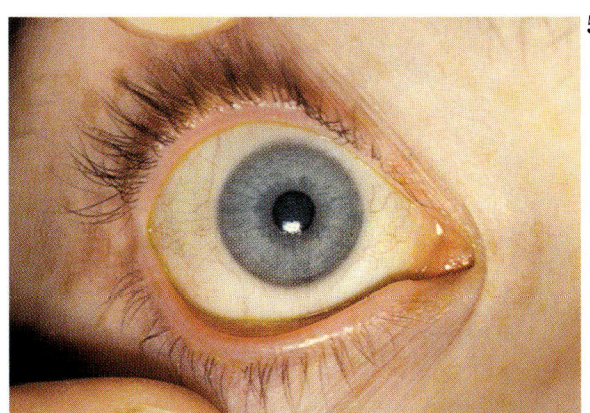

526 More pronounced epithelial oedema after contact lens wear in thyrotoxicosis where tear proteins may be abnormal.

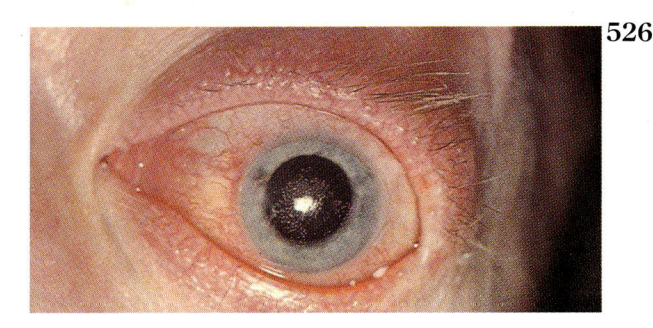

Tear film

Normal tear film is between 5 and 10 µm thick. Several layers have been described but in brief they are the deep, thick mucous layer attached to the epithelial cell surface, then an aqueous mucous layer and superficially a lipid layer some 50 or more molecules thick. The tears are possibly the most important factor in contact lens wear since they provide lubrication and convey to the cornea gases and nutrients as well as removing metabolic and cellular debris.

The quality of the tear film can be investigated by optical methods such as biodifferential interferometry (Hamano), polarized light (J-P Guillon) and specular microscopy (Josephson). Thin films of different refractive indices will by these techniques show interferometry patterns and from these fringes calculations of the thickness of the various phases can be made. The normal tear film can appear by these techniques with marble veining, a regular wave pattern or an amorphous texture. Abnormal films appear broken up or coloured fringes appear suggesting contamination or abnormal lipid. Combinations of all these appearances can occur.

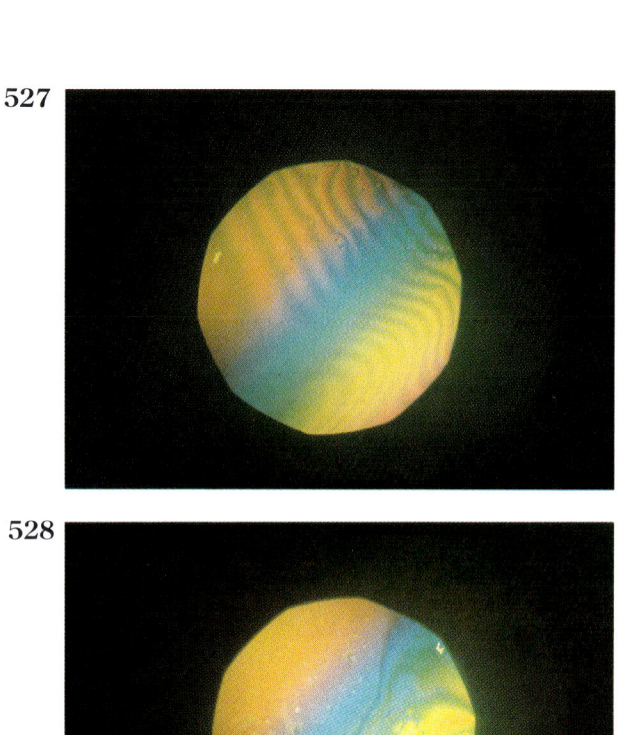

527 Normal wave pattern. Hamano's method illustrating the normal wave pattern.

528 Break-up with some particulate matter.

529 Abnormal appearance on a contact lens surface.

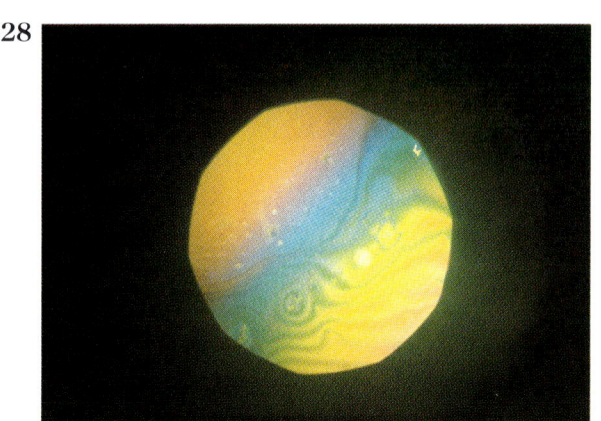

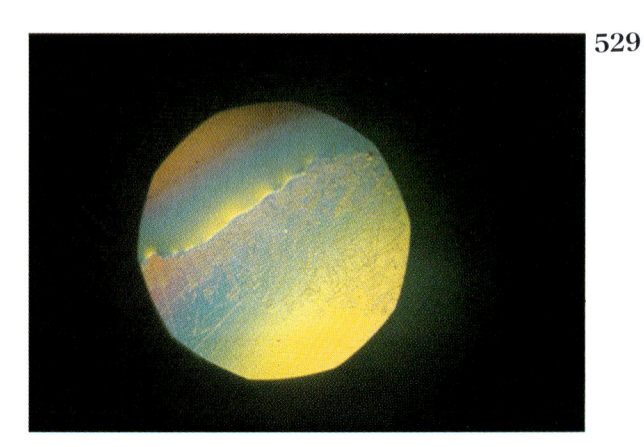

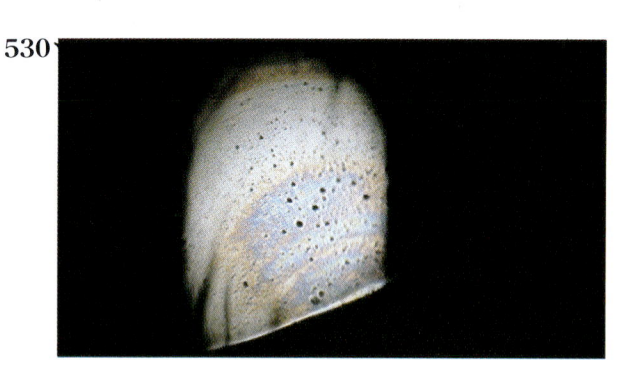

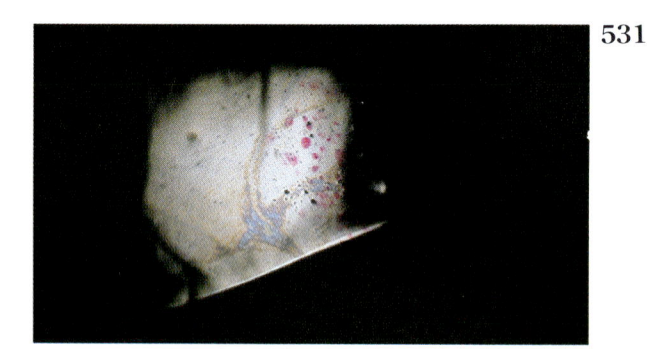

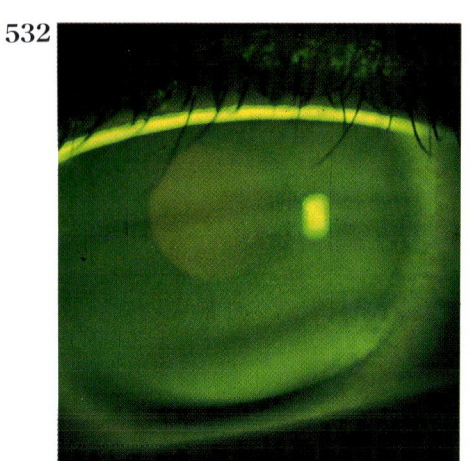

530 & 531   Meibomian secretion of lipid.
Expressed meibomian secretion of lipid forms a thick film initially which, with the closed lid compression, spreads to form waves over the aqueous-mucous film. Eventually the lipid and degraded mucin with cell debris form particulate matter which can form strings in the dry eye syndromes. (J-P Guillon.)

532   The effect of lid pressure during a forced blink will thin the aqueous film and appears as black areas. (J-P Guillon.)

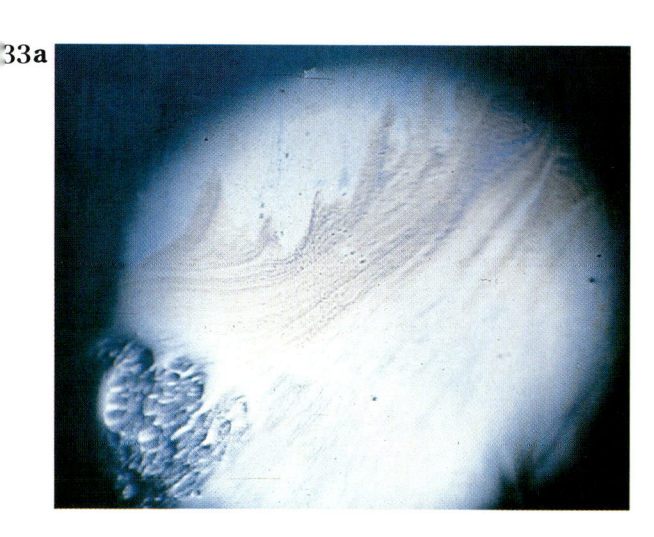

533a **The tear-film break-up time (BUT)** is low (less than 5 seconds) in this eye, which had dry eye symptoms and signs. Localized dry spot formation and abnormal lipid appearance can be seen. (J-P Guillon.)

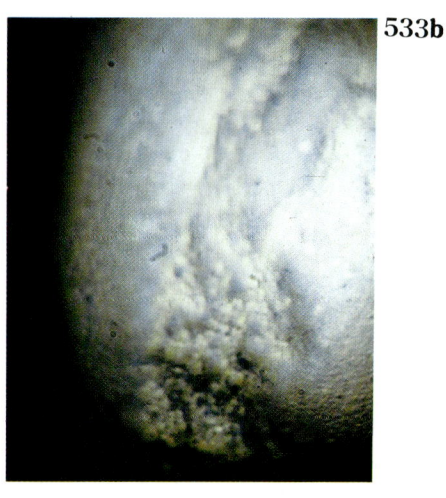

533b **The pre-lens tear film** is often abnormal over lenses. This figure shows a localized dry spot area (lower left portion) and thick lipid as denoted by the marked interferometry colours. (J-P Guillon.)

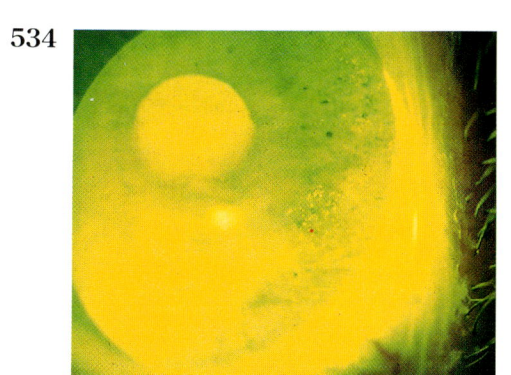

534 & 535 Black areas. The fluorescence cannot be demonstrated in concentrations less than 10^{-6} and, since the molecule is large and the aqueous thickness of the tear film is very thin in some areas, black areas appear with tear film drying and whenever the squamous cell membranes are unable to hold the mucous layer.

The time it takes to form a black area is indicative of the aqueous tear film thickness and is called the break-up time (BUT). Normally this is 10 seconds or more, as measured by biomicroscopic methods of visualization, but is persistently less with diminished lid tear meniscuses. Epithelial dessication is indicative of early tear aqueous deficiency.

Persistent black areas exist over abnormal epithelium (e.g. scar areas, after toxic exposure) and are called dry spots. These can be seen in these figures of toxic keratitis (lens solution induced).

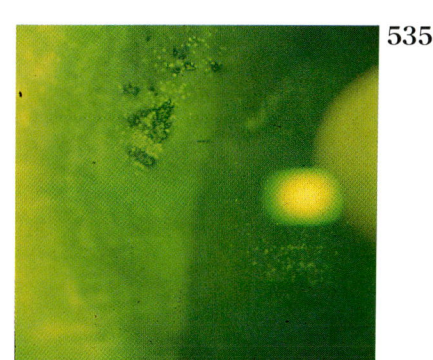

536 Dry spots over RK cornea. Seen over surgical trauma areas.

159

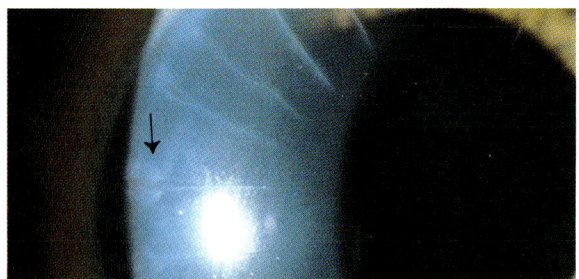

537 Down growth of epithelium. The arrow indicates areas of down growth of the epithelium (RK) where dry spots and contact lens wear erosions are likely to occur—especially with soft lens wear.

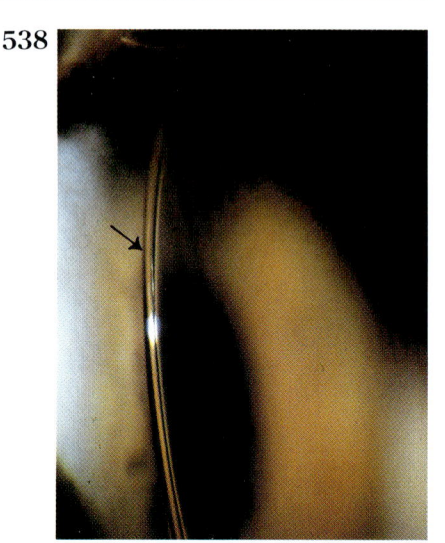

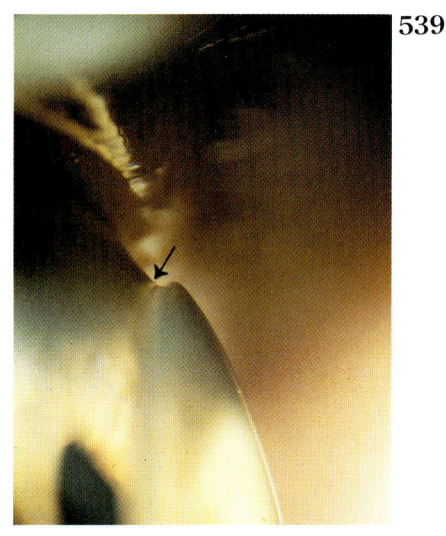

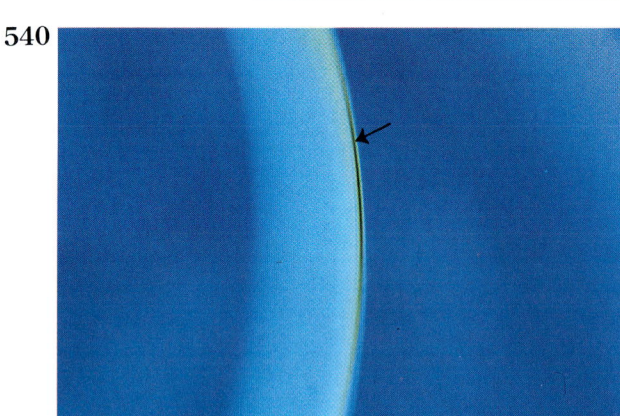

538 The hard lens meniscus is illustrated. Just outside the meniscus is a 'black line' which is an intereference phenomenon of a zone that is light free (arrowed).

539 The very thin tear film zone adjacent to the meniscus can be seen at the point of the arrow.

540 With fluorescein the 'black line' is clearly seen.

(Figures **538-540** by courtesy of W.J. Benjamin.)

Dk/L values

The oedema and pressure effects of contact lenses are related to the thickness distribution. Therefore thickness profile graphs and drawings give important information as to which areas of the cornea are likely to suffer pressure and hypoxia effects and to what degree. (This was shown on pages 20-27 relative to lens design.)

Note to table 15

For a standard lens of 0.1mm thickness the Dk/L is given at 35°C. Note that Dk information by itself is not of great value. Furthermore even Dk/L has to be qualified by lens thickness distribution and the size and fitting characteristics (see page 28).

541 The graph relates the Dk/L values of soft lenses to the degree of corneal oedema as measured by pachometry. The calculated quantity of oxygen at the lens cornea interphase can also be related to the corneal oedema (i.e. stromal thickness). This graph contains data from more than one research worker and is therefore hypothetical but will suffice as a working model. Research findings should not be taken out of their context, though this is done to interpret clinical problems. They are at best a guideline to improve the state of the art.

The graph is only useful if we ask it questions. Suppose that clinically 20 per cent corneal thickness change is our acceptable upper limit, even though it compensates back to normal later or even in some extended wear cases the cornea becomes thinner.

Then the question is: 'What is the lowest acceptable Dk/L?

The graph tells us that all lenses with Dk/L less than 35 $\times 10^{-9}$ (ATVP) are likely to cause more oedema than we allow. Furthermore the graph says that the O_2 at the corneal surface with such a lens is in the region of 7 per cent (approximately 50mmHg).

We know from our physiology that the venous oxygen is of the same order and therefore the closed eye state without a CL must also be about the same.

To apply this knowledge to practice we would have to ask the manufacturer to state for each lens the minimal and maximal Dk/L since the thickness profile, especially for high power lenses, does vary significantly (see page 27).

542 This graph refers to hard gas permeable contact lenses of Dk values possibly between 20 and 50. It is a composite graph showing the spread from the low to high Dk lenses tested. It is taken from the work of R. Hill, S. Brezinski and W.J. Flynn (1985).

We learn from this graph the Dk/L values could be much lower than we know from **541** to produce a comparable corneal O_2 level of 7 per cent.

Thus much thicker hard corneal lenses of these materials could be used before oedema occurs. It is unfair to compare **541** with **542** because the experimental conditions are not known but, nevertheless, it is a guideline.

The inference is easy to make. The soft lens totally covers the cornea whereas the hard lens is smaller and the cornea under the lens obtains almost 50 per cent of its oxygen via the retro-lens tear pump (see page 28).

The real problem is that the atmospheric pressure of O_2 can be suddenly reduced by lid closure and with extended wear this occurs for several hours. Thus thicknesses, sizes and fits considered safe for the open eye are suspect for the closed eye contact lens wearer (see **501**).

Table 15. Permeability of contact lenses to O_2 (using a standard thickness of 0.1mm).

Material	Water %	Dk/L* at 35°C.
PMMA	0.5	0.2
HEMA (B&L)	38	10
Sil/Ac Boston		
III		20
IV		30 plus
Paraperm EW		50 plus
Hydrocurve	50	55
Fluorocarbon	0	70-100
Sauflon gel	75	60

* $\times 10^{-9}$ cm$^{2/s.}$/s.ml O_2/ml $\times$ mmHg.
(Area. Time. Volume. Pressure)

N.B. Because the measurement of O_2 flow is poorly standardized the above figures are not more accurate than ±5.

541

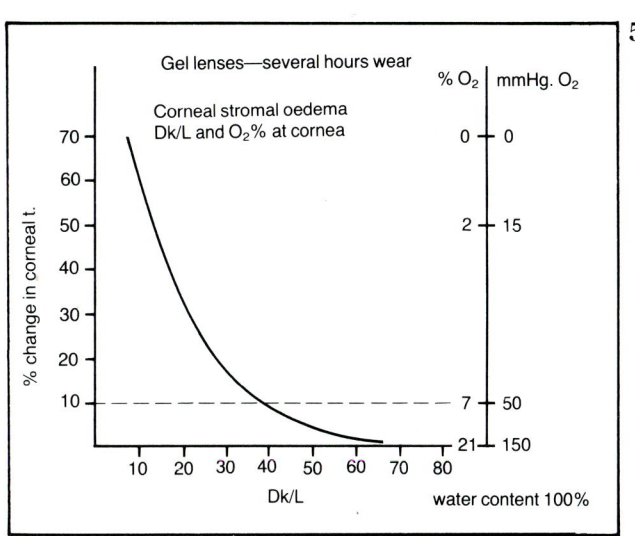

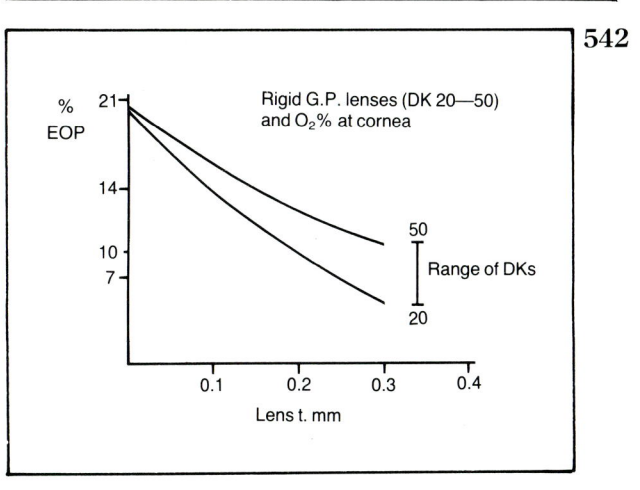

Gel lenses—several hours wear
Corneal stromal oedema Dk/L and O_2% at cornea

542

Rigid G.P. lenses (DK 20—50) and O_2% at cornea
Range of DKs

Punctate keratitis

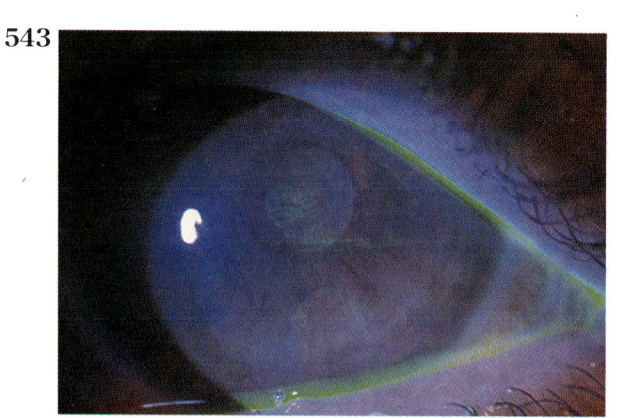

543-547 Punctate keratitis. This complication is often referred to as 'corneal staining' which, while descriptive, is not constructive in the understanding of the condition. This condition has many causes but the end result is loss of superficial cells. Trauma and dessication are the prime causes, but are acerbated by preceding hypoxia, cell oedema and separation.

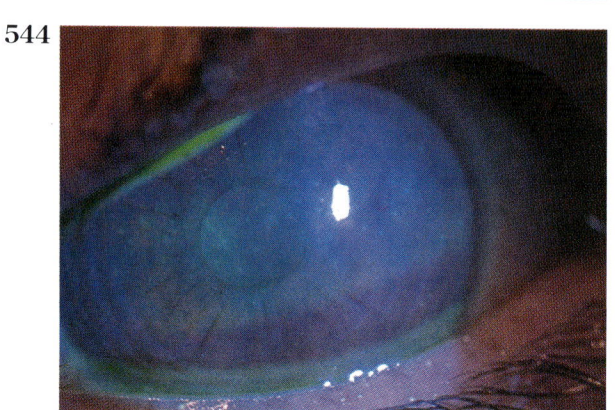

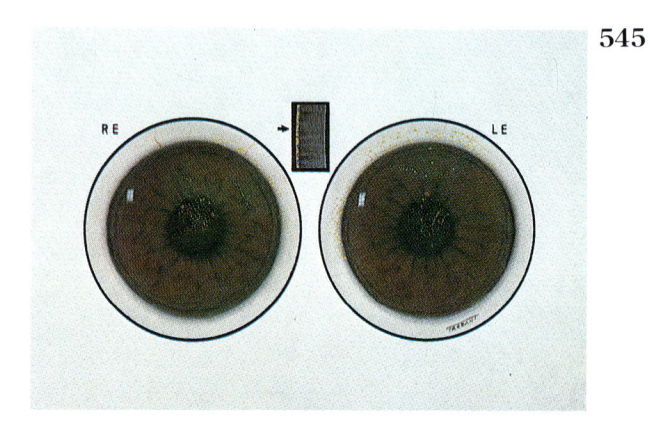

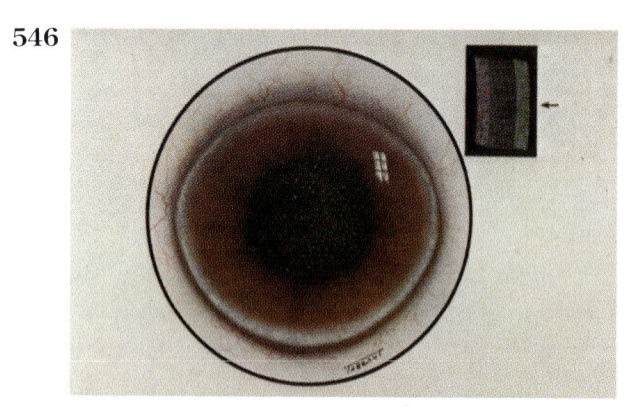

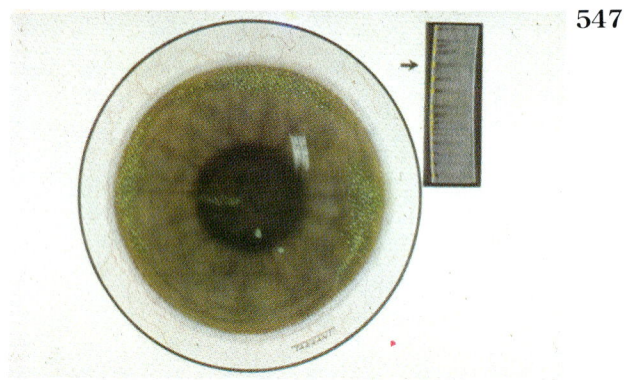

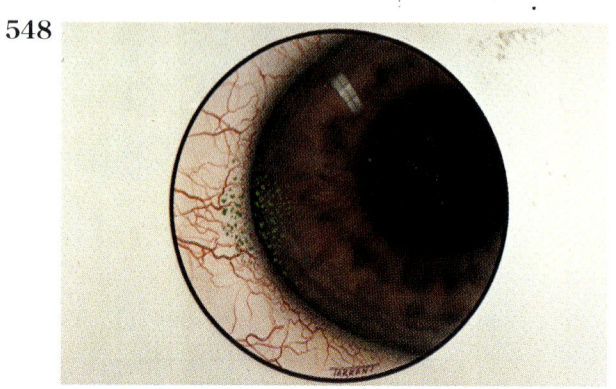

548 Dessication is seen marginally in hard and small, thick soft lenses, in the 9 and 3 o'clock positions.

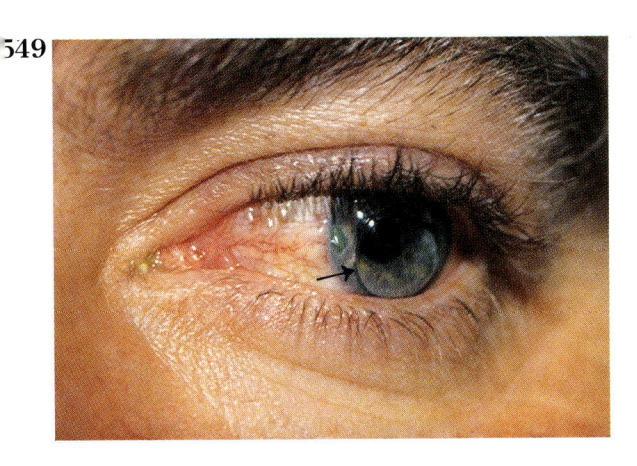

549 The Dellen formation, with stromal thinning—sometimes with extensive marginal ulceration. Healing is rapid once the cause is known and removed.

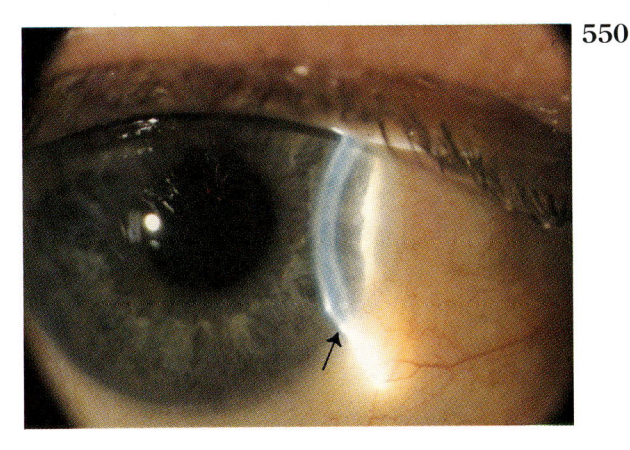

550 Thick, small diameter soft lenses can also cause dessication, as seen here. Dessication can also be seen under high water content thin lenses.

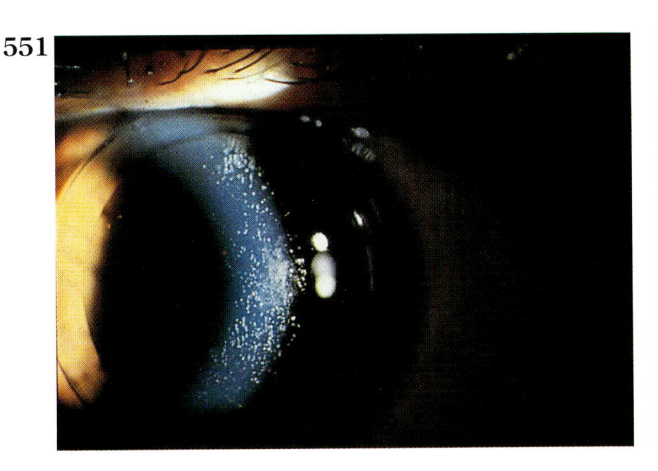

551 & 552 Mucin debris behind GP hard lenses can be associated with punctate keratitis. (W.J. Benjamin)

551 shows the lens *in situ* with mucin behind the lens; when the lens is removed the corneal epithelial trauma can be seen (**552**). Compare with **499 & 500**. Stasis of the retro-lens tear fluid, irrespective of the cause, leads to mucin coagulation.

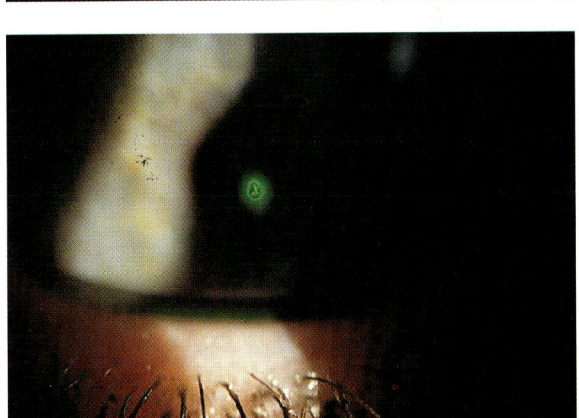

553 Bizarre forms and patterns. The punctate keratitis can take on many bizarre forms and patterns and cause confusion in diagnosis for the uninitiated. Pseudodendritic keratitis (as shown here) has been described. It has to be distinguished from superior limbic keratitis (Theodore), inferior staphylococcal belpharoconjunctivitis and viral keratitis (such as stellate adenovirus and herpes simplex). The contact lens keratitis, when chronic, persists for several weeks, even after cessation of contact lens wear, especially if associated with palpebral conjunctivitis.

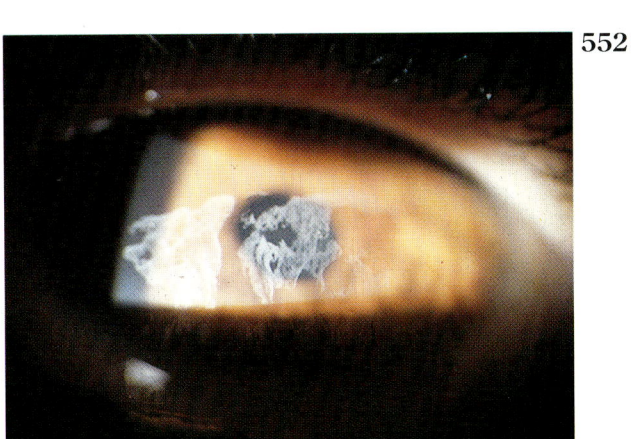

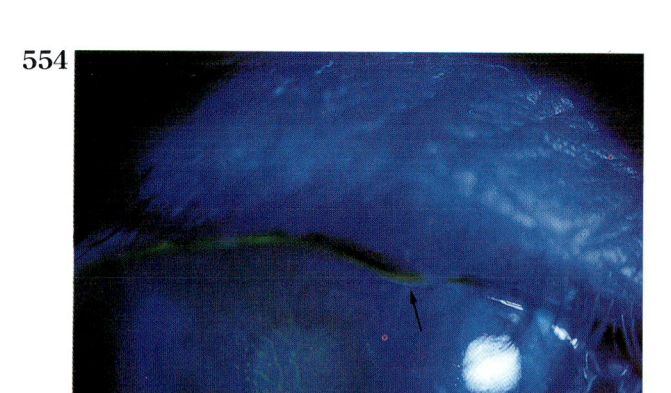

554 Punctate keratitis with confluent linear keratitis due to hard lens wear in a patient with early dry eye syndrome. *N.B.* The 'black line' is present at the edge of the tear meniscus.

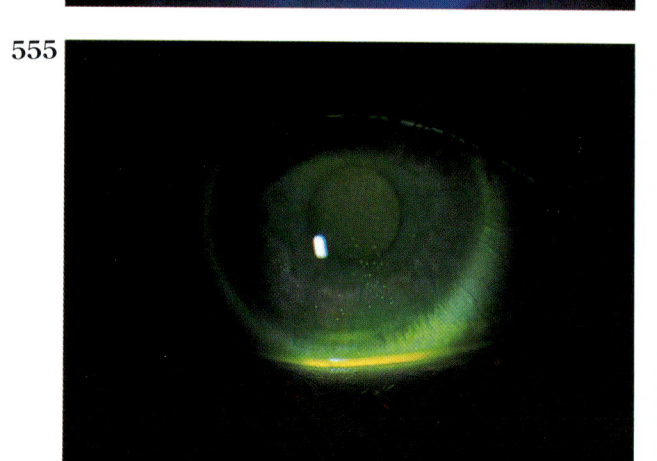

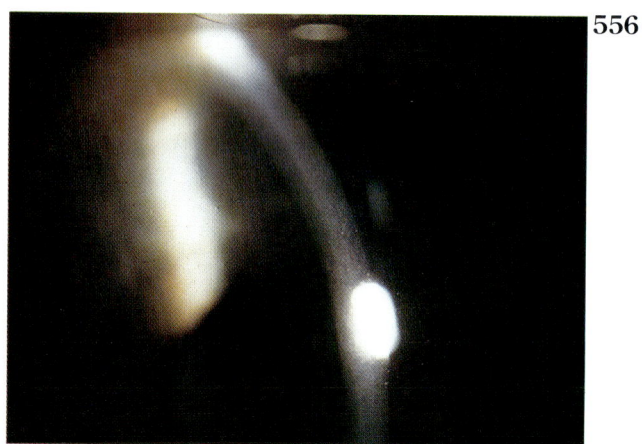

555 & 556 Formation of epithelial microcysts by all types of contact lens wear is not uncommon. Providing there is no deeper pathology to be seen, it is treated by refitting with thinner and higher gas flow lenses. (Graeme Young)

557 The microcysts and vacuoles in the epithelium are best seen in retro-illumination. This drawing indicates that the internal reflection of such abnormalities can be modified by varying the illumination vergence. Such methods in experienced hands may help determine whether a cyst or space is filled with materials higher than the refractive index of water.

558 Epithelial microcysts.

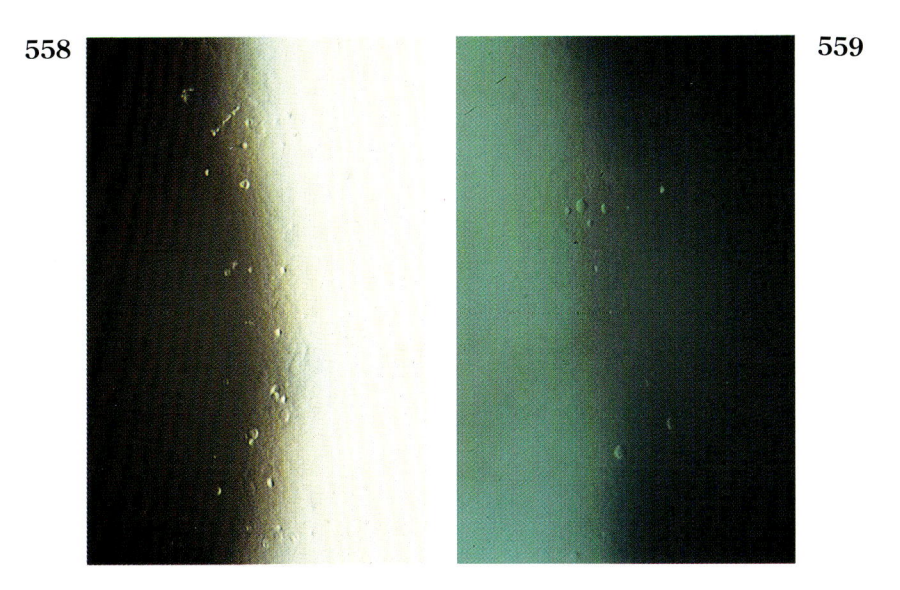

559 Epithelial vacuoles.

(**Figures 557-559** courtesy of Steve Zantos, *Int. C.L. Clinic* 10 (3): 128-144, 1983.)

Corneal reactions

Contact lens wear can induce an inflammatory reaction and, rarely, an infection. When there is coexistent stromal and epithelial oedema there can be infiltration of white cells, immunoglobulins and mediators with, later, fibroblasts and scavenger cells. But the cornea can be infiltrated from within and the movement anteriorly of keratocytes (corneal fibrocytes), and deposition of calcium salts and lipid have been described. The chronicity of the inflammatory reaction is seen by the infiltration of new blood vessels and scar tissue. Metal pigments such as iron from haemosiderin can form deposits. Mercury from CL solutions is known to penetrate the cornea.

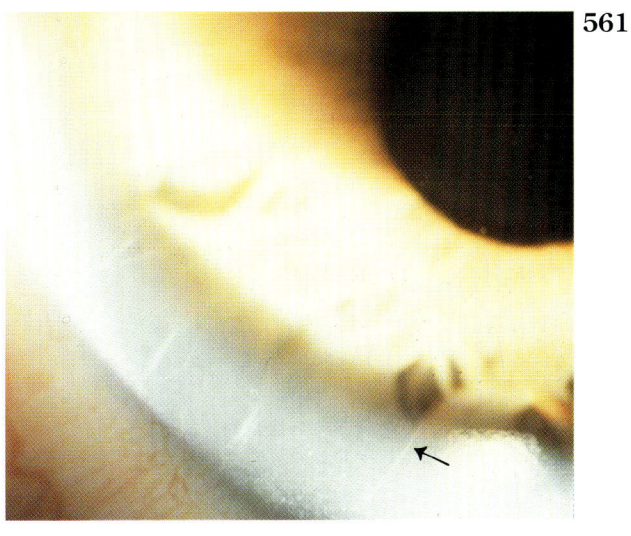

560 & 561 Nerve fibres. It is important for the practitioner to identify the normal from the abnormal. These photographs show nerve fibres medullated and at the periphery of the cornea. They do appear centrally but by then are nonmedullated and in the anterior stroma. (Hans Bleshoy)

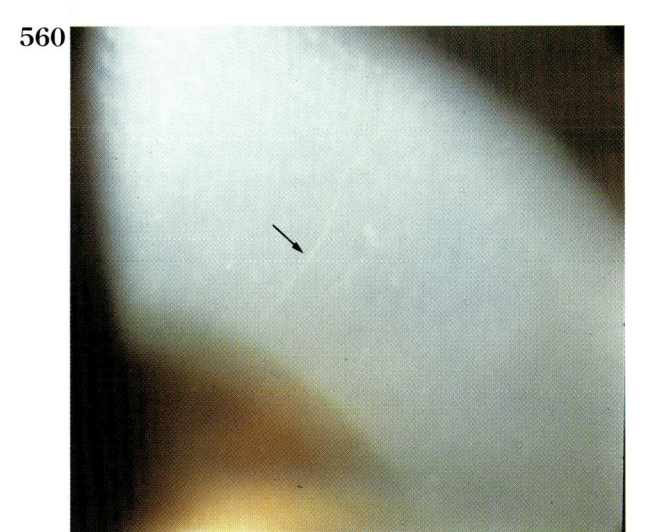

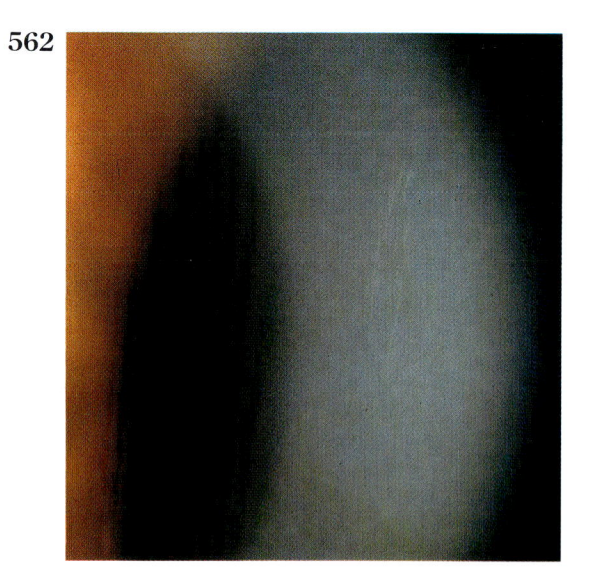

562 Striae from corneal oedema. They are vertical to oblique in direction. (Hans Bleshoy)

563 Striae of the oedematous stroma. They can also be seen in the elderly peripheral stroma and are not necessarily associated with oedema or contact lens wear (arrowed). This specular light photograph also shows the endothelium.

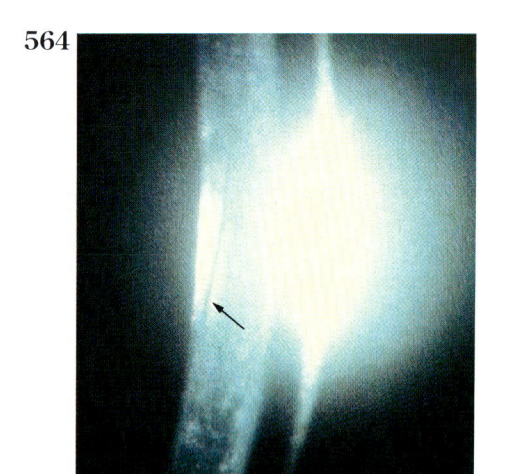

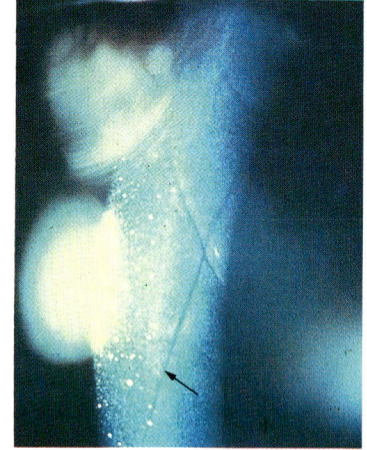

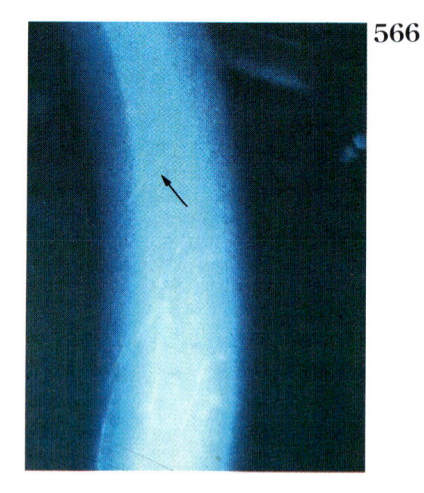

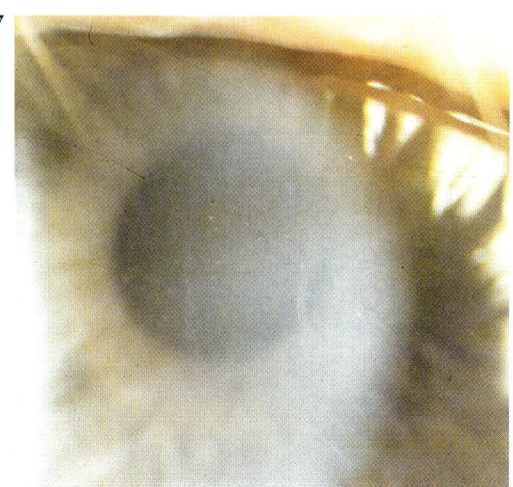

564-566 Striae of oedema. These deep lines in the stroma are indicative of oedema and the vertical lines are at the deeper level. They are called striae of oedema to distinguish them from involutional peripheral stromal striae.

567 Striae from corneal oedema are seen deep and next to Descemet's membrane. The photograph shows striae with corneal oedema and anterior uveitis in a contact lens wearer. (Hans Bleshoy)

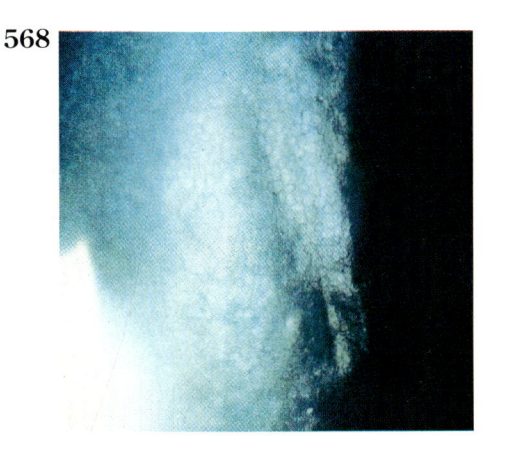

568 Folds or wrinkles in the endothelium seen in a corneal oedema eye.

(Figures **564**, **565**, **566** and **568** are courtesy of Steve Zantos and B. Holden, *Australian J. Opt.* 61:418-426, 1978.)

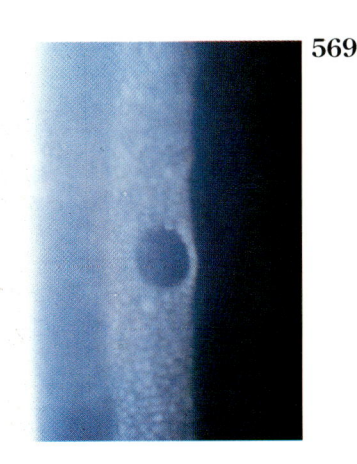

569 Primary endothelial dystrophy (Fuch's) must be noted by the practitioner. It causes stromal oedema, and since it can be inherited it can be diagnosed before signs and symptoms occur. The photograph shows the well-known guttata of the endothelium. (W.J. Benjamin.)

Endothelium and contact lens wear

Under normal conditions, human endothelial cells cannot replicate. However, the cornea will remain transparent even when two-thirds of the cells are absent. This reserve of potential function has to be called into action whenever stromal oedema occurs or cells lose their function. The senile eye has less cells than normal (normal 3000-4000/mm^2 and in the senile state one-third less), but the cornea is not oedematous. The eye, after cataract operations or other invasive trauma, may lose a large number of cells but without loss of corneal transparency.

Changes in the endothelial cell have been noted, such as in size and shape and within the cell itself affecting its metabolism. Separation of the cells and vacuoles, secretory excrescences, secondary effects on Descemet's membrane have been described, even total separation of the endothelium in extreme oedema. However, the practitioner using a biomicroscope at x 40 with specular reflection may not be able to see the detail of the specular microscope. The following photographs of Mr Roger Buckley FRCS will help the student understand the terminology often used to describe changes seen in research with contact lens patients.

570 The normal endothelium in a young male aged 18 years. The cells show well-marked outlines and are all of the same size (homomegathous). Cell density = 3076/mm^2.

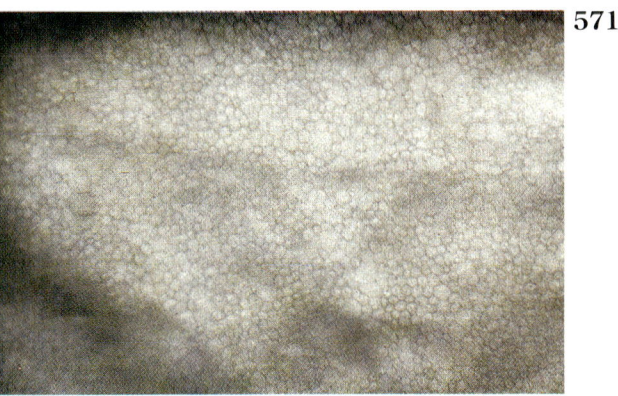

571 Diabetic aphakic wearing a contact lens. There is a differentiation of cell sizes (polymegathous). Some cells are of abnormal shape (poly- or pleomorphous). The cell density is lower than normal, 2309/mm^2.

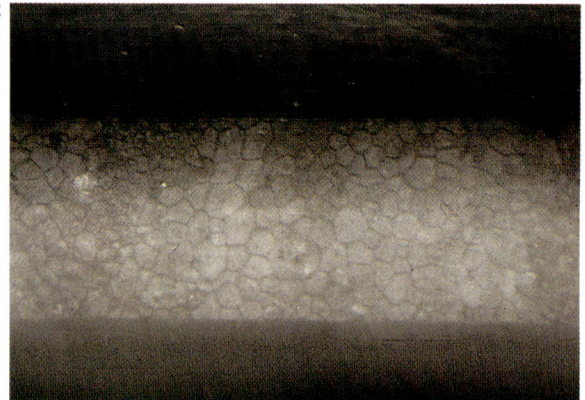

572 Aphakic eye of a male aged 39 years. Intraocular lens of anterior chamber type that was mobile. The endothelium is chiefly pleomorphic and the density is severely reduced, to 709/mm². There is therefore a likelihood of recurrent stromal oedema, especially when senile loss of more cells occurs.

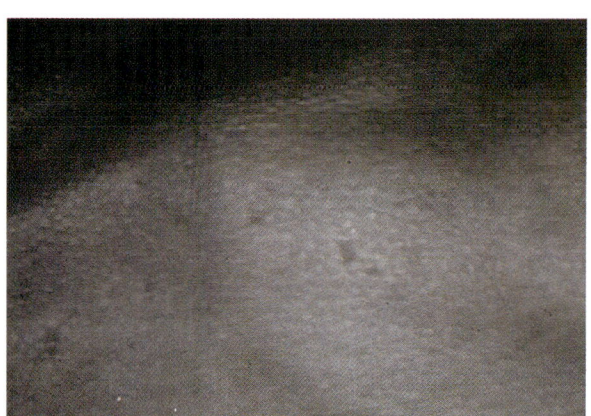

573 Male aged 44 years, normal eye with gel lens of high Dk 75, 0.6 mm thick. Thus the Dk/L = 12×10^{-9} (ATVP), which is too low. Cell density is 2622/mm². The photograph illustrates bleb formation, possibly cell separation.

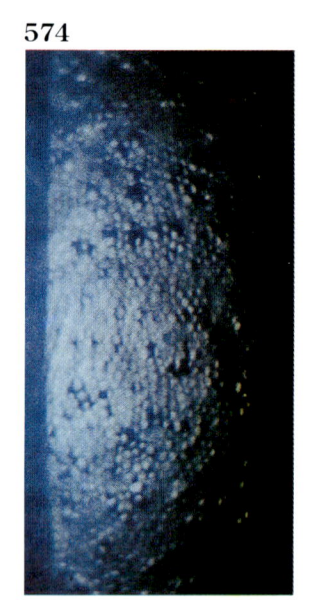

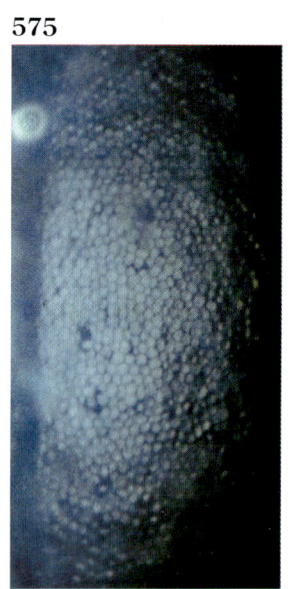

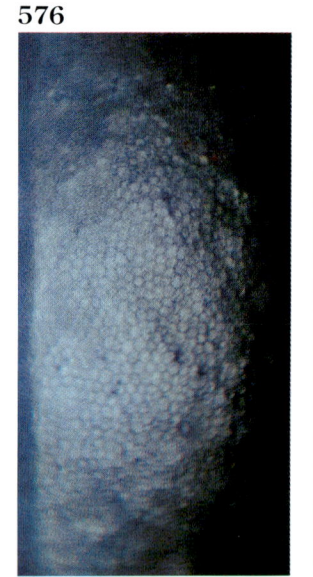

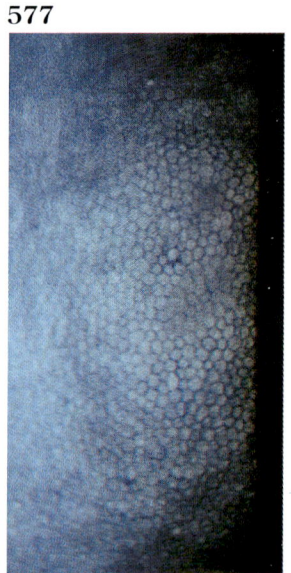

574-577 Hypoxia. The immediate response of hypoxia can be endothelial separation with bleb formation (Holden and Zantos). But the EW lenses show a more protracted picture with cyclic compensation over a time period for the blebs.

The photographs illustrate the bleb response in the morning after overnight wear (to be read from left to right as the first and subsequent nights). Normally the bleb response occurs within 20 minutes and gradually disappears; but this response, present overnight, decreased over the nights it was measured (**577a**).

(Figures are courtesy of L. Williams and B. Holden, *Clin. & Exp. Opt.* 69:3:90-92, 1986.)

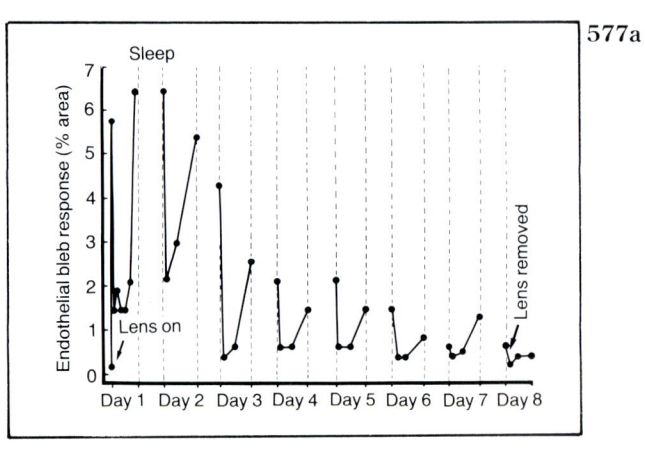

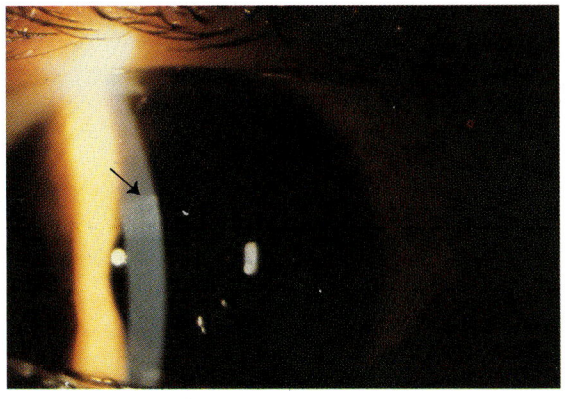

578 & 579 Deep Bowman's infiltration. Gel EW lens—possibly fibrocyte invasion. (Figure courtesy of Dr. Stephani.)

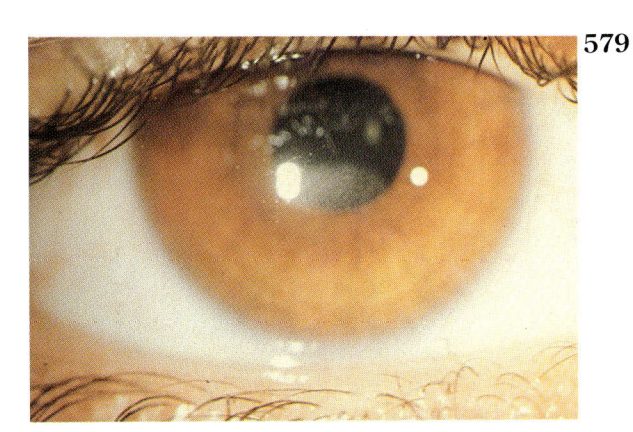

580 Deep Bowman's infiltration. Gel EW lens—possibly fibrocyte invasion.

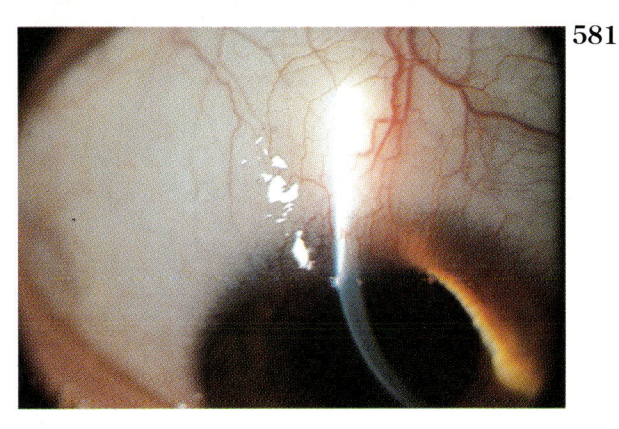

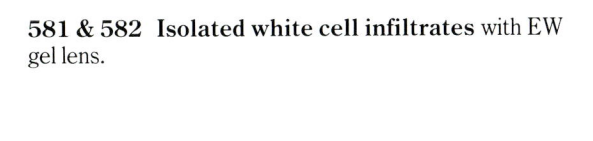

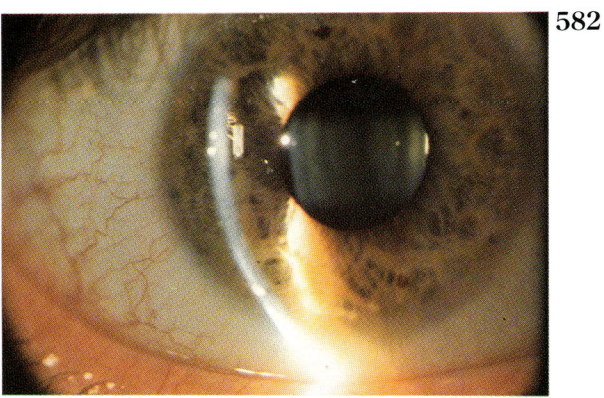

581 & 582 Isolated white cell infiltrates with EW gel lens.

169

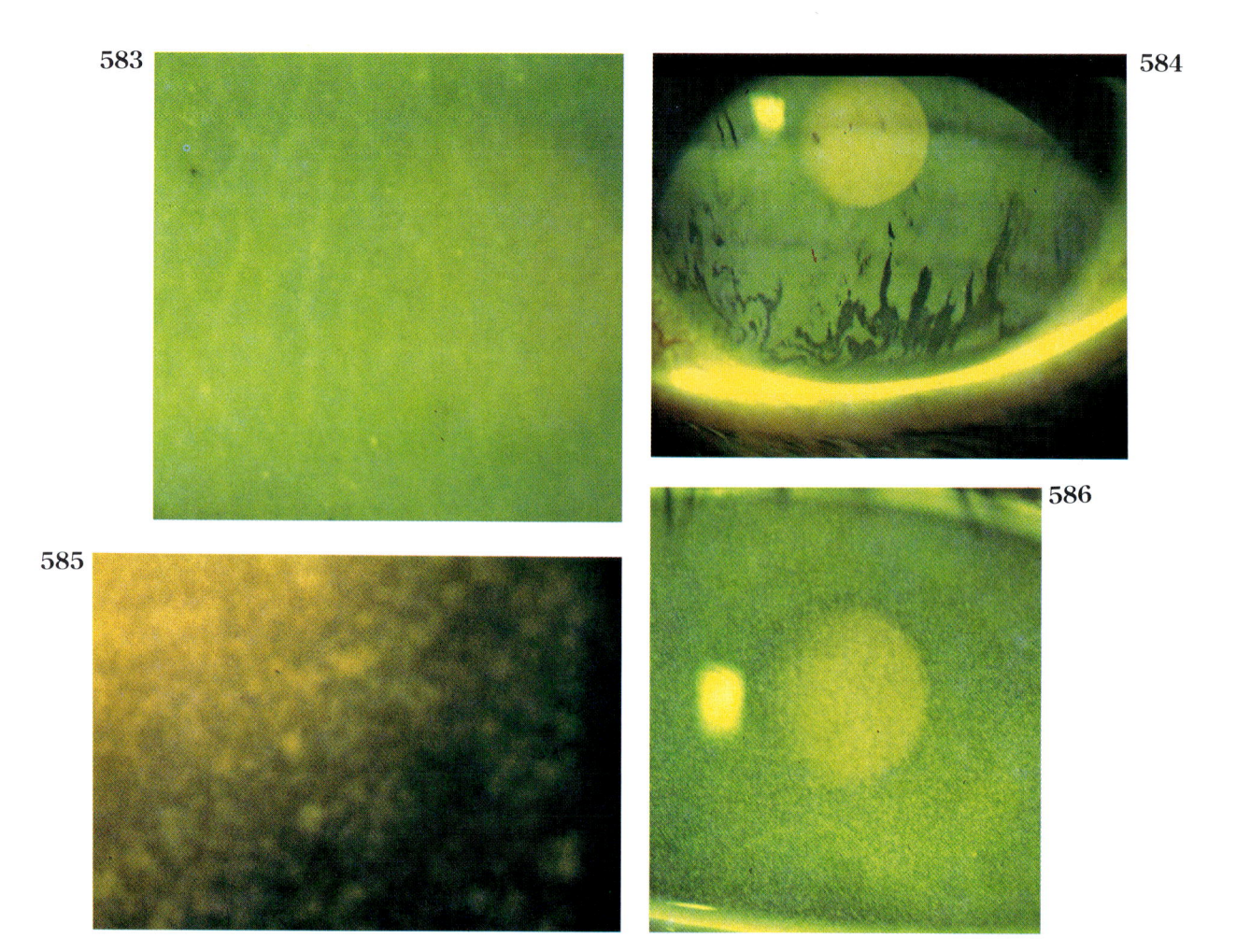

583-586 Toxic keratitis (fluorescein stain). A superficial keratitis, usually widespread and transient, and due to chemical disinfectants in contact lens preparations.

N.B. In **584**, the 'black areas' are where cell damage has occurred (possibly only to the membrane) preventing mucous adhesion and therefore aqueous flow. This was asymptomatic in the patient (see also **535**).

587 & 588 Specular examination of the endothelium. The atlas does not show non-contact lens anomalies but it is worthwhile drawing the practitioner's attention to congenital anomalies seen by the specular examination of the endothelium. Figure **587** shows an abnormality of the endothelium which, on specular photographic microscopy, was shown to be microcysts of the endothelium — they were not likely to affect contact lens wear. (R. Buckley.)

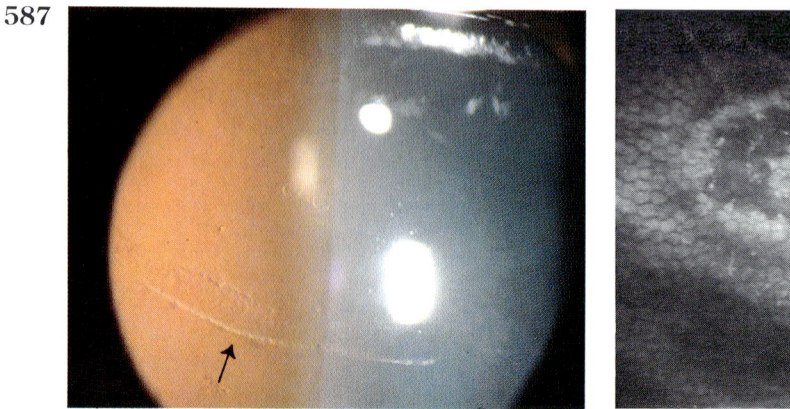

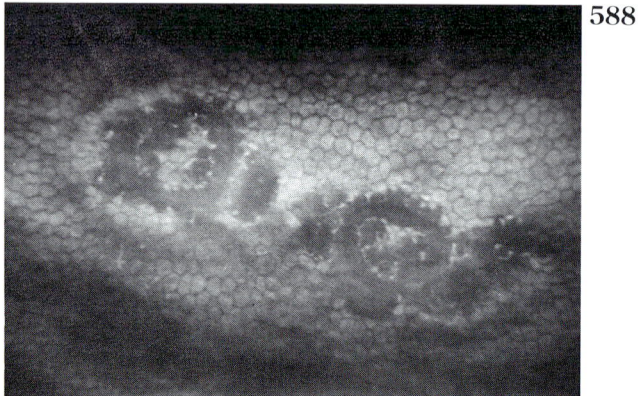

589 Cosmetic visual soft lens wearer (aged 30 years). Wrinkles in the endothelium (arrows) and cell polymorphism can be seen. (N. Ahmed.)

Animal histology—stromal changes with contact lens wear

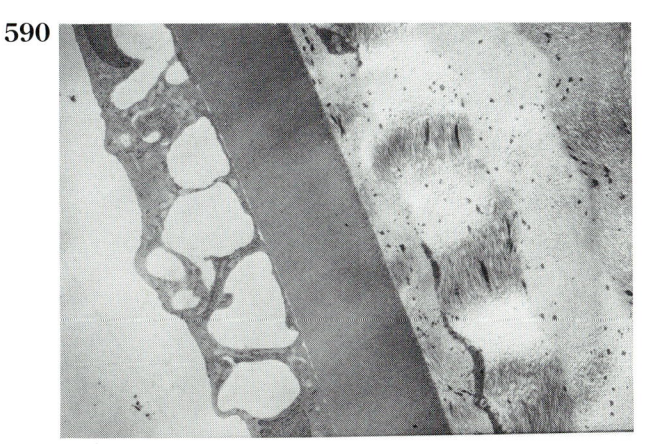

590 EW HGP rabbit. Dk/L = 30×10^{-9} ATVP units. Note the endothelial vacuolation and early separation from the Descemet's membrane.

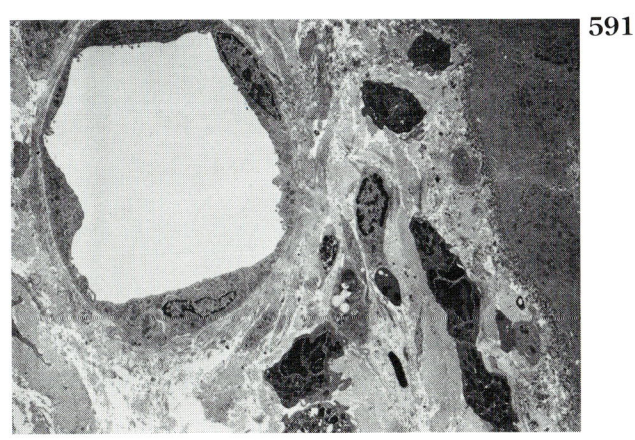

591 New vessels in the stroma. Note the oedema of the stroma.

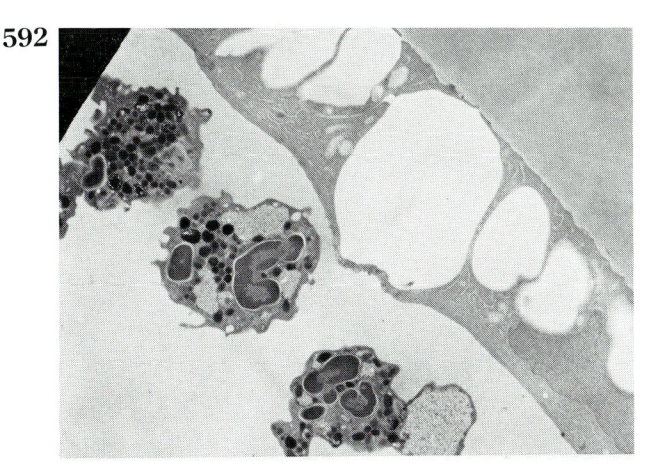

592 The inflammatory response is due to infection. Note the new blood vessels and monocytes in the AC. (L. Chu.)

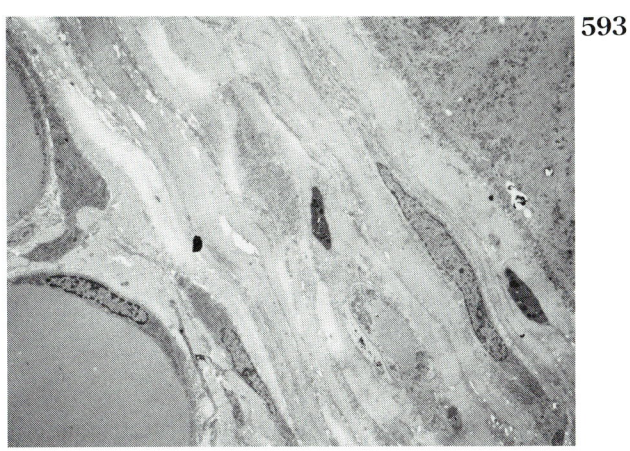

593 Vascularization, stromal oedema and keratocyte degeneration.

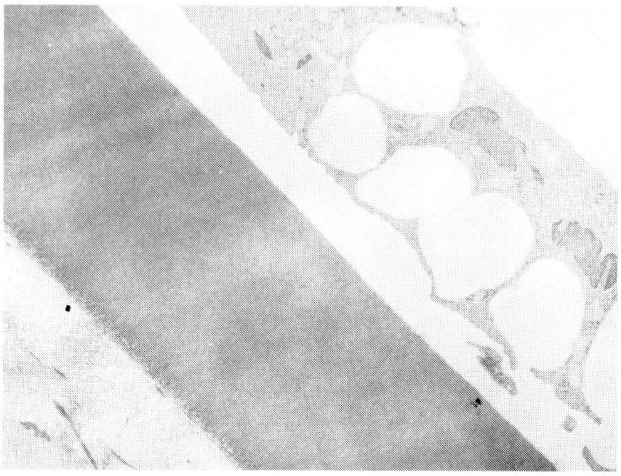

594 & 595 Endothelial vacuolation and separation.

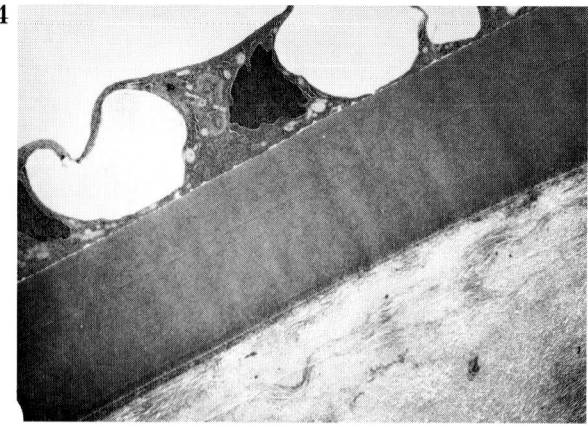

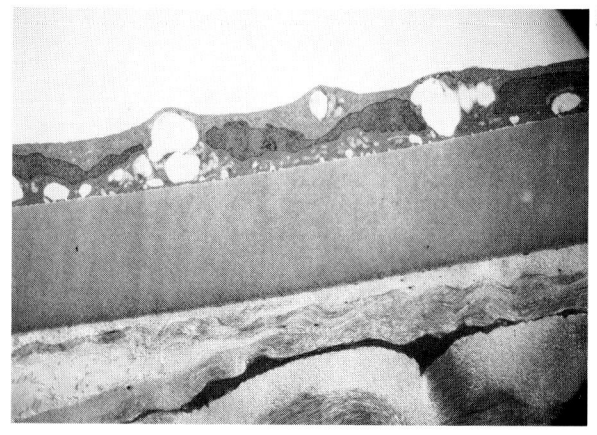

596 Total endothelial separation.

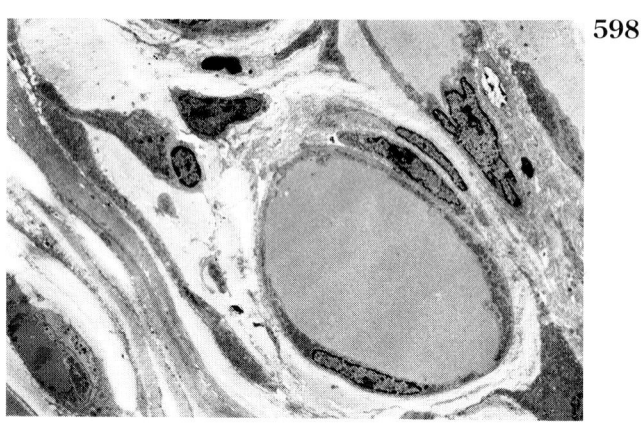

597 & 598 Stromal oedema phagocytes and other cell invasion (note vessels in the stroma). The rabbit histology, with long periods of contact lens wear of different types, indicates that endothelial cell sickness coexists with dysfunction in water transport and the consequent stromal oedema, and sometimes an inflammatory response. In the human the clinical picture is the same but the time relationship different.

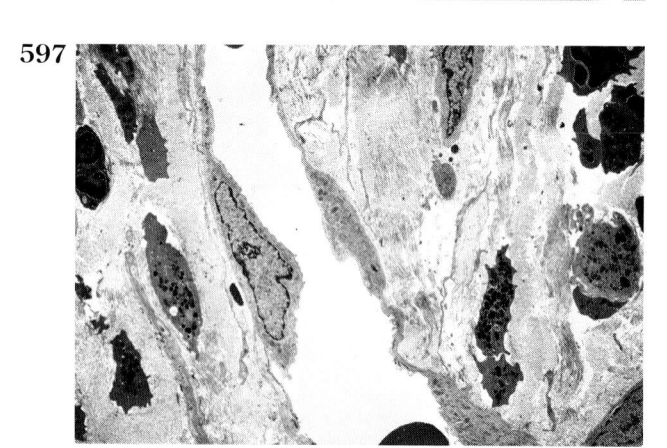

(Figures **590-598** courtesy of J. Bergmanson, M. Ruben and L. Chu.)

Neovascularization

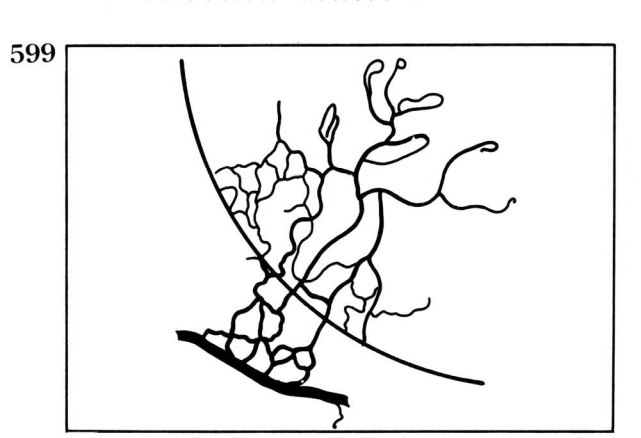

599 Types of vascular pannus formation.

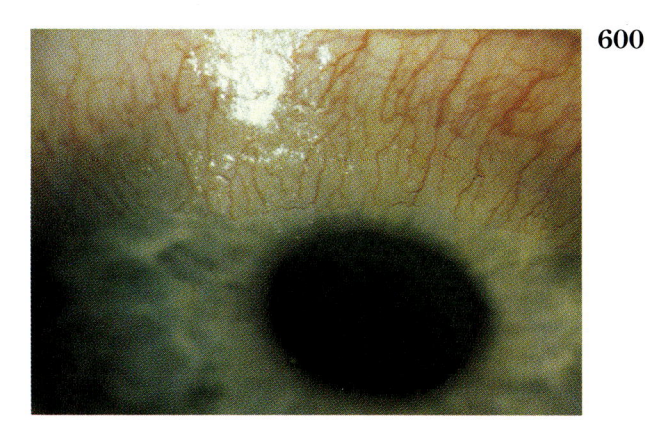

600 Vascular pannus from contact lens wear.

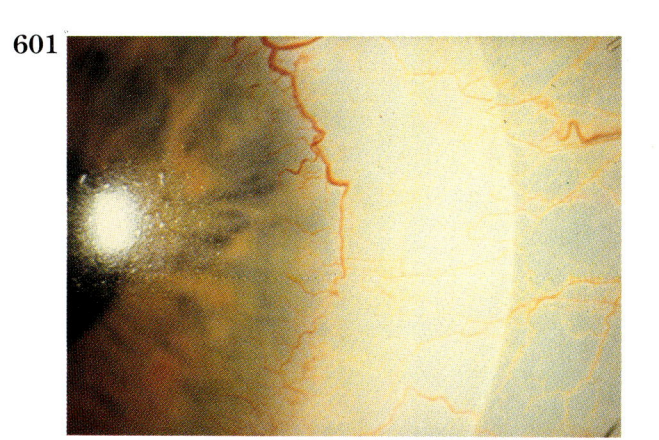

601 Annular vessel from perilimbal plexus.

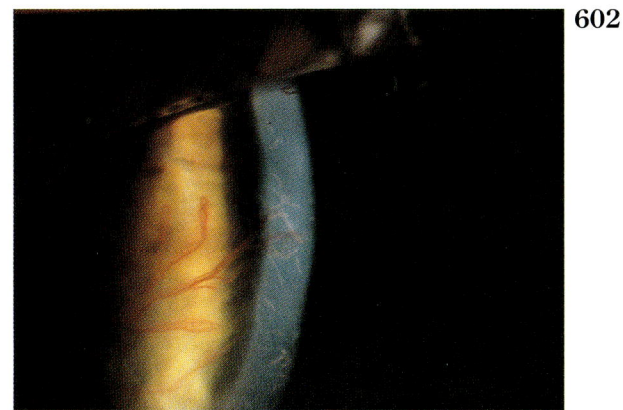

602 Deep stromal vessels.

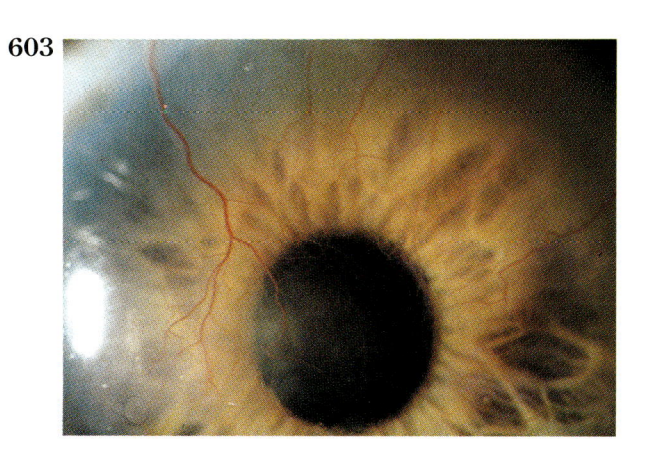

603 Deep stromal vessels.

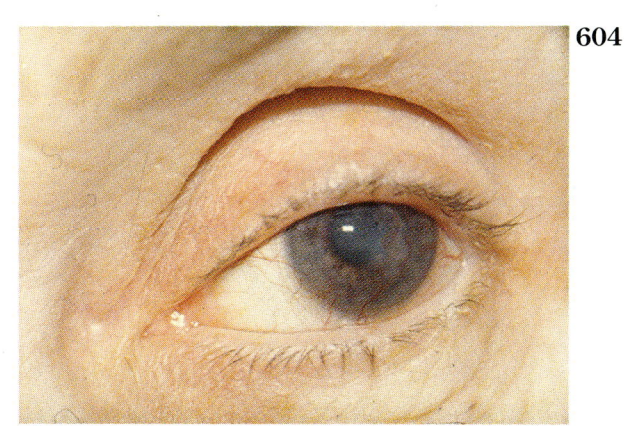

604 Deep stromal vessels.

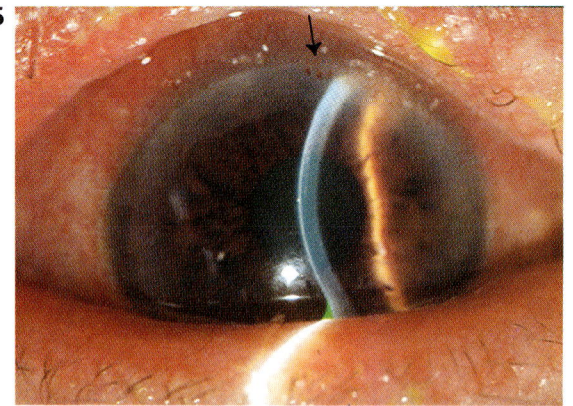

605 Superficial petechial haemorrhages with **conjunctivitis** and contact lens wear.

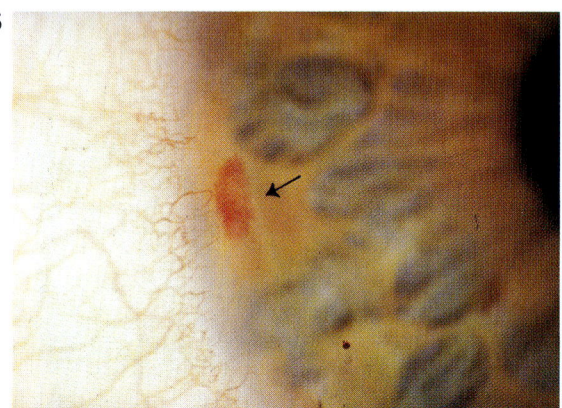

606 Stroma haemorrhage in a gel wearer.

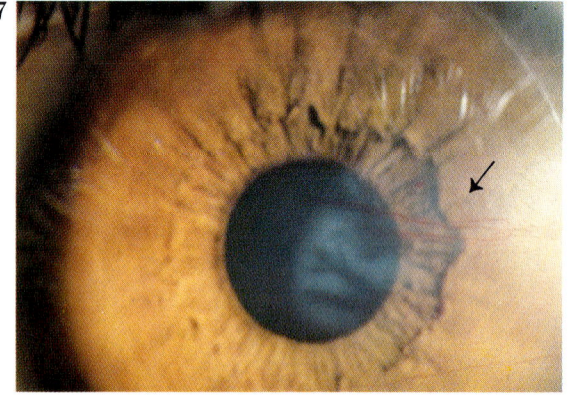

607 The aftermath of **corneal vascularization** can be ghost vessels and a perifibrotic sheathing.

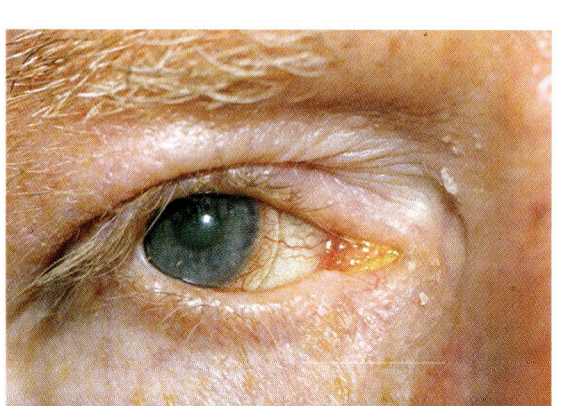

608 & 609 **Exposure keratitis** of seventh cranial nerve origin. It was treated with a gel lens worn continuously and resulted in vascularization and scarring of the cornea. Previous use of scleral lenses was uncomplicated.

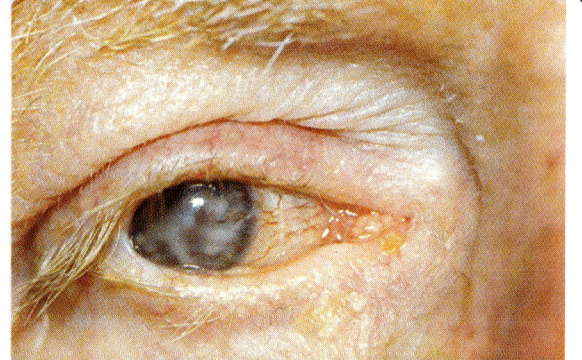

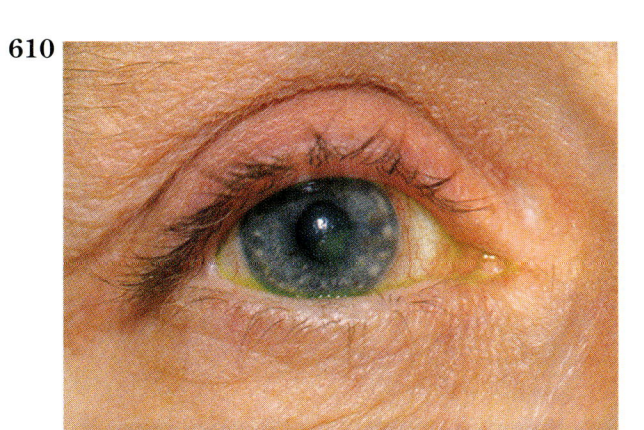

610 & 611 Seventh cranial nerve paresis. Another case of gel lens wear with complications.

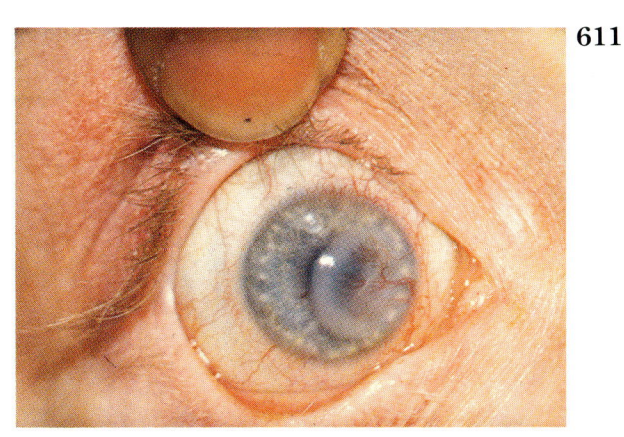

612 Dry eye presenting for cosmetic fitting. (Note the mucus tag).

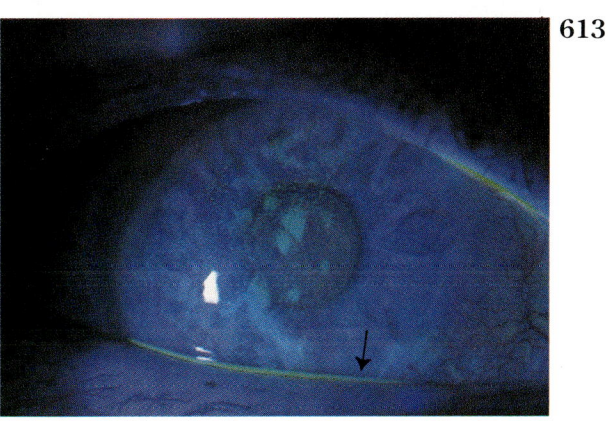

613 Dry eye presenting for cosmetic fitting. (Note the narrow tear lid meniscus).

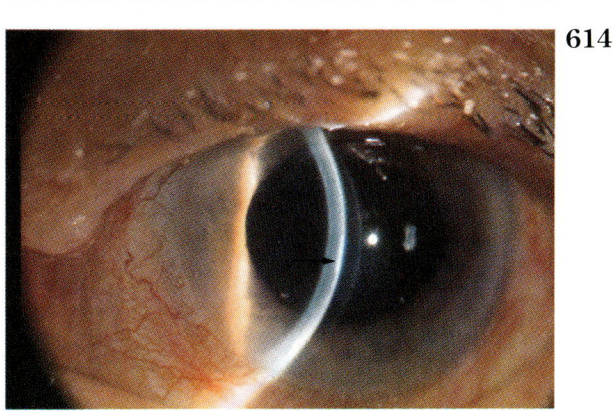

614 Epithelial necrosis with an EW lens in an aphakic diabetic. This may be a membrane abnormality (arrow).

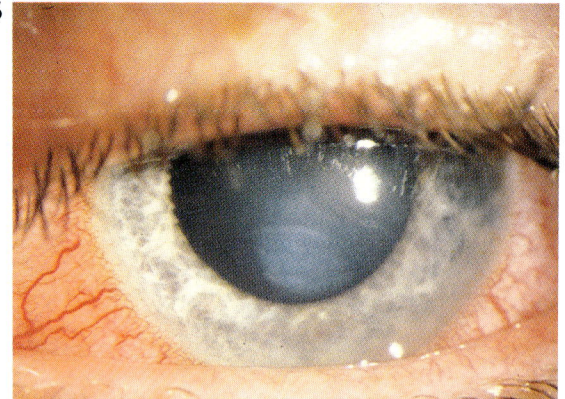

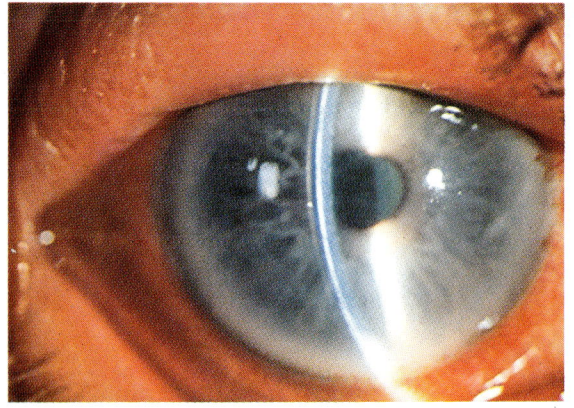

615 & 616 Gross corneal oedema. Sudden onset of gross corneal oedema with Descemet's fold after 24 hours of thick gel lens wear.

617 Slit-lamp section of the above.

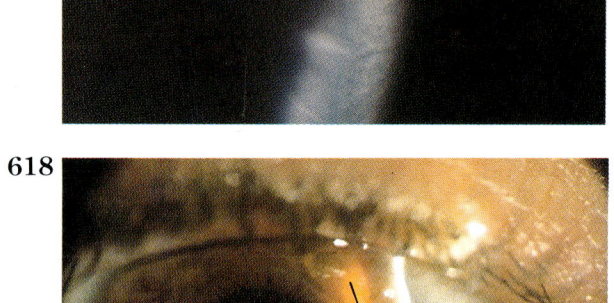

618 & 619 Anterior uveitis, possibly due to daily wear gel lens. It would be difficult to prove the cause (see also **562**).

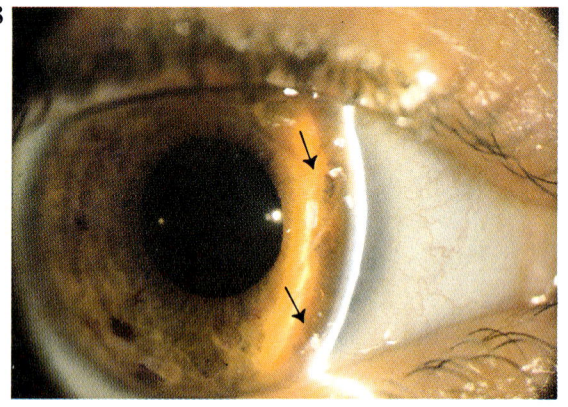

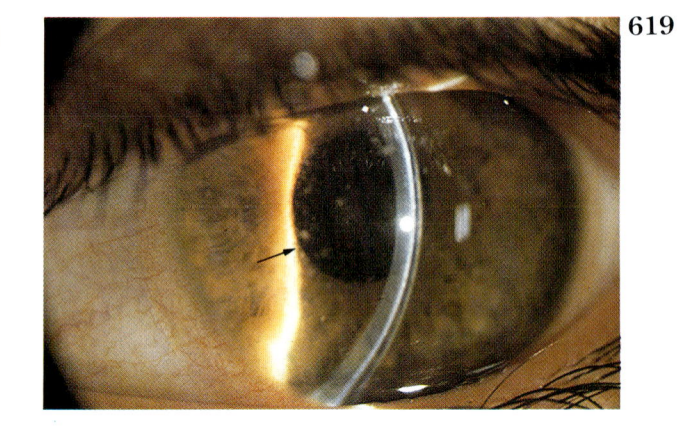

Infection

The contact lens wearer is prone to infection from non-pathogens (opportunist infections) as well as pathogens because the eye and lids are in a compromised state. Furthermore, the use of water without proper disinfection for storage makes the lens a potential source of infection. The eye wearing a contact lens with the residues of disinfectants develops a preference for acid-fast Gram-negative bacteria and therefore serious infections occur with *Bacillus coli*, and pyogenous aerogenosa, rather than with the Gram-positive pathogenic organisms. Even with the use of disinfection methods long-term infections are possible from fungi, especially spores resistant to the disinfectant techniques.

Experience has taught the practitioner that the fewest problems arise from individuals with clean habits who comply with simple directives.

Practitioners themselves can be a source of infection from patient to patient, and effective short-time period methods of cleaning and sterilizing lenses and containers are essential in view of viruses such as the adeno and HIV types (see care of lenses page 47). The organisms most commonly reported as causing vision loss are seratia, *Staphylococcus epidermis*, *B. coli,* fungi (*Candida, Aspergillus*), *Pseudomonas aeruginosa,* and acanthamoeba.

620 Pyocyaneus A. infection. Gel lens wear in a dry eye case—familial dysautonomia. In view of the absence of lysozyme, the dry eye is especially prone to infection, and where a lens is essential as a treatment, prophylactic antibiotics administered locally is advised.

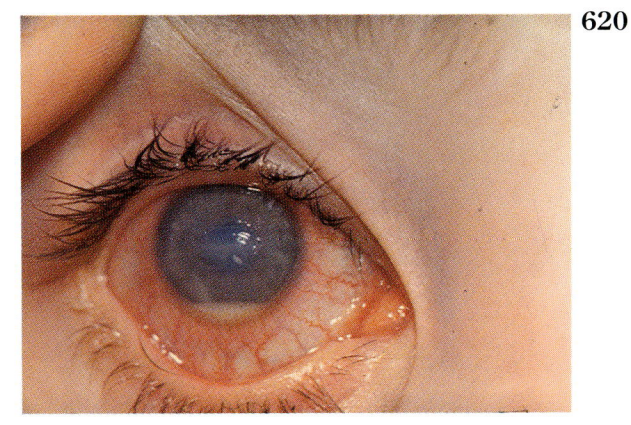

621 & 622 Infection which included yeast, *B. coli* and *P. aeruginosa.*

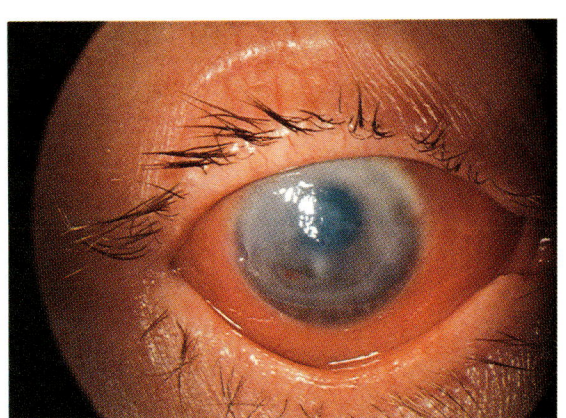

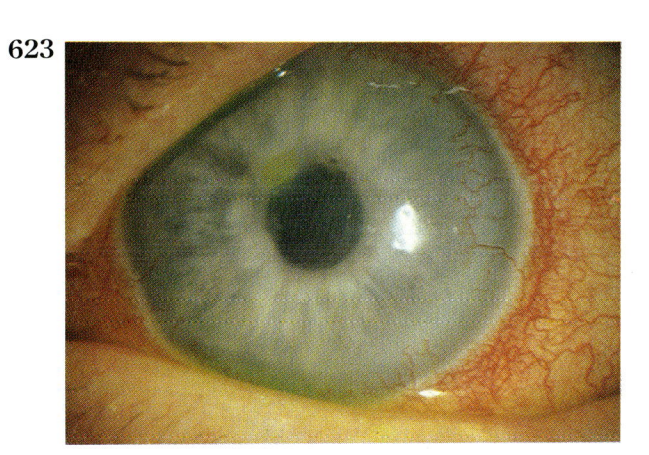

623 & 624 *Staphylococcus* **infection** (suppurative keratitis).

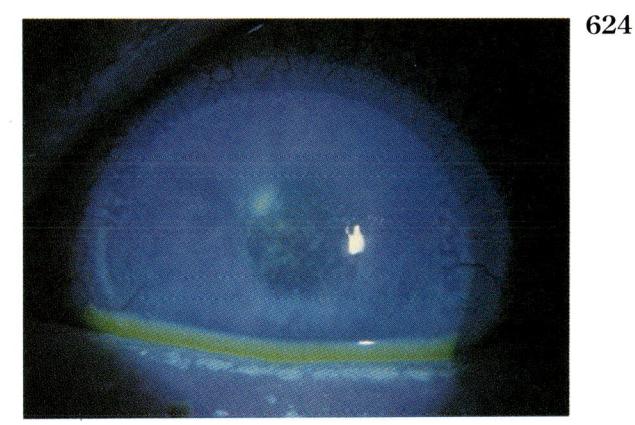

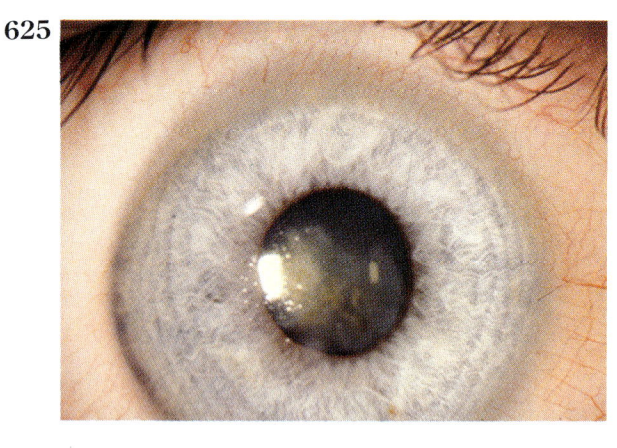

625-627 Suppurative keratitis. Figure **627** is with hypopyon.

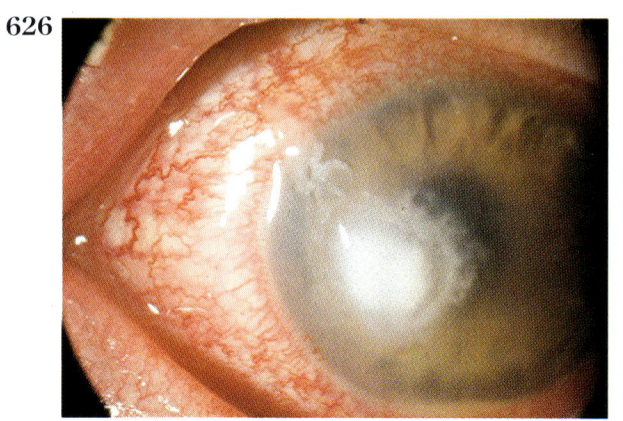

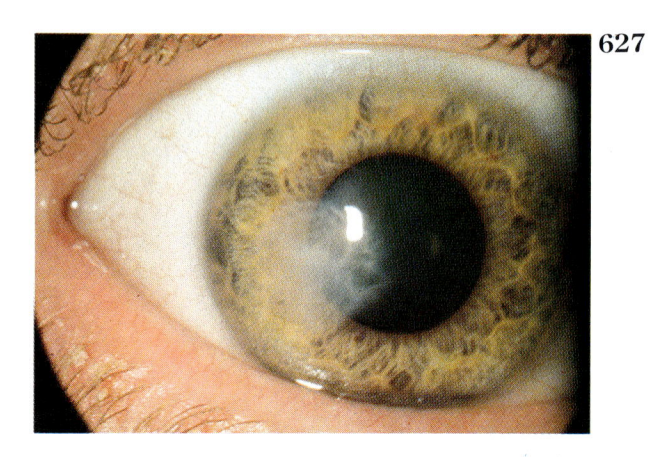

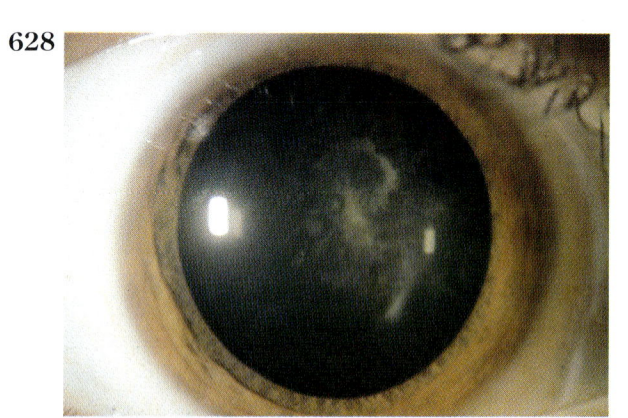

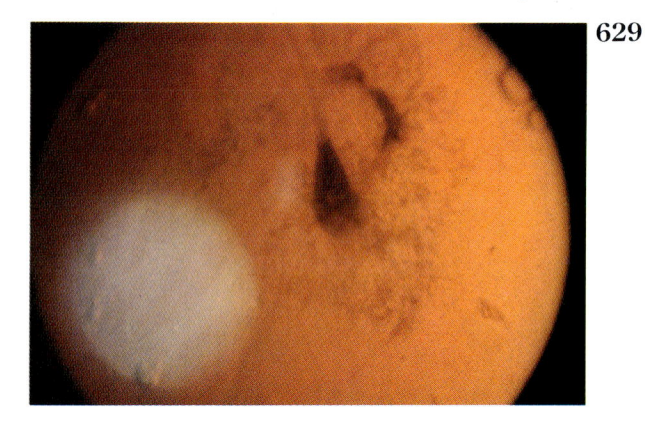

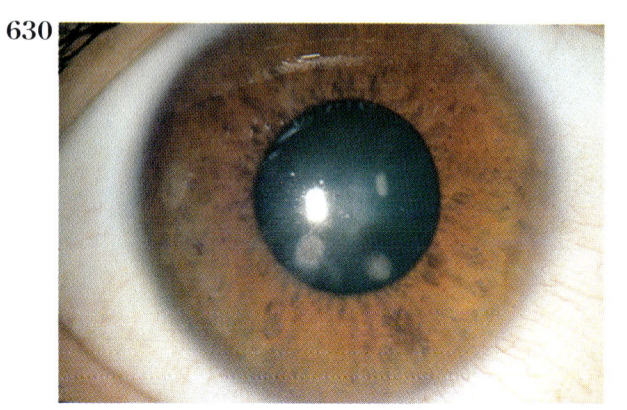

628 & 629 *B. coli* infection.

630 *B. coli* infection producing a nummular type of infection with satellites.
N.B. The fungi infections are the commonest to spoil a lens, but they do not necessarily cause an infective keratitis. Infection does not appear to be related to how often a lens is cleaned, but the incidence in E.W is greater, especially among the debilitated (senile) and diabetic.

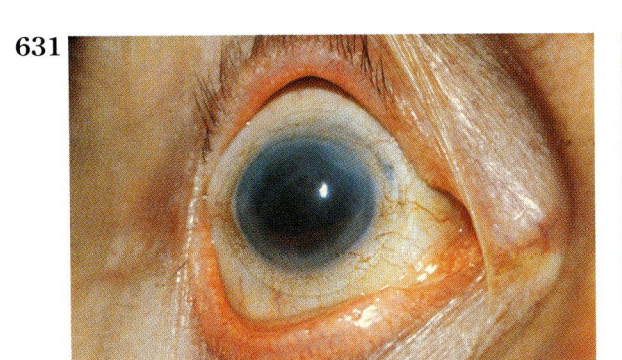

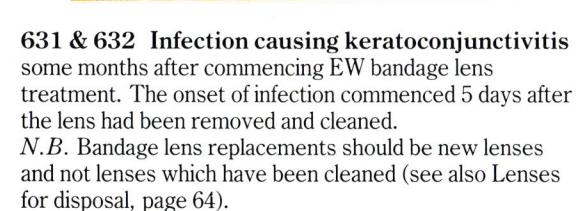

631 & 632 Infection causing keratoconjunctivitis some months after commencing EW bandage lens treatment. The onset of infection commenced 5 days after the lens had been removed and cleaned.
N.B. Bandage lens replacements should be new lenses and not lenses which have been cleaned (see also Lenses for disposal, page 64).

633 Blepharitis is rarely caused by staphylococcal infection but is the commonest complication of contact lens wear. Note associated SPK.

634-636 *Acanthamoeba* **keratitis.** The source of infection can be stagnant water especially heated water, e.g. hot tubs, CL preparations and cases. The organism is a trophozoite and has a cystic form. The infected cornea shows a progressive chronic kerato-conjunctivitis with stromal haze and does not respond to normal treatments.

The differential diagnosis is herpes simplex, but this infection can develop a ring ulcer with perforation and uveitis of some severity. Diagnosis is made from the smear culture and tissue section and investigation of the contact lens and case (and preparations in use).

Figure **634** shows ring keratitis; **635** shows *acanthamoeba* trophozoites ($\times 13,000$) the inset shows trophozoite (arrow) in the corneal epithelium ($\times 230$); and **636** shows cysts in the corneal stroma (ectocysts and endocyst, $\times 9000$; inset bottom left cyst, $\times 850$; inset top right amoebic cyst by indirect immunofluorescence, $\times 540$).

(Figures courtesy of R. Tripathi, R. Monninger and B. Tripathi, Votrag gehaten auf den, 1986. Tagung der Deutschen Opth. Gesellschaft, Berlin.)

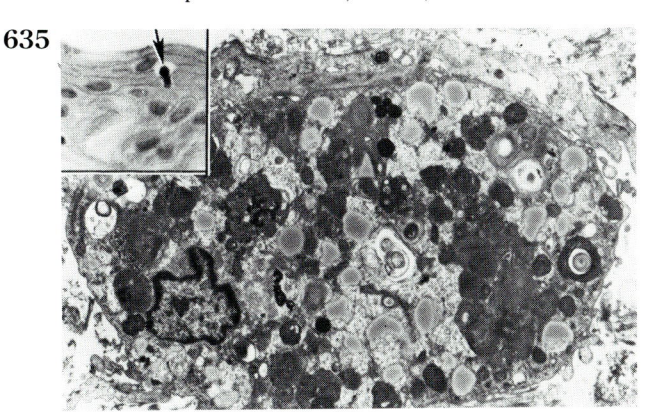

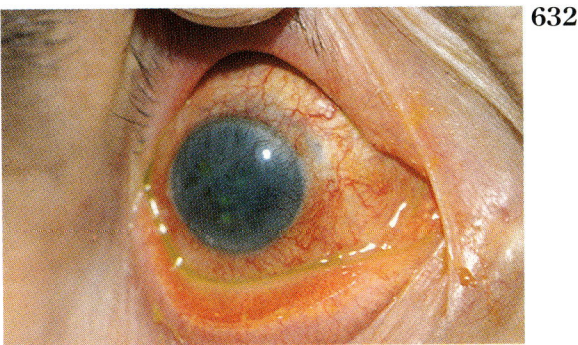

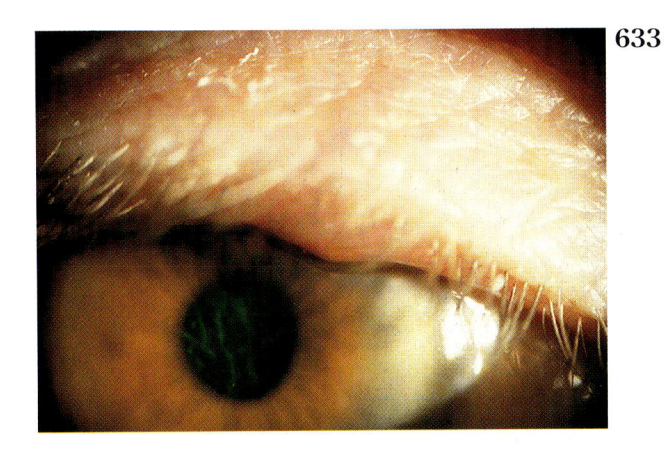

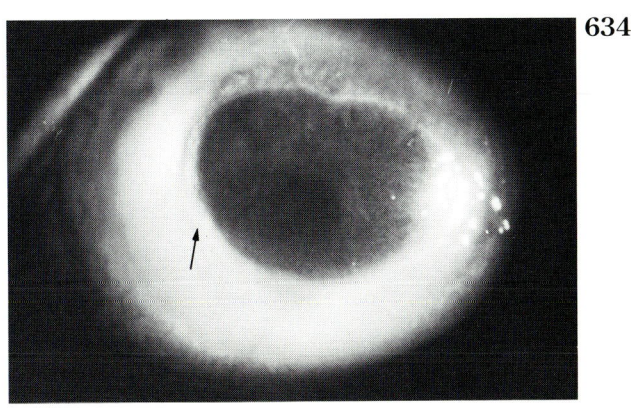

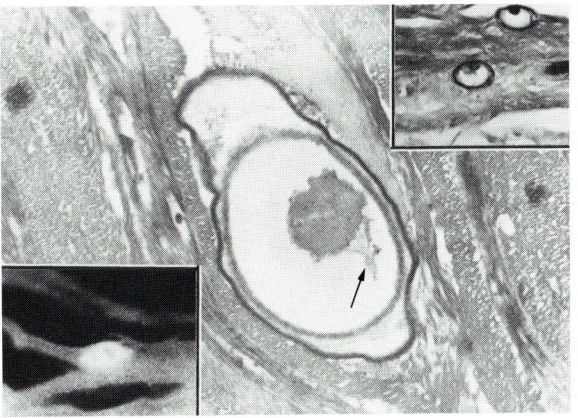

Lids and conjunctival problems

637 Infection of the plica semilunaris.

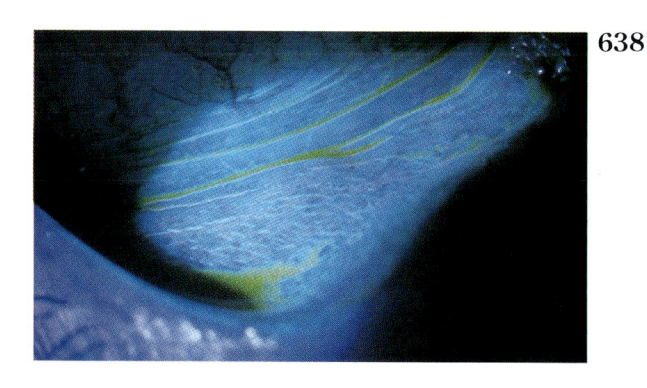

638 Papillary conjunctivitis. Mild, moderate and giant can be useful classifications, rather than measuring the papillae.

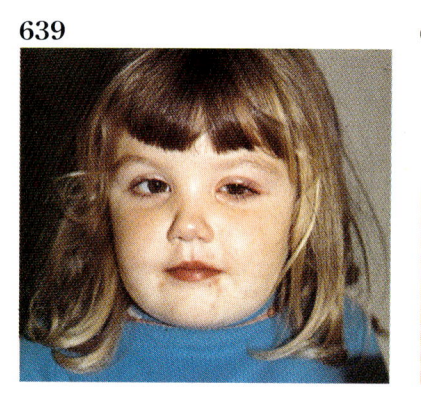

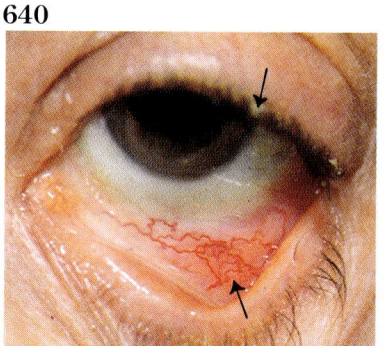

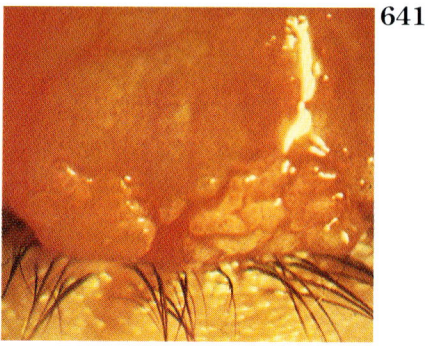

639 Infective blepharitis. Squamous rather than exudative infective blepharitis is the most common complication of contact lens wear.

640 Blepharitis and chronic hyperaemia of the palpebral conjunctivae.

641 Vernal conjunctivitis exacerbated by contact lens wear. The gel lens turned milky-white, possibly due to a lipid emulsion.

642 Giant papillary conjunctivitis from gel lens wear. (Figure courtesy of W.J. Benjamin.) Associated with mucous discharge, irritation, lens coatings, lens-lid adhesion.

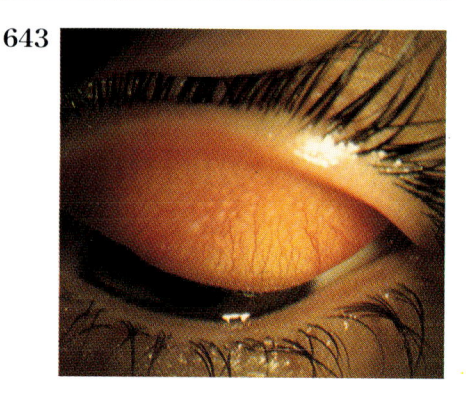

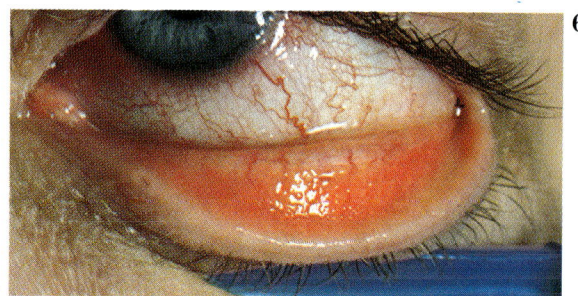

643 & 644 Moderate degree of follicular type conjunctivitis which can affect upper (**643**) and lower (**644**) lids.

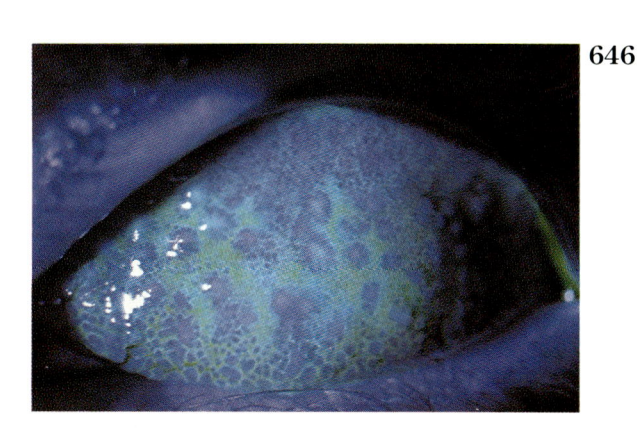

645 & 646 Advanced follicular and papillary conjunctivitis with hyaline changes in the papillae, which can even become calcified.

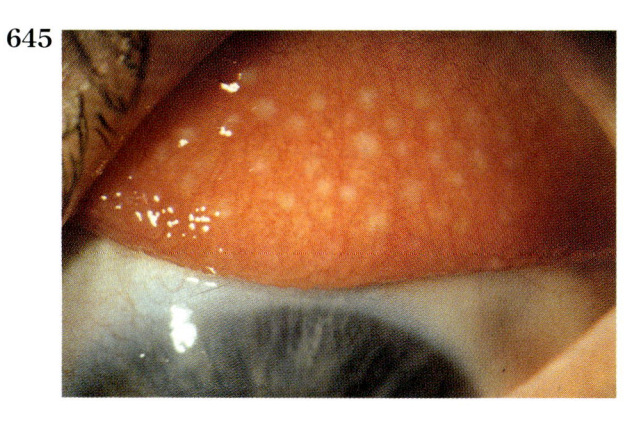

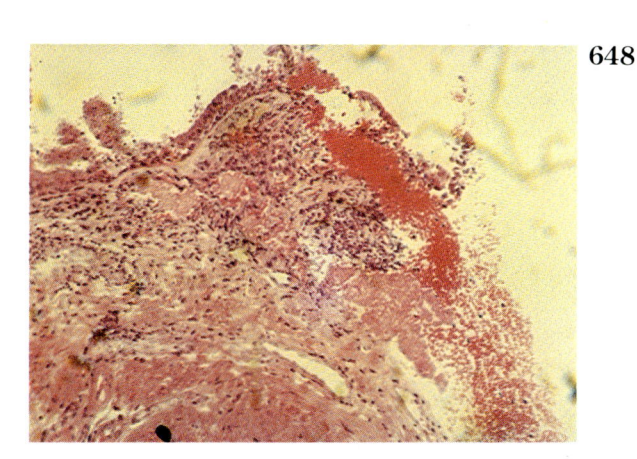

647 & 648 Histology. The conjunctival biopsy shows that the papilla is most likely allergy-related in aetiology. A true papilla has a vascular core and often mast cells are to be seen. The follicular type is an aggregate of lymph cells and other inflammatory agents. Sometimes the reaction appears granulomatous.

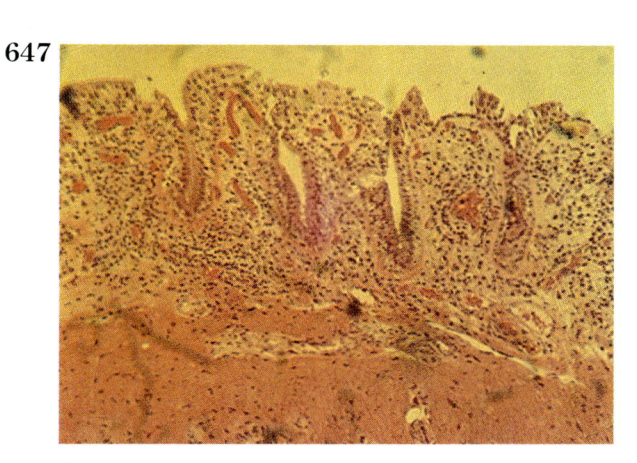

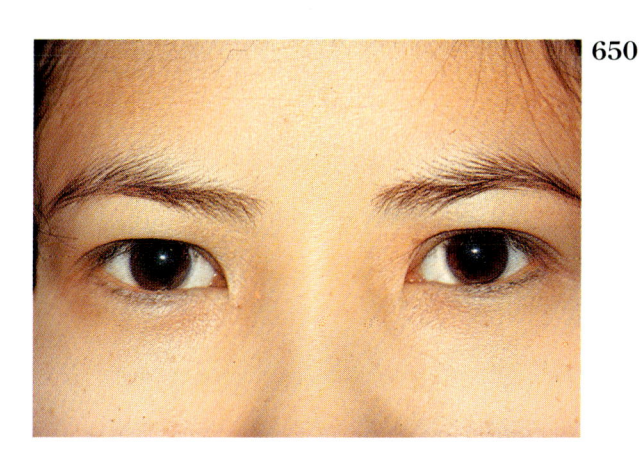

649 & 650 Sudden allergic attack affecting both eyes and due to new solutions, Resolved five days after withdrawl of contact lens wear (**650**).

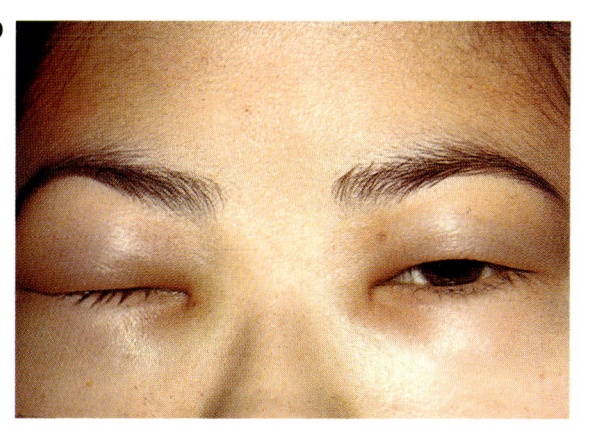

181

Optical problems

651

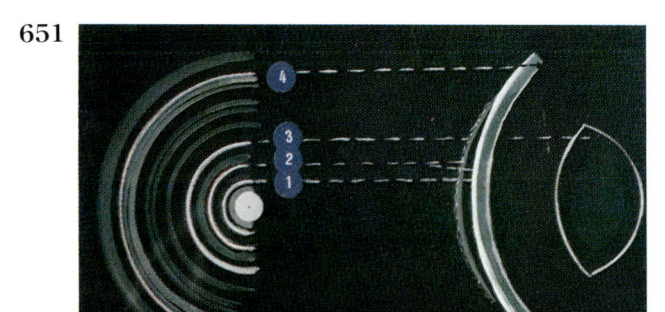

- The oedema of corneal epithelium and endothelium produces a red tinge around lights and
- Lower than normal scoring with contrast sensitivity acuity and mesoptic vision deterioration.
- Image size differences have been illustrated (see figures 314-19) and can present an initial problem.

651 Haloes. These can emanate from the lens or the eye tissues. They can arise from lenses made of two different refractive media (e.g. fused bifocals) or from the scoring with diffraction gratings to produce a change of power. The aetiology is interferometry patterns.

The illustration shows that each refractive interface of the optical system can produce its own type of halo.

652 Excessive lens motility and decentring of the optic is a problem solved by fitting.
- Excessive tearing or lens grease haze are difficult to solve in some patients.
- Residual astigmatism can be a formidable problem.
- Low power corrections (under one dioptre) are difficult to obtain good acuity with.

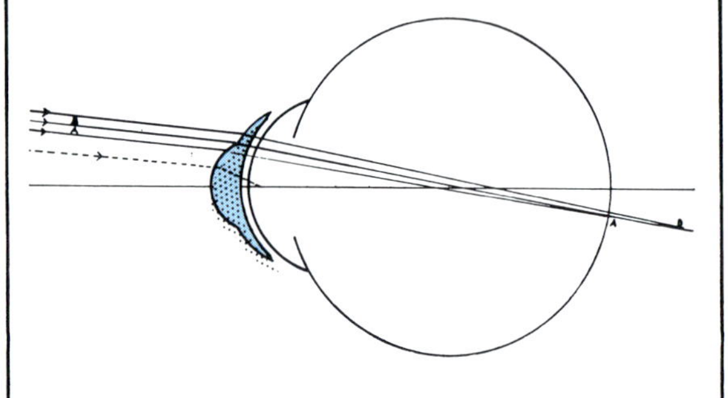

The contact lens acuity tolerance is not as good in low refractive errors as the spectacle lens.

652

Variable prismatic effect with lens sag (reduced optic)

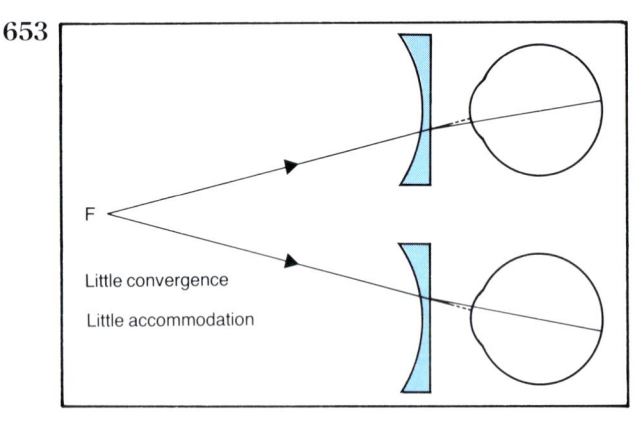

653 Spectacles and myopia. The advantage of a prism's base in the myope with spectacles is lost with contact lenses and the patient may require orthoptic exercises.

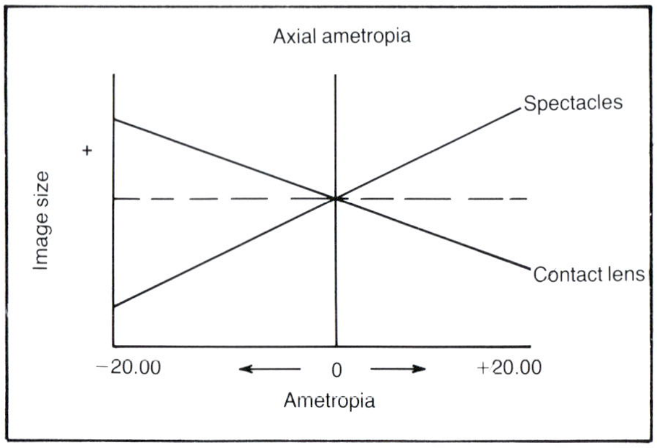

654 Pre-presbyopic (accommodation deficiency of optical origin) state with full myopic correction is a problem for the age group 30-40 years.

653

F

Little convergence

Little accommodation

655 The edge can produce a white flare effect. Other glare effects are due to epithelial oedema and grease haze or dry surfaces of spoilt lenses. They all reduce contrast (especially at night) and sometimes multiple images.

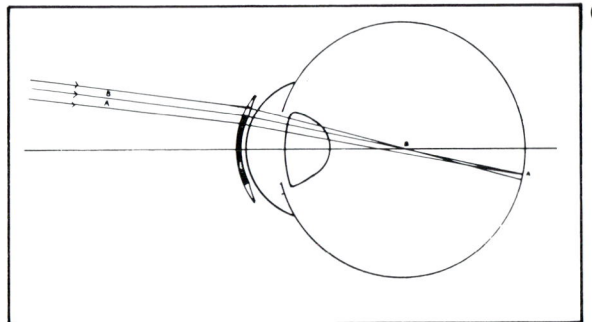

654

Axial ametropia

Spectacles

Image size

Contact lens

−20.00   0   +20.00

Ametropia

655

182

9 Prosthetics

The contact lens that is used to correct physiological ametropia is often called a cosmetic visual contact lens. The word cosmesis means to enhance nature. Thus the contact lens takes away the spectacles and permits the face to look natural. The additional use of coloured contact lens (as with all cosmetics) has to be skilfully used otherwise the effect can be the opposite of that desired and, instead of enhancing nature with a wish to beautify, can make an individual look odd. Use of contact lenses of *abnormal* colour can be considered cosmesis, but only as part of the world of fashion.

Prosthetics are designed to cover or mask disfigurement in such a way that the individual appears normal. Thus the objectives of cosmesis and prothesis are different but the appliances used may overlap in function.

Types of ocular prosthetics

- Contact lenses of different materials and colours to simulate normality. The sizes can vary from corneal to very large scleral lenses.
- Shell prosthesis—a plastic shell made to fit over a residuum of an eye muscle cone implant. The thickness can vary according to the fitting technique.
- Orbital prosthesis or artificial eye.

N.B. The prosthetics practitioner can be a highly-skilled craftsman, but in some parts of the world the only skills available will be those of the contact lens and dental practitioners.

Corneal prosthetic lenses

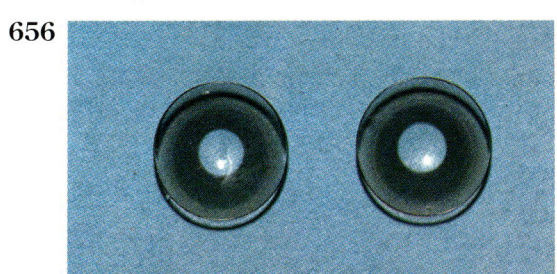

656

657

658

656-658 PMMA corneal lenses. These are all types of PMMA corneal lenses. **656** is coloured fused plastic lens with a clear pupil. **657** is a laminate with the iris painted onto the plastic. Diazo type dyes are used with masks to produce colour effects (as with spectacle lenses).

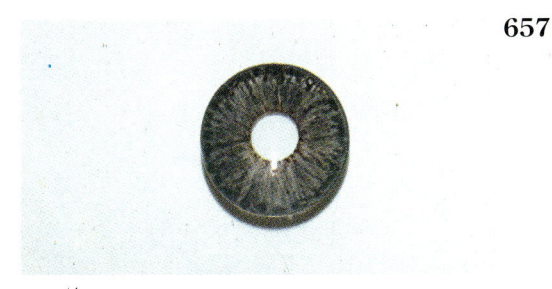

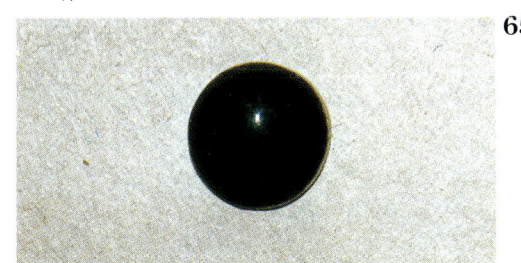

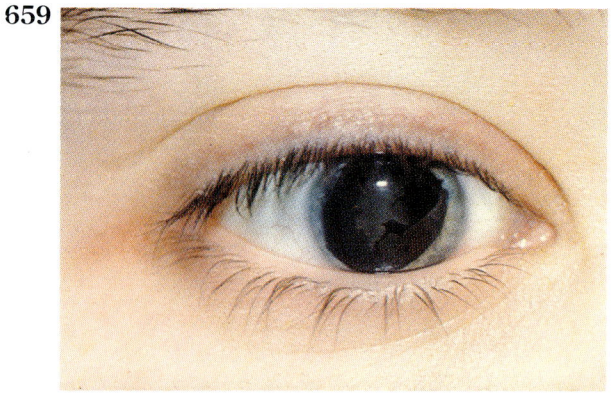

659 & 660 Traumatic aniridia fitted with a stock commercial hard cosmetic lens.

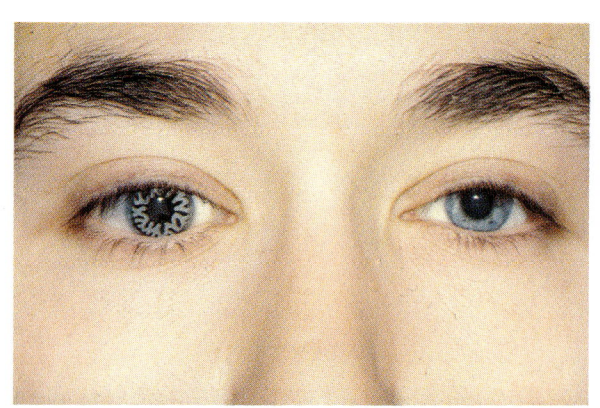

661 & 662 Traumatic aniridia fitted with a prosthetic scleral lens with a painted iris (occlusive).

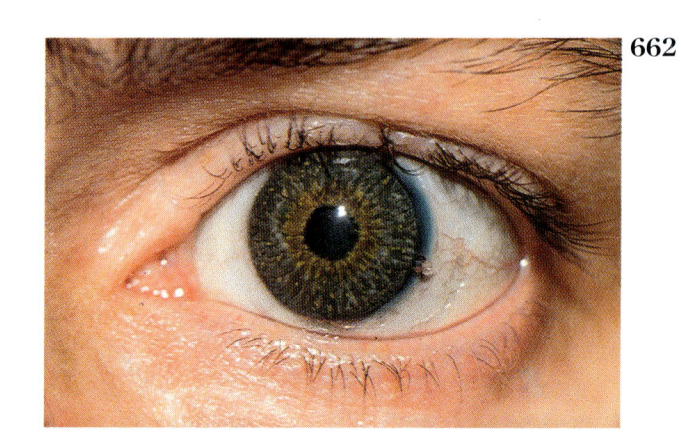

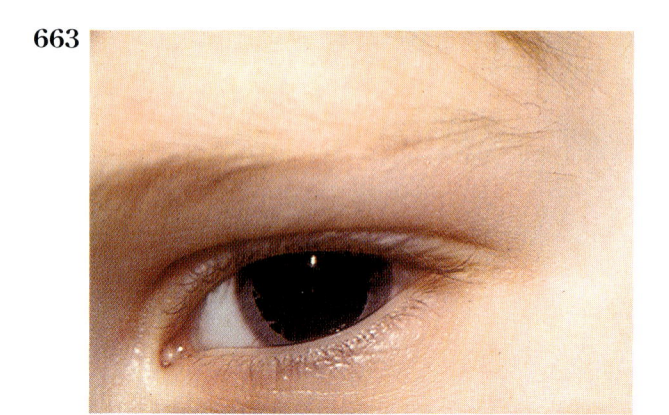

663 & 664 Aniridia fitted with a soft gel coloured lens (opaque colouration).

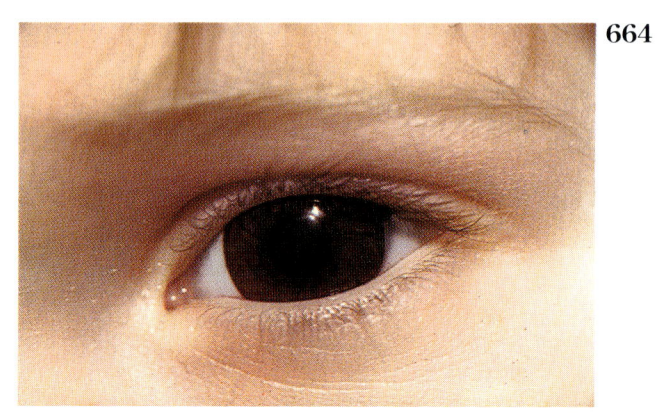

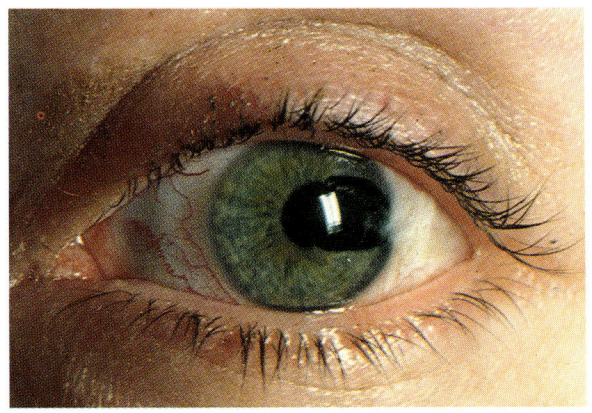

665 & 666 **Traumatic coloboma** fitted with opaque coloured gel lens.

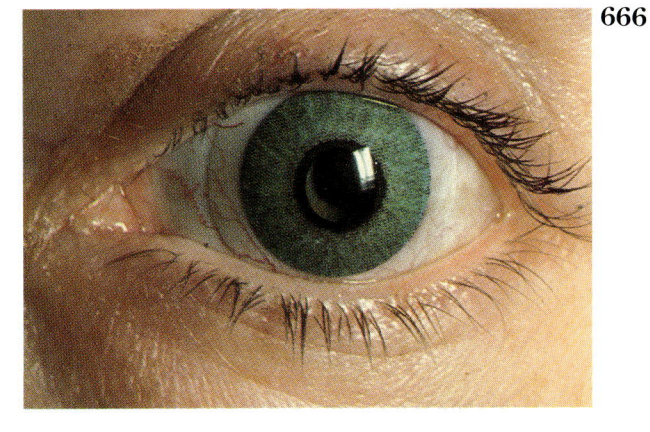

667 **Opaque coloured PHEMA lens** (Hydron).

668 & 669 **Failed keratoplasty** fitted with coloured gel lens.
N.B. To improve the appearance, both eyes can be fitted with coloured lenses to obtain a better match.

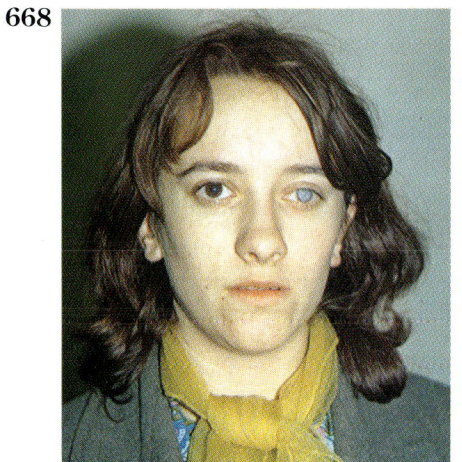

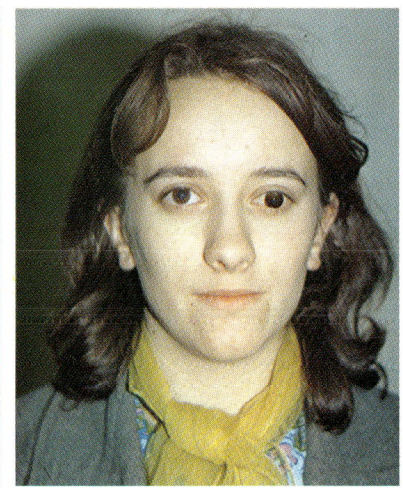

185

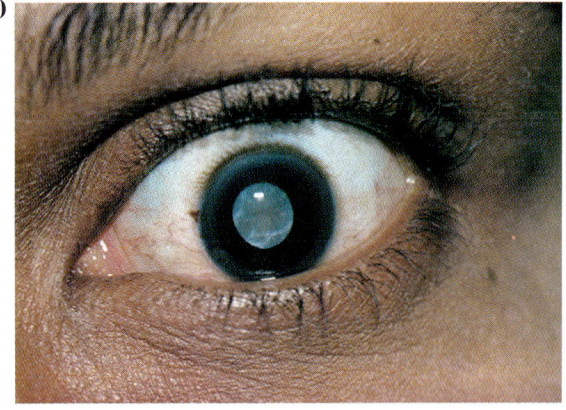

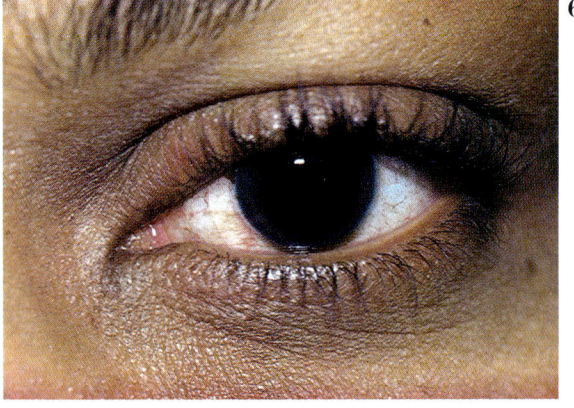

670 & 671 Inoperable cataract covered by a coloured gel lens.

Scleral hard prosthetic lenses and shells

These are fitted using the impression technique described on page 96. Careful centreing is required and the lens has to be proven to be tolerable. In those cases where a clear power optic is desired, the power surface curvatures and thicknesses must all be known. The final stage will be either to remove surface material prior to painting and then graft new plastic over the painting or, with thick shells, to make positive and negative dyes to achieve the new front surface by injection moulding.

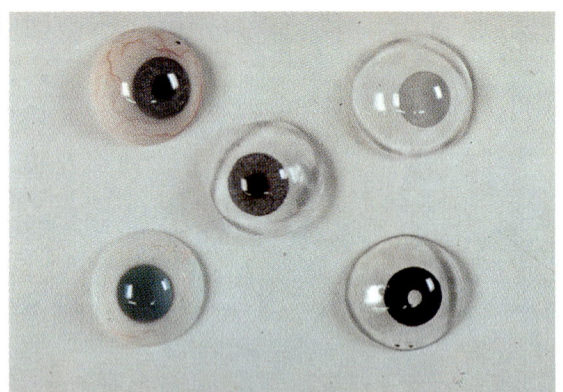

672 Variety of effects possible with scleral lenses and shells.

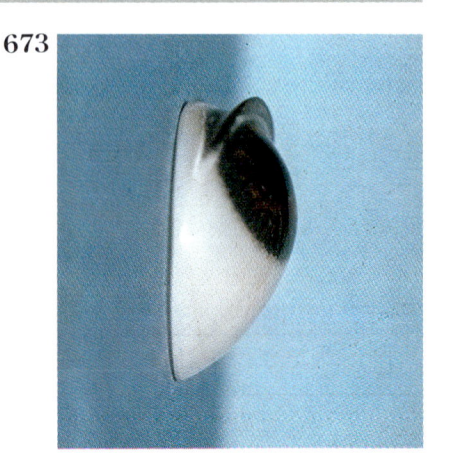

673 Shells with ptosis ledges are possible where there is a coexistent paresis with a disfigured eye.

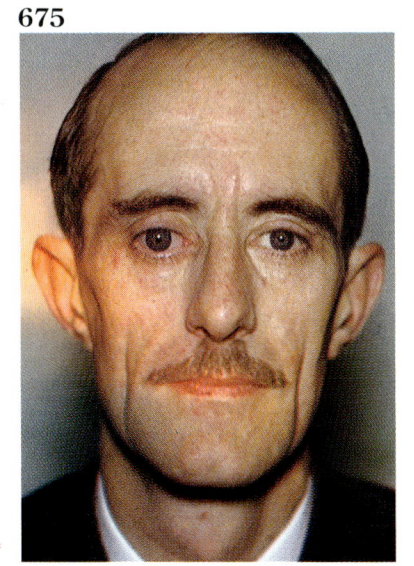

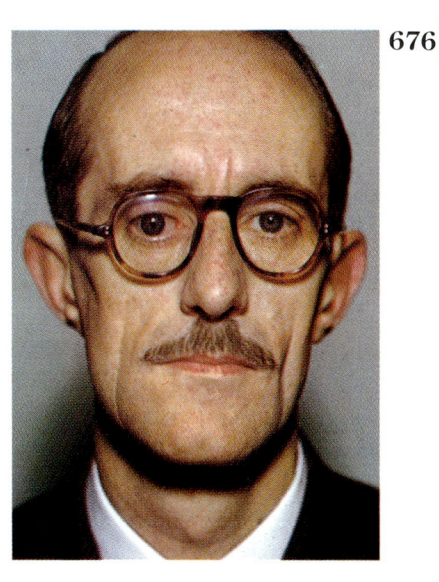

674–676 Spectacle frame. The shell prosthesis can be used with a spectacle frame to diminish the artificial appearance. Furthermore, the spectacle lens over the prosthetic eye can be made a positive or negative power to magnify or lessen the artificial effect and obtain a better balance. Slight tints in the spectacle lenses will also help to mask the disfigurement.

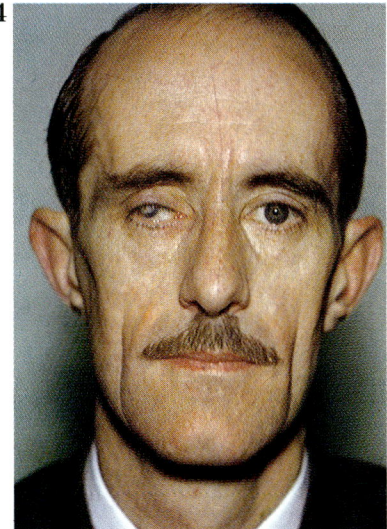

677 & 678 A **dermoid** is hidden by a prosthetic shell.

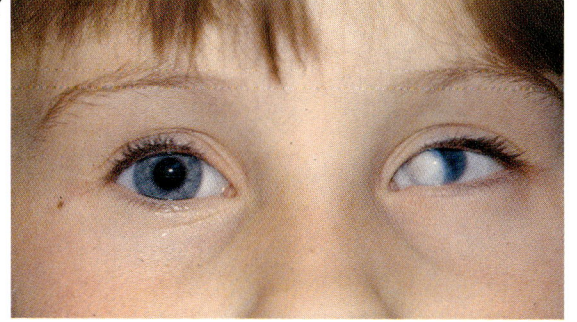

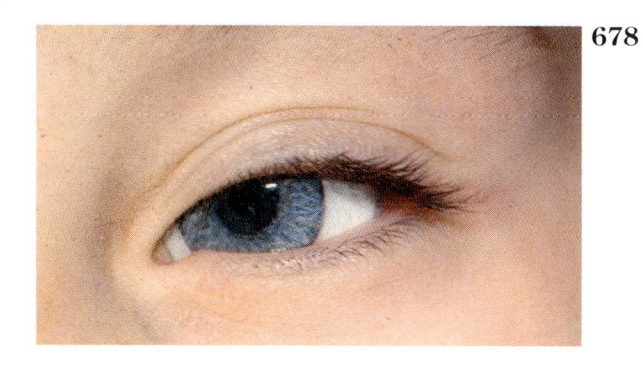

679 & 680 A **convergent strabismus** can be 'corrected' by decentring the shell.
N.B. In some instances, where the strabismus is too great to allow good fitting, corrective strabismus surgery should be done first before fitting.

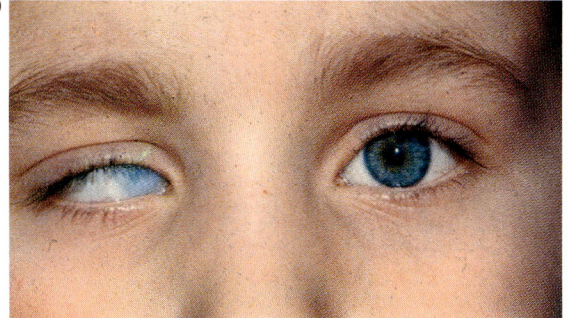

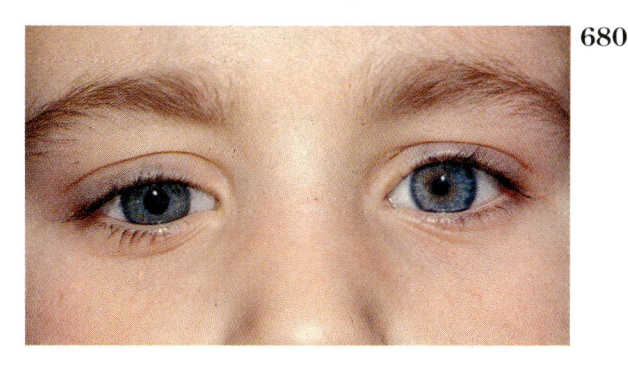

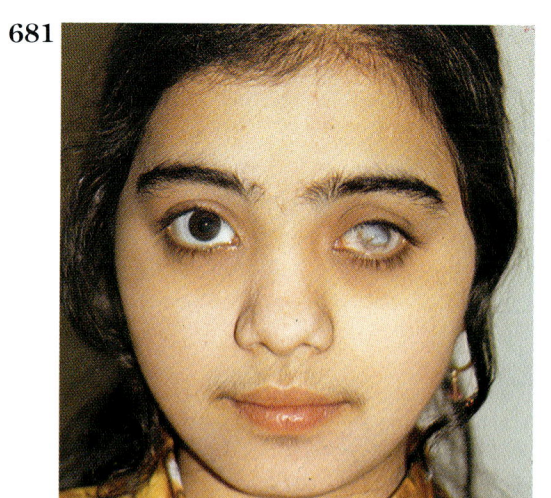

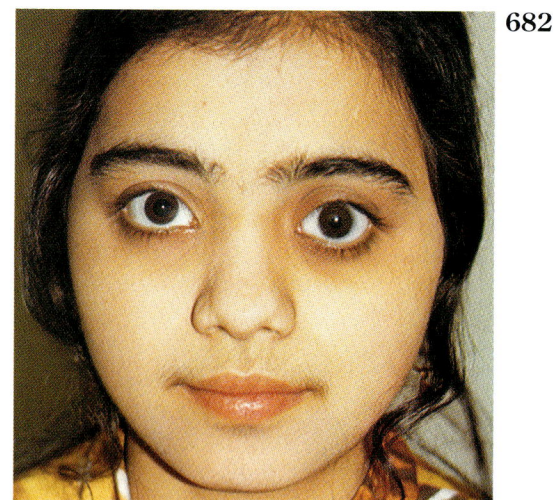

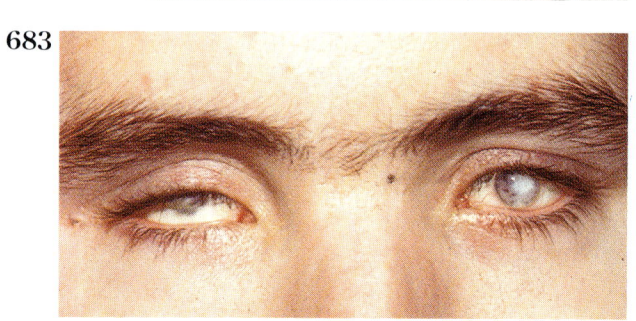

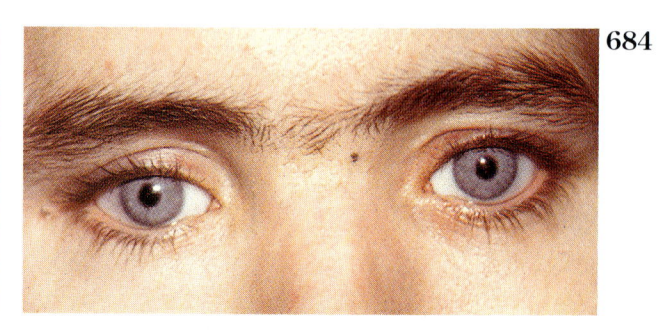

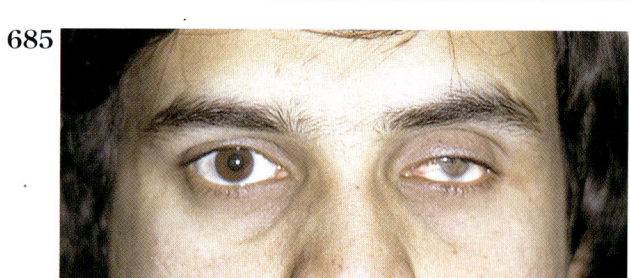

681-686 Disfiguring corneal leukomata covered by prosthetic shells.

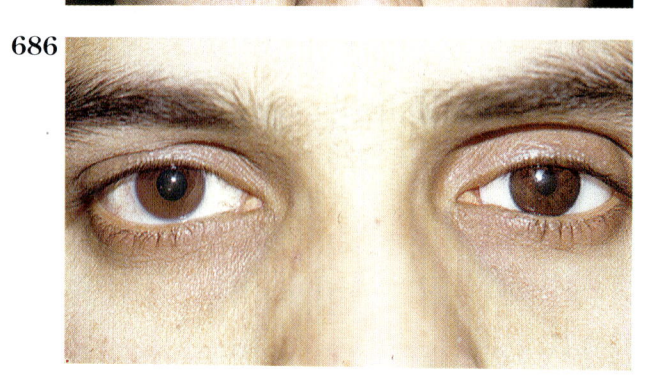

687 & 688 Albinos. While most albinos wish to have contact lenses in the hope of improving vision, various types of coloured opaque lenses can decrease the photophobia and also improve the appearance.

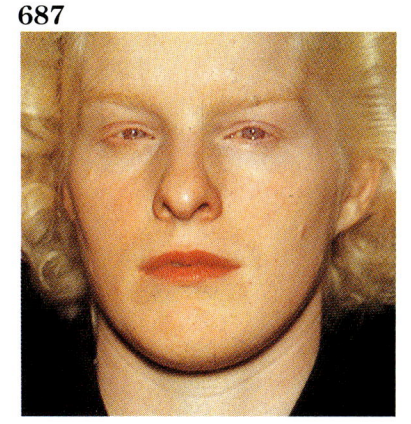

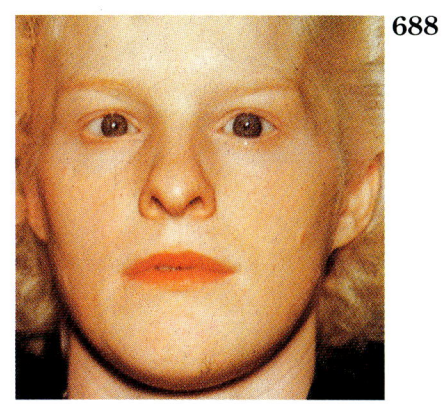

Orbital prostheses

Procedures involving the enucleation and evisceration of the eye have very variable results, often because the procedure may be one of many others in cases of trauma. The young patient would however want the maximal consideration and expertly planned surgery for any of these procedures.

Enucleation problems

- The underlying pathology that led to enucleation may still persist, such as dry eye problem, infection, and recurrent growths.
- The fornices may be shallow or absent and the socket contracted.
- Retro-orbital fat that has retracted, degenerated and been absorbed.
- If a muscle cone implant was placed, it may have been dislodged or not function due to muscle damage or paresis. In any event, muscle cone implants will give restricted movements and a centre of rotation more posterior than normal.
- There can be severe orbital furrow retraction (superiorly) and other lid problems, such as ptosis or abnormalities from trauma and corrective plastic surgery.
- In most instances, it requires the joint efforts of the surgeon and a prosthetic fitter to solve the problem, even with further surgery to the floor or walls of the orbit being necessary.
- The eye evisceration procedure with a ball implant and a scleral graft can give the best results since the end process is to fit a shell prosthesis with almost full eye movement.

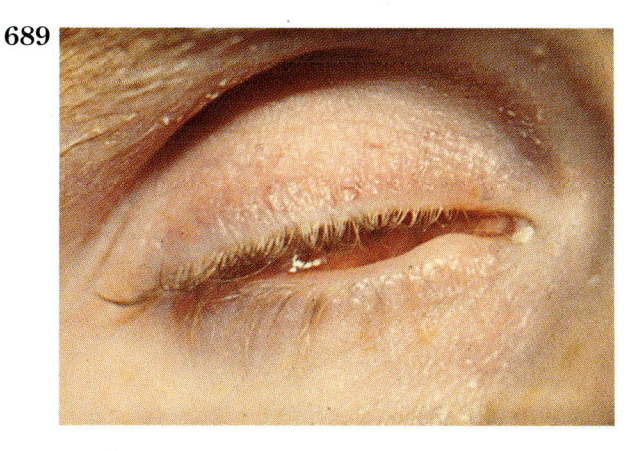

689 & 690 Severe orbital furrow retraction.

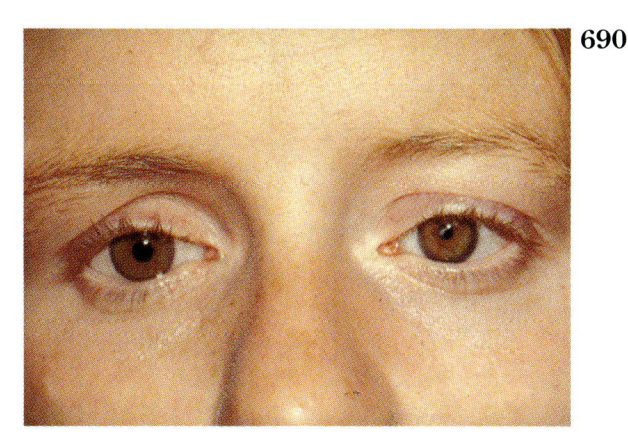

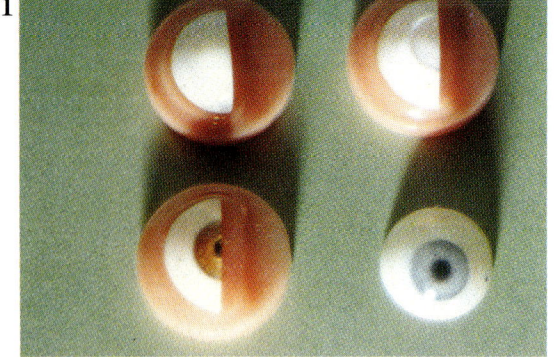

691 Orbital prostheses. A selection of scleral and iris colours, sizes and different conjunctival vessel effects are available as half shells. They can then be cut to shape to obtain the best fit. This type of practice is ideal for one-day fitting and issue providing large stocks are kept.

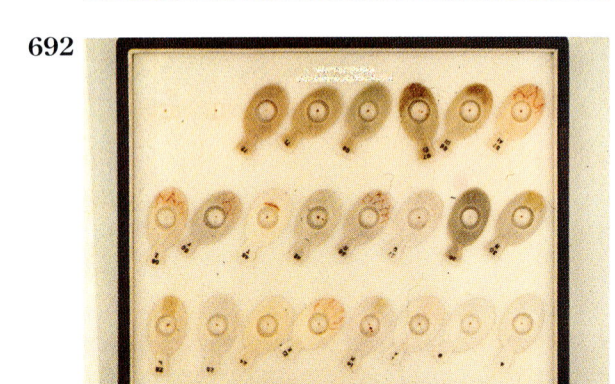

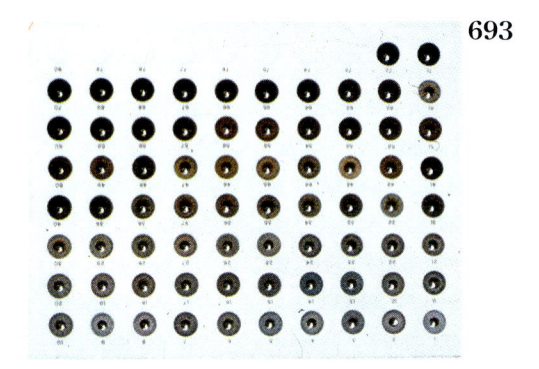

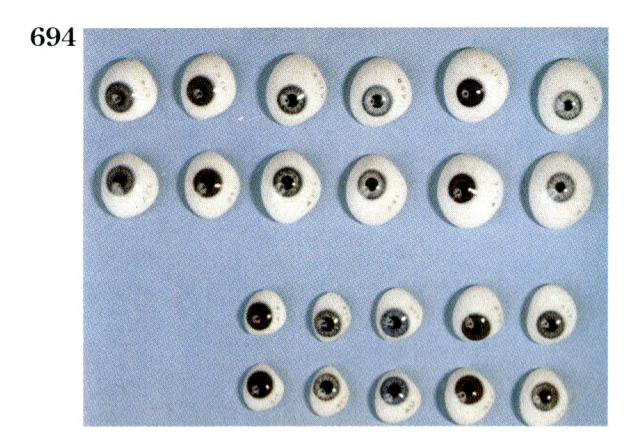

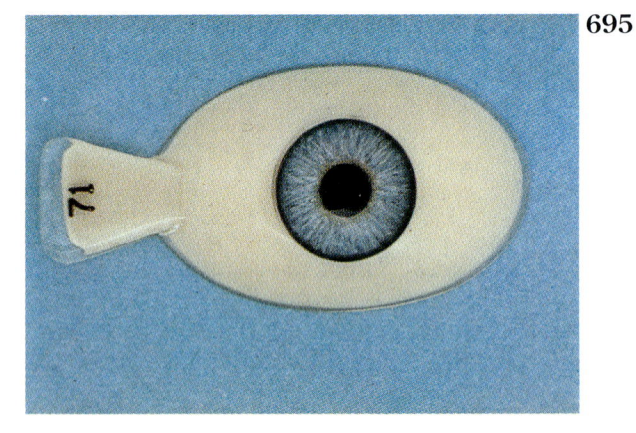

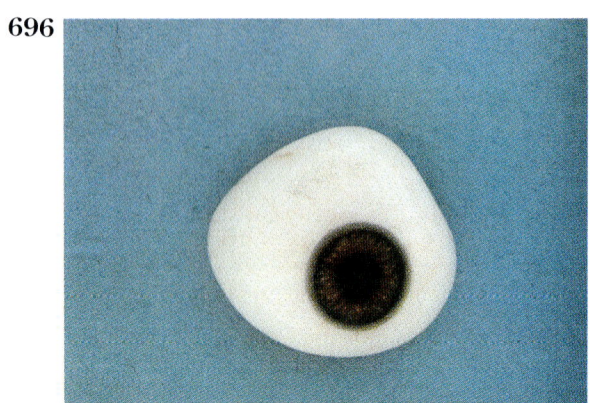

692-696 Fitting set. The alternative to **691** is to have a fitting set of shapes and matching iris and scleral colours (Nissel Artificial Eye). The final eye can then be ordered.

190

Prosthesis stages. The sectioned acrylic models in **691** show the various stages in making the prosthesis.

697-699 Stages in the fitting of an impression prosthesis. 698 is the acrylic model which is modified to obtain a satisfactory fit and then marked and matched for colours.

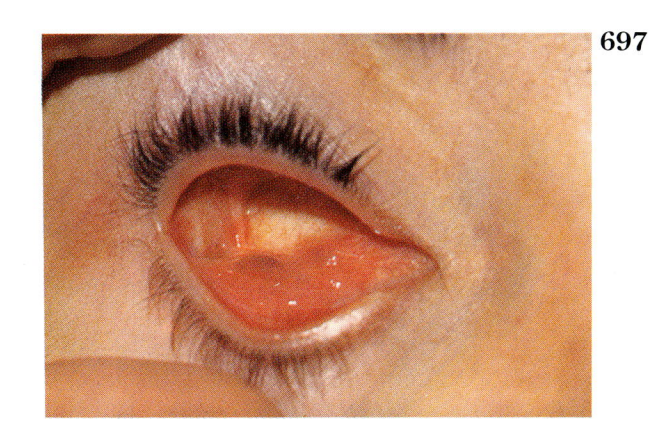

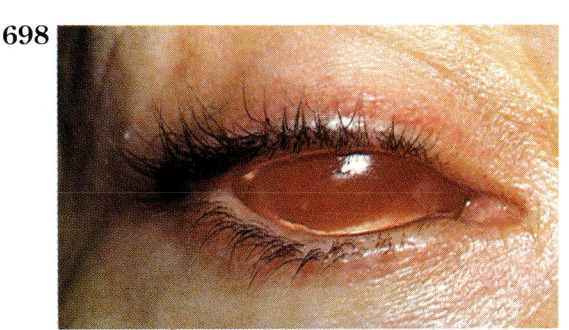

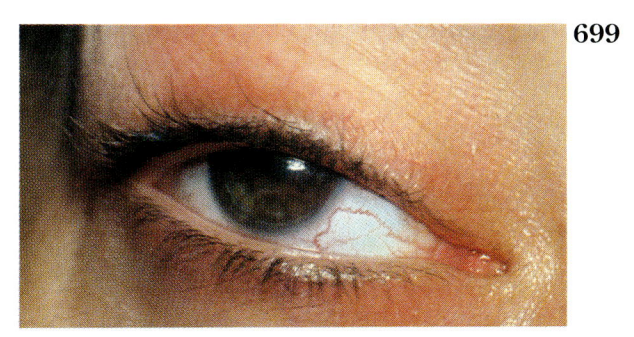

Modifications to the orbital prosthesis

It is perhaps easy to take material away from a prosthesis but the craftsman's skill is to add material. The conventional shape is triangular with the base below. Nasally there is the trochlear notch and temporally material can also be removed (**700**). Posteriorly, material can be removed to lighten the artificial eye but keeping thickness below as ballast. Fitting additions are made at the chairside with soft dental wax heated and moulded to shape. Figs. **701** and **702** show where such additions are usually added.

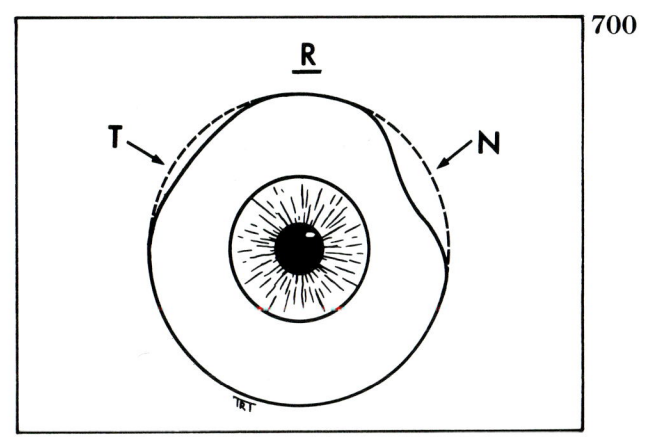

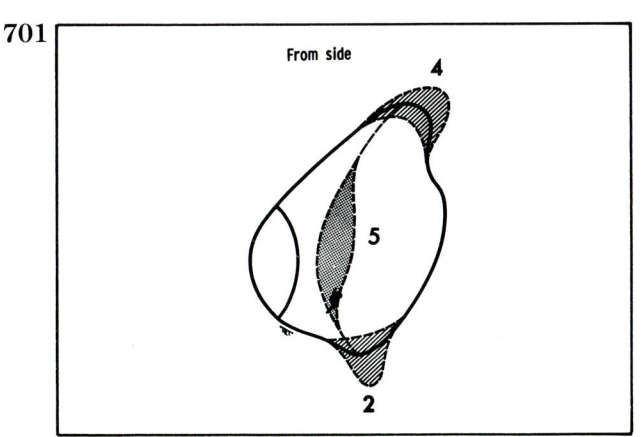

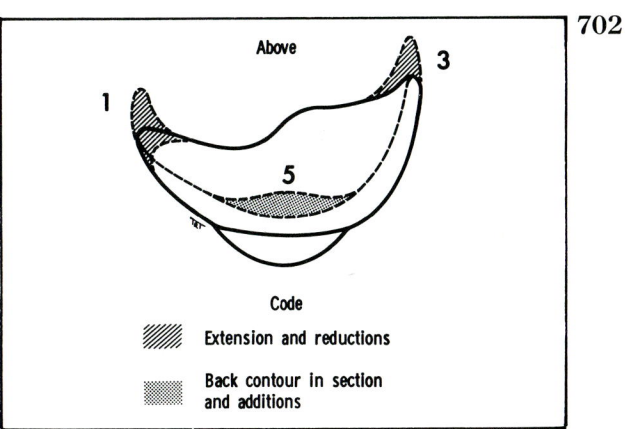

191

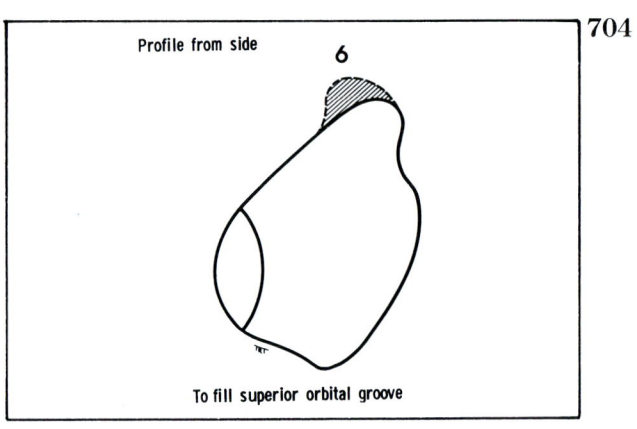

703 & 704 'Lost wax' technique. By the 'lost wax' technique new dyes can be made for the altered eye and acrylic material added or a new eye made. There are many different methods which make this practice a craft requiring training and skill.

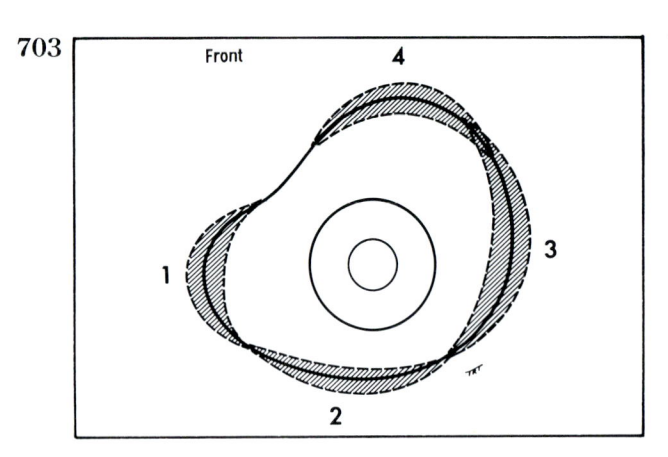

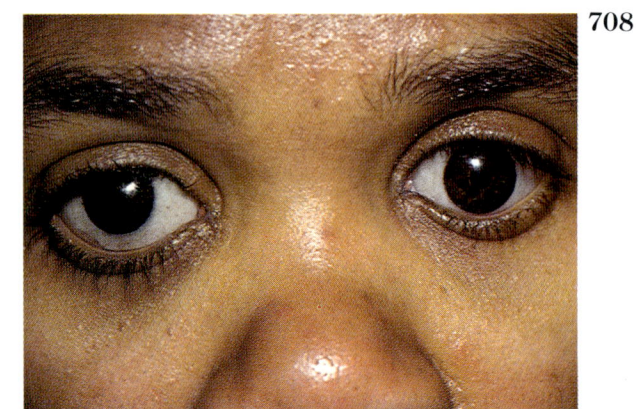

705-708 Poor fit of the right artificial eye. After modifications (**706** & **707**) a remake gave a better result (**708**).

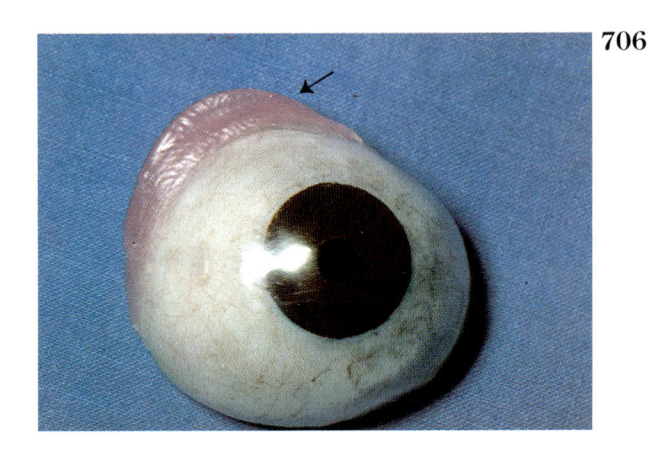

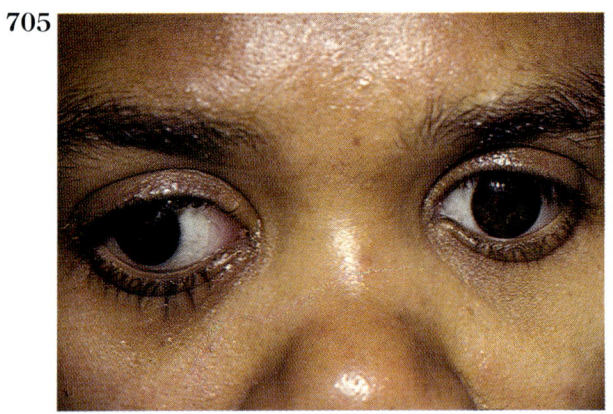

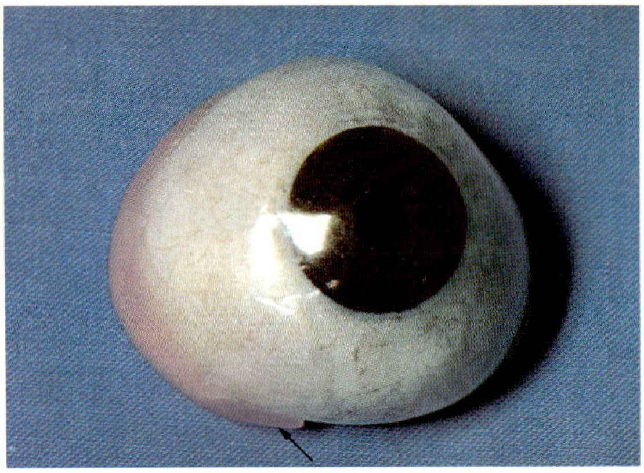

709 & 710 Bilateral anophthalmos with entropion and blepharophimosis—baby. The residual eyes and sockets are funnel shaped and the retention of artificial eyes is very difficult. Black plastic beads of different sizes should be available for fitting and the use of butterfly clear plastic wings to hold the lids apart are an advantage. Every few months the size should be increased.

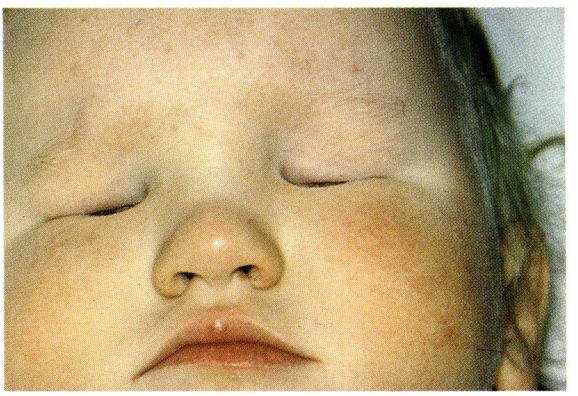

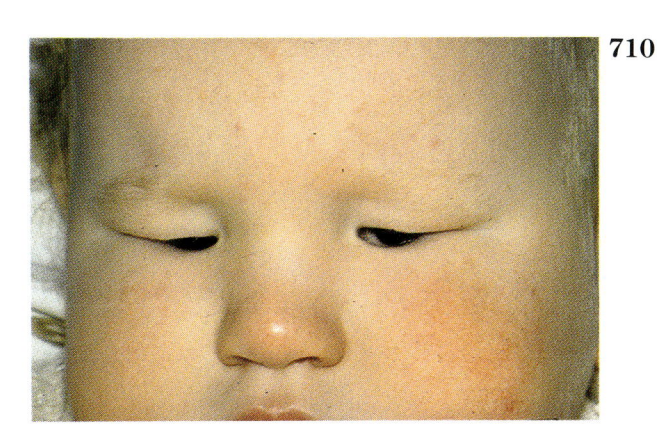

711-713 The 'eye stare' is common to many good fit artificial eyes and simple lid plastic surgical procedures (of which there are many) will overcome this problem (**713**).

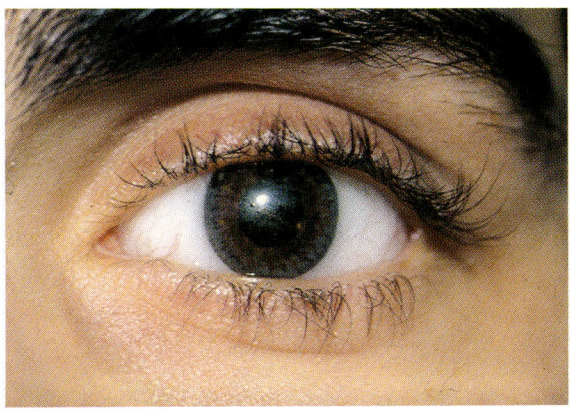

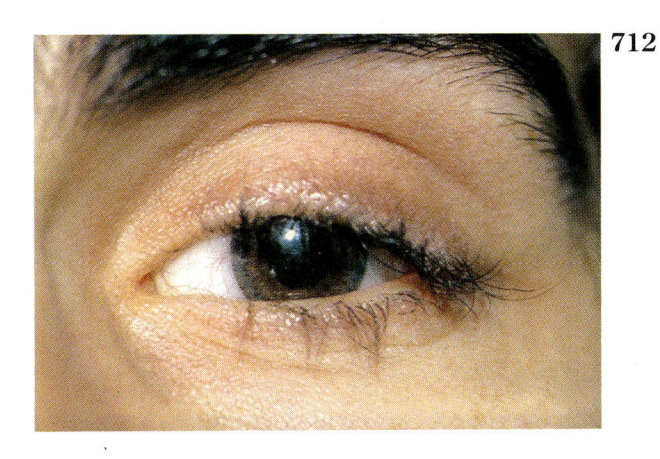

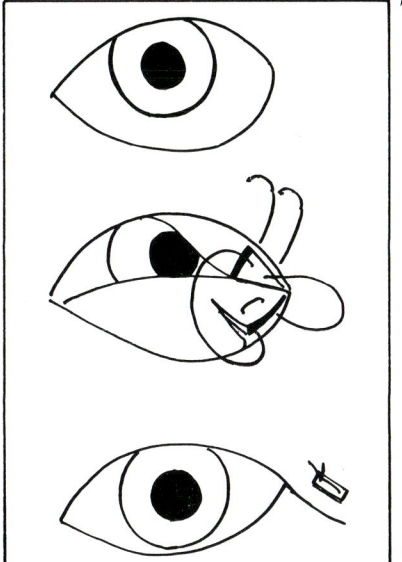

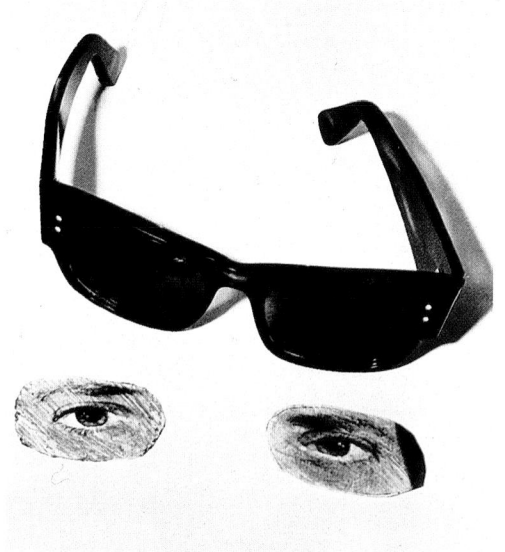

714-716 Acrylic painted shells applied to the skin or supported by a spectacle frame are of use for those cases where an extensive facial disfigurement is present. (Figures courtesy of Reg Wilson.)

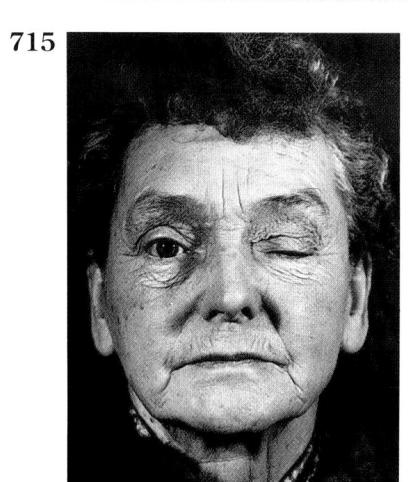

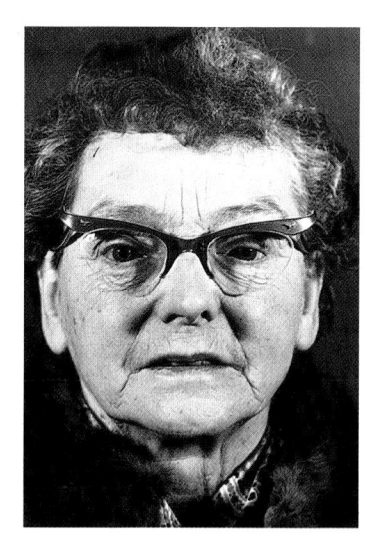

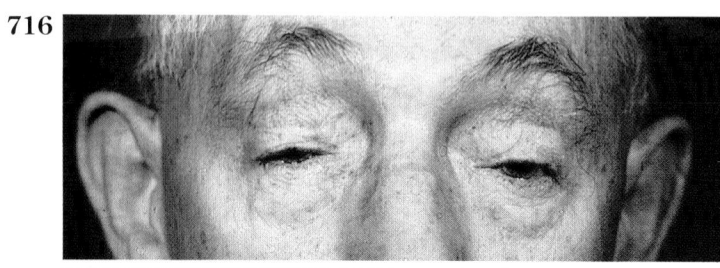

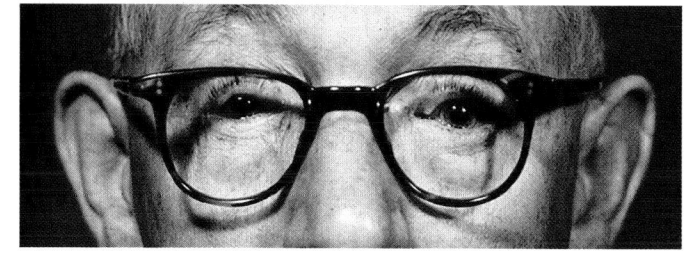

Index

A
Abbreviations, 6
Acanthamoeba infection, 63, 179
Acne rosacea, 138
Adverse reactions
    causes, 151
    conjunctival problems, 180
    Dk/L values and, 160-161
    endothelium, 167-172
    epithelial, 153-155
    gaseous exchange, 151-152
    infection, 176-179, 180-181
    lids, 180
    microcysts, vacuoles, 164-165
    neovascularization, 173-176
    optical, 182
    punctuate keratitis, 162-164
    summary, 150
    tear film and, 157-159
AEL, *see* Axial edge lift
Ageing of lens polymer, 7, 51
Ahmed, N, 170
Albinism, 112, 189
Allergic conjunctivitis, 181
Ammonia burn, 146
Amydo amines lenses, size and thickness, 18
Aniridia
    congenital, 112
    traumatic, 184
Aniseikonia, 105, 107-109
Anisometropia, bilateral, with entropion and blepharophimosis, 193
Anterior chamber
    pathology, 150, 176
    reformation, 148
Anterior uveitis, 176
Aphakia, 113-121
    with bullous keratopathy, 135-136
    choice of contact lenses, 114
    corneal endothelium in, 167, 168
    diabetic, 167, .175
    epithelial necrosis, 175
    in infancy, 118-120
    optics of, 113
    unilateral, 107
Astigmatism
    irregular, 110
    regular, 110
    residual, definition, 79
    toric lenses, 79-80, 93
Axial edge lift (AEL, Z), 19, 20

B
Bacillus coli infection, 176, 177, 178
Bacterial contamination, 62-64
Bandage (protective) lenses, 134-135
    anterior chamber reformation, 148
    infection causing keratoconjunctivitis, 179
    in keratoplasty, 132-133
    ocular burns, 144, 146
Basement membrane disease (recurrent erosion), 137
Benign mucus membrane atrophy (BMMA), 142-143
Benjamin, W J, 14, 155, 163, 167, 180
Bennett, A G, 20
Bergmanson, J, 172
Bifocal lenses, *see* Multi-vision lemses
Binocular vision, contact lens indications, 105-106, 107
Biocompatibility, 7
Bitoric lenses, 80-81

Black areas of tear film, 159, 170
Bleb formation of endothelium, 168
Blepharitis, 179, 180
Blepharoconjunctivitis, inferior staphylococcal, 163
Bleshoy, Hans, 156, 165, 166
Boltz, R, 59, 60, 101
Borates (lipofrin), 50
Bowman's capsule, infiltration of, 169
Brennan, Noel and Efron, N, 45, 46
Bron, A, 156
Buckley, Roger, 16, 170
Bullous keratopathy, 135-137
Bull's eye fit, 124
Buphthalmos, with bullous keratopathy, 137
Burns, ocular, 143-146
BUT (Break-up time), 159

C
Calcium deposits, 57-58
Candida albicans, 60
Cases
    contamination, 62, 63
    lens storage, 50
Cataract
    inoperable, prosthetic lens, 186
    see also Apakia
Cellular hypertrophy, linear, 155
Cellulose acetate butyrate, 15
Checking
    hard lenses, size, 44
    HPG lenses, specific gravity, 46
    lens curvature, 41-42
    magnifiers and microscopes, 38-39
    power, 43
    shadowgraphs, 40
    soft lenses, water content, 45-46
    standards, 38
    thickness gauges, 43
Chemical burns, 144, 145
Chord, curve specification, 20
Chu, L, 171, 172
Cleaners, 50
Coloboma, traumatic, 185
Computerization, 20-26, 100, 101
Congenital aniridia, 112
Congenital endothelial abnormalities, 170
Congenital hyperopia, 109-110
Congenital mesodermal dysplasia, 138
Congenital myopia, 104
Conic section curves, and shape factor, 18, 19
Conjunctivitis, 180-181
    papillary, 180
    vernal catarrhal, 122, 155
    see also Keratoconjunctivitis
Contact (wetting) angle, 8
Contamination, 47, 62-64, *see also* Infections
Cooke, Geoff, 20
Cooper Vision, 35
Cornea
    black areas, 170
    dry spots, 159
    endothelium
        aphakia, 167-168
        Bowman's capsule, infiltration, 169
        congenital anomalies, 170
        folds (wrinkles), 171
        hypoxia, 168
        normal, 167
        toxic keratitis, 170

epithelium
    adverse reactions, 152-157
    down growth, 160
    microcysts, vacuoles, 164-165
    oedema, 150, 151, 152, 154, 156-157
mosaic, superficial, 156
nerve fibres, normal, 165
oedema
    endothelial folds, 167
    gross, 176
    striae, 166
oxygen uptake, 152
puncture wounds, 148
rigidity, 10
staining, *see* Punctate keratitis
stromal changes, in animals, 171-172
Corneal collagen (marginal) dystrophy, 128
Corneal lenses, 17
    albinism, 112
    aphakia, 114, 115
    hard, 68-70
        keratoconus, 122-125
    intermediate sized, 77
    prosthetic, 183-186
Corneal leukomata, prosthetic shell, 187
Corneo-scleral lenses, 17
    aphakia, 116
Cosmesis, definition, 183
Cosmetic visual contact lens, 183
Curves, 18-20
    checking, 41
    fitting, 67

D

Dk, *see* Gas transmission
Dk x 10^{-11} (ATVP), *see* Gas diffusion constant
Dk/L, *see* Gas permeability
Delcourt, J Cl, 154
Dellen formation, 163
Dermoid, prosthetic shell, 187
Descemet's membrane, adverse reactions, 150, 167, 172
Design of lenses
    basic principles, 17-18
    computerized, 20-26, 101
    gas transmission, effect on, 31
Diabetic aphakic, 167, 175
Diffraction lenses, 83-85
Dingeldein, Stephen A, 70
Diplopia, 106-107
Disinfection, 47, 176
    chemical, 49-50
        elution rates, 49
    electrical, 48
    heat, 48
    thermos flask, 48
Disposable lenses, 64-65
    daily wear, 65
    extended wear, 65
Drug dispensing gel lenses, 146
Dry eye, 175
    pathological, 139-141
    polymer damage in, 56
Dry spots, 159
Drysdale's principle (radiuscope), 41
Dyslexia of binocular vision aetiology, 107
Dysplasia, mesodermal, 138
Dystrophy
    heredokerato-, 128
    keratoglobus, 128
    marginal, 128
    myotonic, 149
    primary endothelial (Fuch's), 167
    Reis-Buckler, 128
    Terriens, 128

E

Eccentricity (E), concept of, 18
Echelons (gratings) and diffraction, 3
Edging, 33
EDTA 1%, calcium removal using, 57
Efron, N and Brennan, Noel, 45, 46
Electrical disinfection, 48
Electrodiagnostic scleral lens, 99
Electron spectroscopy (ESCA), 62
Engel, L et al (*An Atlas of Polymer Damage*), 52-54
Enucleation problems, 189
Epikerato problems, 189
Epikerato prosthesis, 120
Equivalent oxygen percentage, 14
Erythema multiforme (Stevens-Johnson syndrome), 141-142
Exophoria, 105
Exposure keratitis, 140, 174
Eye stare with prosthesis, 193

F

Familial dysautonomia (Riley-Day syndrome), 139, 177
Fifth cranial nerve ganglion ablation (neuropathic keratitis), 140
Fitting
    assessment, 72-74
    computer programs, 101
    corneal hard lenses, 68-70
    corneal intermediate sized lens, 77
    directional forces affecting, 66
    dynamic, 66
    finding lens curve from eye model, 67
    general principles, 66
    hard lens centration, 74-76
    infant aphakia, 120
    interpalpebral lens, 74
    keratoconus, 122
    lens power, 71
    lid-lens adhesion, 78
    maintenance (lens stability), 66, 67, 81-82
    multi-vision (bifocals, multifocals), 83-86
    prescriptions, writing, 100
    scleral (haptic), 96-99
    soft lenses, 87-96
        examples, 89-92
        toric, 93-96
    static, 66
    toric lenses, 79-81, 93-96
    trial lenses, 71-72
Fleischer's ring, 122
Flexure, 17
Fluorocarbons, 16
    gas flow, 12, 27
Focimeter, 43
Fuch's (primary endothelial) dystrophy, 167
Fundus viewing lenses, 99
Fungal contamination, 62-64

G

Gas diffusion constant (Dk x 10 (-11) (ATVP)), 6, 12
Gas (oxygen) probe, 13
Gas permeability (Dk/L), 6, 12-14
    measurement, 12
    values, 160-161
Gas-permeable lenses (GP, HGP, RGP)
    Dk/L values, 161
    gas flow, and thickness, 27
    polymer damage, 55
    specific gravity, 46
    trial, 71, 72
    ultrastructural damage, 52
Gas transmission (Dk), 12
Gel lenses
    aphakia, 114, 117, 119
    BK corneal vascularization with, 136
    checking, 39

drug dispensing, 146
dry eyes, 139-140
iris, 112
keratoconus, 125-127
occlusive therapy, 106-107
polymer damage, 55-56, 58-59
prosthetic, 184-186
surface degeneration, 59
see also Hydrophilic lenses
Glare effects, 182
Glycerine 2%, 51
Gonioscope lenses, 99
Gratings (echelons) and diffractions, 83
Guillon, J P, 158, 159

H

Haemorrhage, 174
Haloes, 182
Haptic lenses, *see* Scleral lenses
Hard (rigid) lenses, 17
    centration, 74-77
    corneal, fitting, 68-70
    meniscus, and tear film zone, 160
    size, checking, 44
    stability factors, 67
Healon, 51
Heredokeratodystrophies, 128
Herpes simplex
    drug dispensing gel lens, 146
    infection, 179
Heterophoria, 105
Hill, R, 14
HIV disinfection, 47, 177
Hydrophilic lenses
    fitting
        examples, 89-92
        keratometry, 92
        principles, 87
        thickness and size, 87
    range of, 88-89
    thickness gauges, 43
    water content, checking, 45-46
    see also Gel lenses; Soft lenses
Hydrops of cornea, 127
Hyperopia
    and alternating convergent strabismus, 105-106
    congenital
        adult hypermetrope, 110
        small eye (hereditary form), 109
Hypoxia, 168
Hysteresis, 11, 55

I

Infections
    keratitis, 177-179
    lids and conjunctival problems, 180-181
    see also Contamination
Inflammatory keratoconjunctivitis, 138
Injection moulding, 34
Insertion, 47
Interferometry patterns (Moire fringes), 41, 70, 83, 85
Interpapebral lenses, 74
Iron foreign body deposit, 59

J

Janes, Joseph A, 133

K

Keratitis
    exposure, 140, 174
    infective, 177-179
    neuropathic, 140
    pseudodendritic, 163
    punctate, 162-165
    ring, 179
    superior limbic, 155, 163
    suppurative, 171, 172
    toxic, 170
    viral, 163
Keratoconjunctivitis
    infection causing, 179
    inflammatory, 138
Keratoconus, 121-122
    hard corneal lenses, 122-125
    hydrops, 127
    lens fitting, 122
    soft lenses, 126-127
    superficial corneal mosaic, 156
Keratoglobus, 128
Keratometry, 68, 92, 96, 121
Keratopathy, bullous, 135
Keratoplasty, 122, 129-133
    bandage lenses, 132-133
    failed, prosthetic lens, 186
Klyce. Stephen D, 70

L

Lathe cutting, 32-33
Lathe generation method, 37
Lens
    physical properties, 7
    surface degeneration
        future investigations, 62
        microscopy, 59-61
Lens order form, 100
Lid-lens adhesion 66, 67, 74, 77, 78, 82
Lids
    adverse reactions, 150, 180
    black areas and pressure of, 158
    closure, corneal changes and, 151
Lipase preparations, 50
Lipid
    haze, 56, 57
    Meibomian secretion, 158
Lipofrin (borates), 50
Low power lenses
    rigidity, 29
    thickness, 28, 29
Lubricant drops, 51

M

Magnifiers, 38-39
Manufacture
    lathe cutting, 32-34
    moulding, 34-35
    pressure grinding, 34
    scleral lens, 36-37
Marechal-Courtois, Ch., 154
Marfans syndrome, 115
Marginal dystrophy, 128
Marginal inflammatory ulceration, 138
Meibomian secretion of lipid, 158
Menicon, GP, 77
Mesodermal dysplasia, 138
Mesodermal dystrophy, 138
Metal burn, 144, 146
Methacryloxypropyltris (trimethylsiloxanyl) silane (MOPS), 16
Microscopy, 38
Modification, 34
Moire fringes, *see* Interferometry patterns
Monniger, R, 63, 179
Mooren's ulcer, 138
MOPS, *see* Methacryloxypropyltris (trimethylsiloxanyl) silane
Motility, excessive, 182, *see also* Stabilization
Moulding
    injection, 35
    spin, 34
Mucin debris, and punctate keratitis, 163

Mucus tag, 175
Mulberries (small mucolipid conglomerates), 60-61
Multi-vision (bifocal, multifocals) lenses, 83-86
    segment design, 85-86
    simultaneous vision, 83-85
Mustard gas burn, 143
Myopathies, ocular, 148-149
Myopia, 103-104
Myotonic dystrophy, 149

N
Negative peripheral carrier design, 25-26
Neovascularization, 173-176
Neuropathic keratitis (5th cranial nerve ganglion ablation), 140
Nissel, Artificial Eye, 190
Nystagmus, 113

O
Occlusive coloured ptosis, 149
Occlusive therapy, 106-107, 112
Ocular burns, 143-146
Ocular myopathies, 148-149
Optical problems, 182
Orbital prostheses, 189-194
Over-refraction, 71
Oxygen (gas) probe, 13
Oxygen percentage, equivalent, 14

P
Pachometer, 43
Pamnametrics, 42
Paralytic strabismus and diplopia, 106
Partially sighted, 111
Peroxide disinfection, 50
PHEMA, see Poly-(2-hydroxymethylmethacrylate)
Photokeratography, keratoplasty, 129
Photokeratometry, 68-69, 122
    colour-coded, 70
Photokeratoscopy, 110
Physical properties, 7
Piccolo, M, 59, 60
Pierre Robin syndrome, 104
Pilkington diffraction lens, 84
Pilocarpine, lens release, 147
Plica semilunaris, infected, 180
PMMA, see Polymethylmethacrylate
Poly (2-hydroxymethymethacrylate) Phema
    chemical formula, 15
    gas permeability, 12, 27
    iron foreign body deposit, 59
    phase-contrast microscopy of surface, 58
    polymer degeneration in rheumatoid arthritis, 59
    properties, 15
    prosthetic lenses, 183
    rigidity, 10
    size and thickness, 18, 27
    symblepharon prevention, 144
    trial, 71
    ultrastructural damage, 52
Poly (dimesthylsiloxane), 16
Poly (diphenyl-dimethyl-methylvinyl siloxane), 16
Polymer damage, 55-62
    surface degeneration, microscopy, 59-61
Polymethylmethacrylate (PMMA)
    chemical formula, 15
    corneal lenses, 183
    gas permeability, 12
    guide to trial fitting sets, 72
    properties, 15
    rigidity, 10
Power, 71
    checking, 43
Pre-presbyopia, 103, 182

Prescription
    computer programs and, 100
    writing, 100
Pressure grinding, 34
Primary endothelial (Fuch's) dystrophy, 167
Prism ballast, 81, 85, 94, 127
Prosthetics
    corneal lenses, 183-186
    orbital, 189-194
    scleral hard lens, 186-189
    shell, 145, 186-189
    types of ocular, 183
Protease preparations, 50
Protective lenses, see Bandage lenses
Protein coating, 55, 56, 57, 59
    cleaners, 50
Pseudo-conic surfaces, 30
Pseudodendritic keratitis, 163
Pseudomonas aeruginosa, 62, 176, 177
Pterygium, 155
Ptosis lens, 148
Punctate keratitis, 162-165
Puncture wounds, corneal, 148
Pyocyaneus A infection, 177

R
Radiation effects, 7
Radiokeratotomy, 133-134
Radiuscope (Drysdale's principle), 41
Recurrent erosions (basement membrane disease), 137
Reduced optic design, 22-24, 28, 29
Refojo, M, 15, 46
Refractometer, soft contact lens, 45
Reis-Buckler dystrophy, 128
Reproducibility, 7
Retro-illumination, 164
Rheumatoid arthritis, soft lens degeneration, 59
Rigidity, 10, 17, 29
Riley-Day syndrome (familial dysautonomia), 139, 177
Ring keratitis, 179
Ruben, M, 172

S
Sagitta (S), curve specification, 20
Sattler's veiling, 157
Scleral (haptic) lenses, 17
    acne rosacea, 138
    albinism, aniridia, 112
    aphakia, 114, 116
    dry eyes, 140-143
    electrodiagnostic, 99
    fitting, 96-99
    manufacture, 36-37
    ocular myopathies, 148-149
    preformed geometric, 99
    prosthetic, 184, 186
    Trodd type, 148
Secondary 10n mass spectrometry (SIMS), 62
Seventh cranial nerve paresis, 141, 175
SF, see Shape factor
Shadowgraphs, 40, 67
Shape factor (SF), 18, 19, 20
Shell prostheses, 145, 186-189
Silanes, 16
Silicone acrylates, gas permeability, 12
Silicone rubber lenses
    aphakia, 118, 120
    chemical formulae, 16
    dry eyes, 143
    fitting
        examples, 89-92
        keratometry, 92
        principles, 87
        range of, 88-89

thickness and size, 87
gas permeability, 12
polymer damage, 56-57
properties, 16
rigidity, 10
size and thickness, 18
Siloxanes, 16, 18
Size of lens, 17
    factors affecting, 17-18
    lens specification by, 17
Small eye (hereditary form of hyperopia), 109
Soft lenses, 17
    contamination, 63
    design
        low water content, 22
        negative peripheral carrier, 25-26
        reduced optic, 22
        thickness, control of, 24
        tri-curved spherical and aspheric, 21
    disposable, 64-65
    Dk/L values, 161
    drying during wear, 63
    fitting, 87-96
    keratoconus, 126-127
    measurement, acceptable tolerances, 44
    polymer degeneration in rheumatoid arthritis, 59
    stability factors, 67
    toric, 93-96
    see also Gel lenses; Hydrophilic lenses; Silicone rubber lenses
Spectacle frame, with shell prosthesis, 187, 194
Spin moulding, 34
Spoilage, 51
Stability, lens, 66, 67, 81-82
Staphylococcus infection (suppurative keratitis), 171, 172
Sterilization, 47
Stevens-Johnson syndrome (erythema multiforme), 141-142
Strabismus
    convergent, prosthetic shell, 187
    hyperopia and alternating convergent, 105-106
    paralytic, and diplopia, 106
Stromal haemorrhage, 174
Stromal oedema, 171, 172
Stromal vascularization, 171-174
Subnormal vision aids, 111
Superior limbic keratitis, 155, 163
Suppurative keratitis, 171, 172
Surface tension, 8
Surface wettability, 8-10
Symblepharon, 143-145

T

Tank/minor device (Chaston), 42
Taylor, D, 119
Tear film
    black areas, 159
    break-up time (BUT), abnormal, 159
    contact angle, 8, 51
    interferometry patterns, 157
    investigations, 157
    normal, 157
    pre-lens, 159
    surface tension, 8, 66
Tear flow, under contact lens, 73
Tear pump mechanism, lens design and, 28
Telechelic perfluoropolyether, 16
Tensile modules, 12
Terriens dystrophy, 128
Thermos flask disinfection, 48
Thickness
    factors, 17
    gas flow and, 27
    gauges, 43
    high minus powers using reduced optics, 24
    low power design and, 28

Thyrotoxicosis, corneal oedema, 157
Tobacco smoking, lens discoloration due to, 56
Toposcope, 41
Toric lenses, 30, 79-81, 93-95, 96
Toxic keratitis, 170
Transparency, 11
Tri-curved spherical and aspheric lenses, design, 21
Trial lenses, 19, 71-72
Trimethylsiloxanyl (methacryloxypropyltris) silane (MOPS)
Tripathi, B J, 63, 179
Tripathi, R C, 61, 63, 64, 179
Trodd type ptosis lenses, 148
Tropias, 105
Truncations, 82, 85, 93, 95

U

Ulceration
    marginal, 138
    methaherpetic, 147
Ultrasound sagittometer, 42
Ultrasound tank, for cleaning lenses, 50
Ultrastructure, damage to, 52-54
Unilateral aphakia, 107
Uveitis, anterior, 176

V

V-slot gauge, 44
Vascular pannus formation, 173
Vinylpyrrolidone, (VP)
    chemical formula, 15
    properties, 15
Vinyls
    gas permeability, 12
    size and thickness, 18
Viral keratitis, 163
VP, *see* Vinylpyrrolidone

W

Warp of lens, 17
Water absorption, 7
Weicon, 107, 112
Wesley-Jesson system, 42
Wetting angle, *see* Contact angle
Wilson, Reg, 194

X

X-ray photoelectroscopy (XPS), 62

Y

Yeast infection, 60, 64, 177
Young, Graeme, 164

Z

Z factor, *see* Axial edge lift
Zantos, Steve, 165